QUICK REFERENCE CARD

Important Apothecaries' Equivalents and Abbreviations

Volume (Liquid)

60 minims (M or ♏) = 1 fluid dram (fl dr or fl ʒ)

16 fluid ounces (fl oz or ʒ) = 1 pint (O or pt)

2 pints (O or pt) = 1 quart (qt)

4 quarts (qt) = 1 gallon (C)

Weight

60 grains (gr) = 1 dram (dr)

8 drams (dr) = 1 ounce (oz)

Important Metric Equivalents

Volume (Liquid)

1 milliliter (mL) = 1 cubic centimeter (cc)

1000 milliliters (mL) = 1 liter (L)

Weight

1000 micrograms (mcg or μg) = 1 milligram (mg)

1000 milligrams (mg) = 1 gram (G)

1000 grams (G) = 1 kilogram (kg)

Important Liquid Equivalents

1 minim = 0.06 milliliter (mL)

15 or 16 minims = 1 mL

1 fluid dram = 4 mL

1 fluid ounce = 30 or 32 mL

16 fluid ounces = 500 mL

1 quart = 1000 mL or 1 liter (L)

Important Volume Equivalents

1 grain = 60 milligrams

15 or 16 grains = 1 gram

1 dram = 4 grams

1 ounce = 30 or 32 grams

2.2 pounds = 1 kilogram

Common Celsius and Fahrenheit Body Temperature Equivalents

Celsius	Fahrenheit
35°	95°
36°	96.8°
37°	98.6°
38°	100.4°
39°	102.2°
40°	104°
41°	105.8°

Computing Dosage

$$\frac{\text{Desired Dosage}}{\text{Have Dosage}} = \frac{\text{Desired Amount}}{\text{Have Amount}}$$

or

Desired Dosage : Have Dosage =
Desired Amount : Have Amount

Determining Number of Drops per Minute

- If the drop factor is 10 drops = 1 mL, divide the hourly amount of fluid by 6.

- If the drop factor is 15 drops = 1 mL, divide the hourly amount of fluid by 4.

- If the drop factor is 20 drops = 1 mL, divide the hourly amount of fluid by 3.

- If the drop factor is 60 drops = 1 ml, divide the hourly amount of fluid by 1.

Determining Hourly Rate when the Drop Factor and the Drop Rate Are Known

- If the drop factor is 10 drops = 1 mL, multiply the drop rate of fluid by 6.

- If the drop factor is 15 drops = 1 mL, multiply the drop rate of fluid by 4.

- If the drop factor is 20 drops = 1 mL, multiply the drop rate of fluid by 3.

- If the drop factor is 60 drops = 1 mL, multiply the drop rate of fluid by 1.

Comparison of Standard and 24-Hour Time

Standard	24-Hour
Midnight	2400
1:00 am	0100
2:00 am	0200
3:00 am	0300
4:00 am	0400
5:00 am	0500
6:00 am	0600
7:00 am	0700
8:00 am	0800
9:00 am	0900
10:00 am	1000
11:00 am	1100
Noon	1200
1:00 pm	1300
2:00 pm	1400
3:00 pm	1500
4:00 pm	1600
5:00 pm	1700
6:00 pm	1800
7:00 pm	1900
8:00 pm	2000
9:00 pm	2100
10:00 pm	2200
11:00 pm	2300

Commonly Used Abbreviations

Meaning	Abbreviation	Meaning	Abbreviation
after	p̄	intramuscular	IM
after meals	pc	intravenous	IV
ampule	amp	intravenous piggyback	IVPB
as desired	ad lib	intravenous push	IVP
at once, immediately	stat	keep vein open	KVO
before	ā	left eye	OS
before meals	ac	left ear	AS
both eyes	OU	liquid	liq
both ears	AU	nasogastric tube	NGT
by mouth	PO	nothing by mouth	NPO
drops per minute	gtt/min	of each	aa
discontinue	dc	once if necessary	sos
elixir	elix	quantity sufficient	qs
*every day, once a day	qd or od	right ear	AD
every hour	qh or q1h	right eye	OD
every 2 hours	q2h	solution	sol
every 3 hours	q3h	subcutaneous	SC
every 4 hours	q4h	sublingual	SL
every 6 hours	q6h	suspension	susp
every 8 hours	q8h	three times a day	tid
every 12 hours	q12h	tincture	tinct
*every other day	qod	topical	T
fluid	fl	total parenteral nutrition	TPN
four times a day	qid	twice a day	bid
hour of sleep	hs	when necessary; as needed	prn
hypodermic	H	with	c̄
inhalation	I or INH	without	s̄
intradermal	ID		

Abbreviations for Measurement of Medications

Meaning	Abbreviation
capsule	cap
cubic centimeter	cc
dram	dr or ʒ
drop	gtt
fluid dram	fl dr or fl ʒ
grain	gr
gram	g
kilogram	kg
liter	L
microgram	mcg or µg
milligram	mg
milliequivalent	mEq
milliliter	ml or mL
millimole $\left(\frac{1}{1000} \text{ of a mole}\right)$	mmol
minim	m or M
one-half	ss̄
ounce	oz or ʒ
fluid ounce	fl oz or fl ʒ
teaspoon	tsp
tablespoon	Tbs
tablet	tab
*unit	U

*The Joint Commission on Accreditation of Healthcare Organizations (JCAHO) issued a safety goal to prohibit the use of certain abbreviations that are considered unacceptable due to their tendency to be misread and lead to medication errors. The JCAHO has asked that health care organizations begin phasing out these unacceptable abbreviations. Because many of these are still in use, it is important that nurses recognize these abbreviations and understand the alternatives to their use. JCAHO recommends that "unit" be used instead of "U," "every day" be written instead of "q.d." and that "every other day" be written instead of "q.o.d."

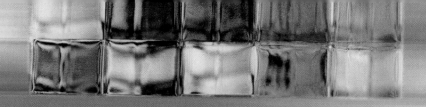

MATH
AND MEDS
FOR NURSES

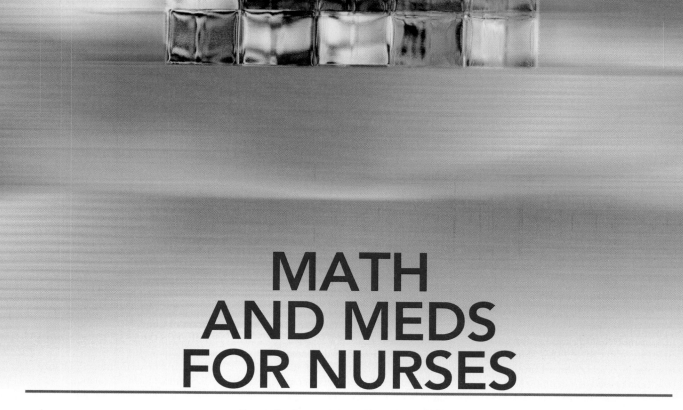

MATH AND MEDS FOR NURSES

SECOND EDITION

Dolores F. Saxton, RN, BSEd, MA, MPS, EdD (Deceased)

Norma Ercolano O'Neill, RN, MS

Professor Emeritus
Nassau Community College
Garden City, NY

Colleen Glavinspiehs, DNSc, RN, BS, MSN, FNP

Professor
Burlington County College
Pemberton, NJ

THOMSON

DELMAR LEARNING

Australia   Canada   Mexico   Singapore   Spain   United Kingdom   United States

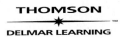

THOMSON

DELMAR LEARNING

Math and Meds for Nurses
Second Edition
by Dolores F. Saxton, Norma Ercolano O'Neill, and Colleen Glavinspiehs

Vice President, Health Care Business Unit:
William Brottmiller
Editorial Director:
Cathy L. Esperti
Senior Acquisitions Editor:
Matthew Kane
Marketing Director:
Jennifer McAvey

Developmental Editor:
Maria D'Angelico
Editorial Assistant:
Erin Silk
Technology Director:
Laurie Davis
Technology Production Coordinator:
Sherry Conners

Production Manager:
Barbara A. Bullock
Art and Design Specialist:
Jay Purcell
Production Coordinator:
Kenneth McGrath
Project Editor:
David Buddle

Library of Congress Cataloging-in-Publication Data
Saxton, Dolores F.
    Math and meds for nurses / Dolores F. Saxton, Norma Ercolano O'Neill, Colleen Glavinspiehs.—2nd ed.
        p.   cm.
    Includes index.
    ISBN 1-4018-3456-6
    1. Nursing—Mathematics—Handbooks, manuals, etc.
    2. Pharmaceutical arithmetic—Handbooks, manuals, etc.   I. Ercolano-O'Neill, Norma.
    II. Glavinspiehs, Colleen.   III. Title.
RT68.S29 2005
615'.14—dc22

2004049788

ISBN 1-4018-3456-6

Notice to the Reader

In Memoriam

Dolores F. Saxton, RN, BS, MA, MPS, EdD

It is with deep sorrow that we mourn the loss of our dear friend and colleague, Dr. Dolores F. Saxton, who died suddenly on May 25, 2003, following complications from vascular surgery.

For those of us who knew her, Dr. Saxton was not only a beloved sister and aunt, but she was also a woman who excelled as a nurse, as an educator, as an author, and as an active community member. A woman before her time, Dr. Saxton epitomized the definition of a professional nurse.

She was born and raised in Brooklyn, New York and attended New York City schools. Following her graduation from Norwegian Hospital School of Nursing in Brooklyn, Dr. Saxton enlisted in the U.S. Army during the Korean War. Following her discharge, she was active in the Army Reserve, where she attained the rank of Major. Her higher education in nursing included a baccalaureate degree in nursing and a master of arts in nursing from New York University and a doctorate in education from Columbia University.

As an educator, Dr. Saxton taught at St. Vincent's School of Nursing in New York City and at Nassau Community College in Garden City, New York. While teaching at Nassau Community College she achieved the rank of professor. She also served as Chairman of the Nursing Department and later was appointed Dean of Health Sciences and Physical Education. During her tenure at Nassau Community College, she was the recipient of the Chancellor's Award for Excellence in Teaching. In 1972 Dr. Saxton was one of the cofounders of the New York State External Degree program in nursing, a nontraditional nursing program that is now a division of Excelsior College. After retiring from Nassau Community College in 1989, she served as Chairman of the Nursing Department of Burlington Community College in Pemberton, New Jersey.

Dr. Saxton was known throughout the United States as an author of nursing textbooks. Her creativity and her demand for excellence and accuracy made her a lead author and lead editor of a myriad of nursing education publications. She had a knack for wording complex material very simply. Her first endeavor with writing was a very understandable text entitled "Programmed Instruction in Arithmetic, Dosage and Solutions." The text contained about 70 pages.

Since 1977 we co-authored a number of texts relating to the computation of dosage. The first published work we co-authored for Delmar Learning was *Math and Meds for Nurses*. It was by far the most inclusive and the most detailed book we jointly wrote. Dr. Colleen Glavinspiehs joined us for the second edition of the book to add the most recent developments in drug administration and to aid us in deleting outdated material. She worked with us from 2002 until 2003.

To say that Dr. Saxton was an active participant in the community is an understatement. Some of her community activities included a three-year tenure as an active member and trustee of the Board of Education in Farmingdale, New York. In addition she served as a volunteer at the local elementary school for many years. Her involvement in the Gift of Life Program raising funds to sponsor children with heart defects was inspiring and will be missed by the community.

On the lighter side, Dr. Saxton had a wonderful sense of humor and an unforgettable laugh. She was an avid New York Mets fan who regularly attended Mets games. Dr. Saxton was a collector *par excellence*. She collected Coca Cola memorabilia, Precious Moments, and Toby mugs, but her most treasured collection was her teddy bears, a collection that filled every room in her home. At the time of her death she was in the process of writing a price guide reference book for teddy bear collectors.

It was an honor to have known Dolores and to have worked so closely with her. She was our very dear friend and will be sorely missed.

Norma E. O'Neill
Colleen Glavinspiehs

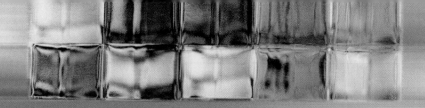

Contents

Preface

This text is designed to enhance the learner's understanding of basic mathematics skills and their application to accurate calculation of dosages of drugs and solutions. The authors realize that the administration of medications is only one small aspect of the nurse's responsibility; however, it is one aspect of care that can move rapidly from life-saving to life-threatening if even a minute error is made in calculation.

In Unit 1 we have used numbers solely to demonstrate and review principles, without regard to nursing situations. We recognize that the nurse would not encounter these numbers in patient care settings. Aside from Unit 1, we have attempted to use as examples those numbers, fractions, decimals, percents, drugs, and solutions most commonly confronted by the nurse in today's health care environments.

ORGANIZATION

The text is divided into eight units. Unit 1 is a review of basic mathematics related to dosage computation. Unit 2 reviews systems of measurement. Unit 3 prepares the learner for the safe administration of medications. Unit 4 demonstrates the use of the ratio-and-proportion method of calculating dosage of oral and parenteral medications. Unit 5 focuses on intravenous fluids and intravenous medications. Unit 6 presents the computation of dosages for infants and children. Although our emphasis throughout this text is on the use of the ratio-and-proportion method to solve computation problems, in Unit 7 the formula method and the dimensional analysis method have been included so that the learner can explore alternate methods of computation. Unit 8 reviews medication orders and medication records and concludes with a comprehensive posttest that provides an opportunity to measure the level of dosage calculation knowledge achieved.

ASSISTIVE TOOLS

A quick reference card for use in the clinical area is included. This card contains abbreviations, conversion equivalents, common body temperature equivalents, the 24-hour clock, and IV flow rates and infusion times.

The **CD-ROM** is an interactive multimedia presentation that includes sample problems, review questions, and a testing component. The program provides scoring, helpful hints, animations, and color photos and illustrations. It is designed for individual, self-paced learning at home or in the computer lab.

CHAPTER HIGHLIGHTS

Learning Outcomes open each chapter and detail what the learner should be able to do after completing the chapter.

VIP (Very Important Principles) **Boxes** simplify and reinforce essential data.

Calculation Alert Boxes offer succinct steps for conducting calculations.

Note Boxes bring mathematical facts to the reader's attention.

Tests

Several different types of tests are offered within the text.

A **Pretest** is offered in Chapter 1. It allows learners to test their math skills before beginning a review of basic math skills. Answers are provided following the test.

Posttests are offered in Chapter 8 and Chapter 25. The Chapter 8 test allows learners to test their math skills after they have had a chance to review basic math skills. The Chapter 25 test allows learners to test their dosage calculation skills. Answers are provided following each test.

The **Problem Sets** offered within the chapters allow learners a chance to practice each concept after it has been discussed. Answers are provided after each test.

Self-Evaluation Tests are offered in Chapters 2 through 7 and Chapters 9 through 13 to allow learners to check their understanding of several concepts before moving on to the next section. Answers are provided so learners can check their work.

Review Tests are presented at the end of Chapters 13 to 23 to allow learners to test themselves on all the concepts discussed within the chapters. Answers are provided following each test.

Solutions for the Self-Evaluation Tests from Chapters 9 through 13 and Review Tests from Chapters 16 through 23 can be found in the Appendix. The answers to the Posttest in Chapter 25 are also repeated in the Appendix.

ACKNOWLEDGMENTS

We wish to extend our sincere thanks to our families for their support, to our students and colleagues for pointing out areas of need, and to Irene Elber, who helped turn our pages into a manuscript.

We would like to thank the following accuracy reviewer:

Cheryl L. Graff, RN, MSN
Instructor, Adult Medical-Surgical Nursing and Pharmacology
Highland Community College
Freeport, IL

We would like to thank the following content reviewers for their invaluable feedback:

Marty Bachman, PhD, RN
Associate Professor
Front Range Community College, Ft. Collins, CO

Vicki Barclay, MLT, CMA, MS
West Kentucky Technical College, Paducah, KY

Elizabeth Battalora, MSN, RN
Assistant Professor of Nursing
Louisiana College, Pineville, LA

Susan Beggs, RN, MSN
Austin Community College, Austin, TX

Diane Creed-Kern, RN, MSN
Professor of Nursing
Moraine Valley Community College, Palos Hills, IL

Betty Earp, BSN, RN
Nurse Assistant Coordinator
Mesa Community College, Sun Lakes, AZ

Rebecca Gesler, RN, MSN
Director of Nursing
St. Catherine College, Louisville, KY

Vicky Parker, MS, RN, CNP
Assistant Professor of Nursing
Ohio University, Frankfort, OH

Josy Petr, RN, MS
Educational Testing Director
Indiana University School of Nursing, Northwest Campus, Gary, IN

Russell Shipley, MA, RN, MSN
Instructor, Program of Nursing
Laramie County Community College, Cheyenne, WY

Mary Ellen Symanski, PhD, RN
Associate Professor of Nursing
University of Maine, Bangor, ME

The many technical data, photographs, syringes, drug labels, package inserts, package labels, and packaging were reproduced with permission of:

Abbott Laboratories, Abbott Park, IL (Reproduced with the permission of Abbott Laboratories):

aminophylline, atropine sulphate, 5% dextrose and 0.225% sodium chloride injection, 5% dextrose and 0.45% sodium chloride injection, 5% dextrose and 0.9% sodium chloride injection, epinophrine, EryPed 200, gentamicin, Omnicef oral suspension, 50% magnesium sulfate, 0.9% sodium chloride injection, Synthroid, potassium chloride, various IV solutions

Alaris Medical Systems, San Diego, CA

Medley Medication Safety System

American Medical Association, Chicago, IL

Nomograms

Aventis Pharmaceutical Inc., Kansas City, MO

Claforan sterile

Bayer Pharmaceutical Division, West Haven, CT (Courtesy of Bayer Corporation):

Adalat CC, Avelox, Cipro, Precose

Bristol-Myers Squibb, Princeton, NJ

packing inserts for Megace and Cytoxan

Eli Lilly and Company, Indianapolis, IN (Labels reproduced with permission of Eli Lilly and Company):

heparin sodium, Humulin L, Humulin N, Humulin R, Humulin U, Humulin 70/30, NPH Iletin II pork, Regular Iletin, Mandol, Nebcin, phenobarbital, Seconal, Vancocin HCl, V-Cillin K

Elkins-Sinn, Inc., Cherry Hill, NJ (Courtesy of ESI Lederle, a Business Unit of Wyeth Pharmaceuticals, Philadelphia, PA):

Ativan, fentanyl citrate injection, heparin sodium, meperidine, morphine

Forest Pharmaceuticals, St. Louis, MO (Label reproduced with permission of Forest Pharmaceuticals):

Elixophyllin Elixir

GlaxoSmithKline, Philadelphia, PA (Labels reproduced with permission of GlaxoSmithKline):

Amoxil, Ancef, Augmentin, Compazine, Lanoxin, Purinethol, Tagamet, Zantac, Zofran, Zyloprim

Hoffman-LaRoche, Inc., Nutley, NJ

Bactrim, Bumex, Klonopin, Klorepin

ICN Pharmaceuticals, Costa Mesa, CA (Reproduced with permission of ICN Pharmaceutical Inc.):

Librium

Merck & Co. Inc., North Wales, PA (Labels used with permission of Merck & Co., Inc.):

Cogentin, Cozaar, Decadron, Fosamax, Mefoxin, Pepcid

Novartis Pharmaceuticals, Summit, NJ

Neoral, Slow-K

Pfizer, Inc., New York, NY (Label reproduced with permission of Pfizer, Inc.):

Cerebyx, Dilantin, Nitrostat, Pfizerpen, Unapen, Unasyn, Vistaril

Pharmaceutical Associates, Inc., Greenville, SC (Courtesy of Pharmaceutical Associates Inc.):

aluminum hydroxide, hydrocodone bitartrate, potassium chloride oral solution 10%

Pharmacia Corporation, Peapack, NJ and Kalamazoo, MI (Courtesy of Pharmacia Corporation):

Adriamycin PFS, Cleocin Phosphate, Depo-Medrol, Halcion, Lomotil, Micronase, Solu-Cortef, Solu-Medrol, Xanax

Roche Laboratories, Inc.

prefilled, single dose syringe

Roxane Laboratories, Inc, Columbus, OH (Labels used with permission of Roxane Laboratories, Inc.):

codeine, Digoxin Elixir, furosemide, Lactulose, lithium citrate syrup, PredniSONE

Schering Corporation, Kenilworth, NJ (Reproduced with permission of Schering Corporation. All rights reserved.):

Proventil Syrup

Wyeth Pharmaceuticals, Philadelphia, PA (Courtesy of Wyeth Pharmaceuticals, Philadelphia, PA):

Ativan, fentanyl citrate injection, heparin sodium, merperidine, morphine sulfate

Permission for the use of the hospital records appearing in Chapter 24 was graciously given by the Long Island Jewish Medical Center in New Hyde Park, New York, and by St. Francis Hospital in Roslyn, New York, for illustrative purposes only. Neither the Long Island Jewish Medical Center nor St. Francis Hospital in Roslyn, New York, warranty the outcome or performance achieved by the use of these documents.

NOTE: The product information contained in the package insert for each drug should be consulted before administering any medication.

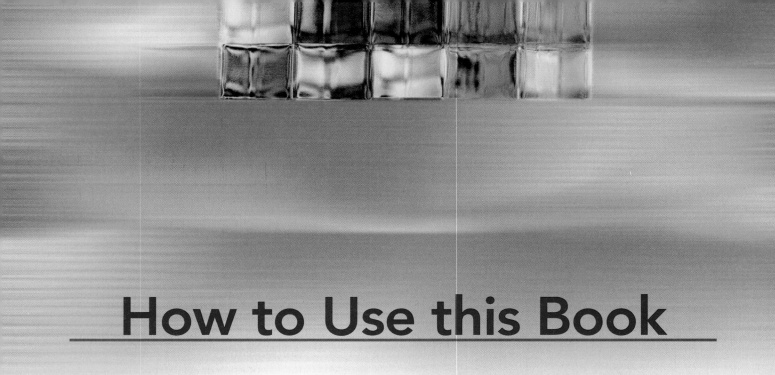

How to Use this Book

This text accommodates the needs of students at various levels of proficiency. It begins with basic concepts and progresses to more complex dosage calculations. There are three levels of testing to sharpen your skills.

PROBLEM SETS

Appear after each new concept to allow you to practice problems. Answers are provided after each set for immediate feedback.

COMBINED SYRINGE AND LABEL QUESTIONS

Problems require you to perform dosage calculations and then indicate correct dosages on the syringes. Combined questions ensure that knowledge is integrated and applied.

SELF-EVALUATION TESTS

Offered in Chapters 2–7 and Chapter 9. They allow you to check your understanding of several concepts before moving on to the next section. Answers are provided at the end of each test.

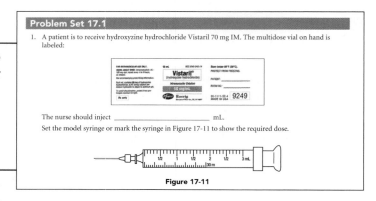

Problem Set 17.1

1. A patient is to receive hydroxyzine hydrochloride Vistaril 70 mg IM. The multidose vial on hand is labeled:

The nurse should inject _____ mL.

Set the model syringe or mark the syringe in Figure 17-11 to show the required dose.

Figure 17-11

Self-Evaluation Test 4.5
Multiplying and Dividing Decimals

1. 9.2×3	9. 64.5×0.375
2. $18 \div 2.4$	10. $2.003 \div 0.16$
3. $15 \div 0.25$	11. $0.166 \div 0.125$
4. 0.8×0.4	12. $0.125 \div 0.025$
5. $0.75 \div 15$	13. $0.325 \div 0.125$
6. 7.5×3.75	14. 1.066×0.0625
7. $0.1 \div 0.375$	15. 0.156×0.03215
8. 0.001×0.2	

Answers 1. 27.6 2. 7.5 3. 60 4. 0.32 5. 0.05 6. 28.125 7. 0.267 8. 0.0002 9. 24.188 10. 12.519 11. 1.328 12. 5
13. 2.6 14. 0.067 15. 0.005

REVIEW TESTS

Offered in Chapters 13–23. Provide a comprehensive review of the chapter topics. Answers are provided at the end of each test.

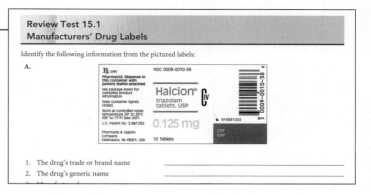

EXAMPLES AND SOLUTIONS

Each new concept is followed by an example problem with step-by-step solution to show you the logical approach in solving the problem.

VIP (VERY IMPORTANT PRINCIPLES)

Provide a concise overview of key principles and safety considerations.

VIP

- Always read the manufacturer's label or the drug insert before mixing the drug.
- Follow directions for the type and amount of diluent to be added, if provided by the manufacturer.
- When reconstituting powdered medication for intramuscular use, and the amount of diluent to be added is not stated by the manufacturer, try to limit the amount of diluent to be added so that the desired dose of medication is contained in between 1 mL and 2 mL of the resulting solution. This limits the amount of fluid that must be injected.
- If the drug has a displacement factor, use the manufacturer's figures of drug strength in setting up the proportion.
- Label the vial of mixed medication with the type and amount of diluent added, strength of the reconstituted solution, the date and time mixed, and the nurse's initials.

CALCULATION ALERT

Provide hints and reminders for performing dosage calculations.

Calculation Alert

When dividing decimals, carry the results out to four decimal places. If the digit in the fourth decimal place is equal to or greater than 5, add 1 to the digit in the third decimal place; if the digit in the fourth decimal place is 4 or less, drop it.

NOTES

Highlight important mathematical principles.

NOTE

The difference using either of the two approaches (mL or minims) is extremely small and well within the 10% conversion factor; therefore, either approach can be used for setting up this type of problem.

LABELS

Actual, full-color labels are used to support the problems. The problems challenge you to read and interpret information on the labels.

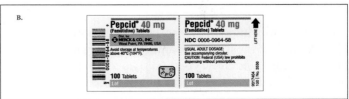

SYRINGES

Drawings of syringes are depicted in actual size to allow you to practice reading intricate calibrations.

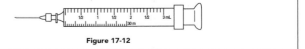

Figure 17-12

How to Use
the Practice Software

We hope you enjoy the interactive CD that accompanies this book. Every attempt has been made to make it a fun, attractive, and effective learning environment. Careful attention was paid to providing step-by-step solutions in a consistent format. Through the use of this software, you will continuously expand your skills and confidence in performing dosage calculations.

ORGANIZATION AND FEATURES

Main menu

The main menu is organized by content areas and further divided by more specific topics of study. Each topic includes a VIP (very important principle) and review sets.

Review Sets

Each chapter includes review sets that incorporate labels and syringes for the most realistic and challenging practice experience. Review sets allow you two tries to obtain the correct answer. If the correct answer is not obtained on the second try, the answer and solution appears on the screen.

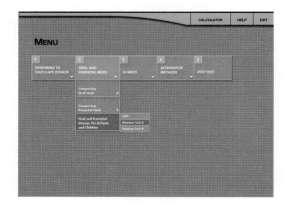

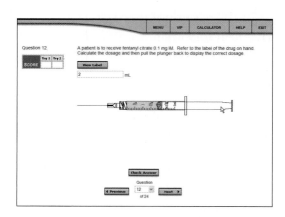

Scoring

Most of the problems are scored so that you can assess strengths and weaknesses and determine which topics need further study.

Labels and Syringes

Real full-color labels are provided to aid recognition and readability of information needed to perform a calculation. Photos of real syringes are also provided.

Interactive syringes

Some questions include interactive syringes. You use the mouse to click and drag the syringe plunger to the correct syringe measurement. All syringes are presented in actual size.

Posttest

A comprehensive test allows you to practice all previously studied topics. You have one opportunity to answer correctly, simulating a true testing environment. Answers and solutions are provided.

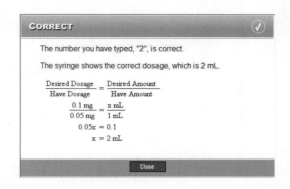

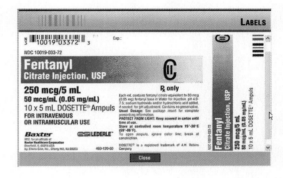

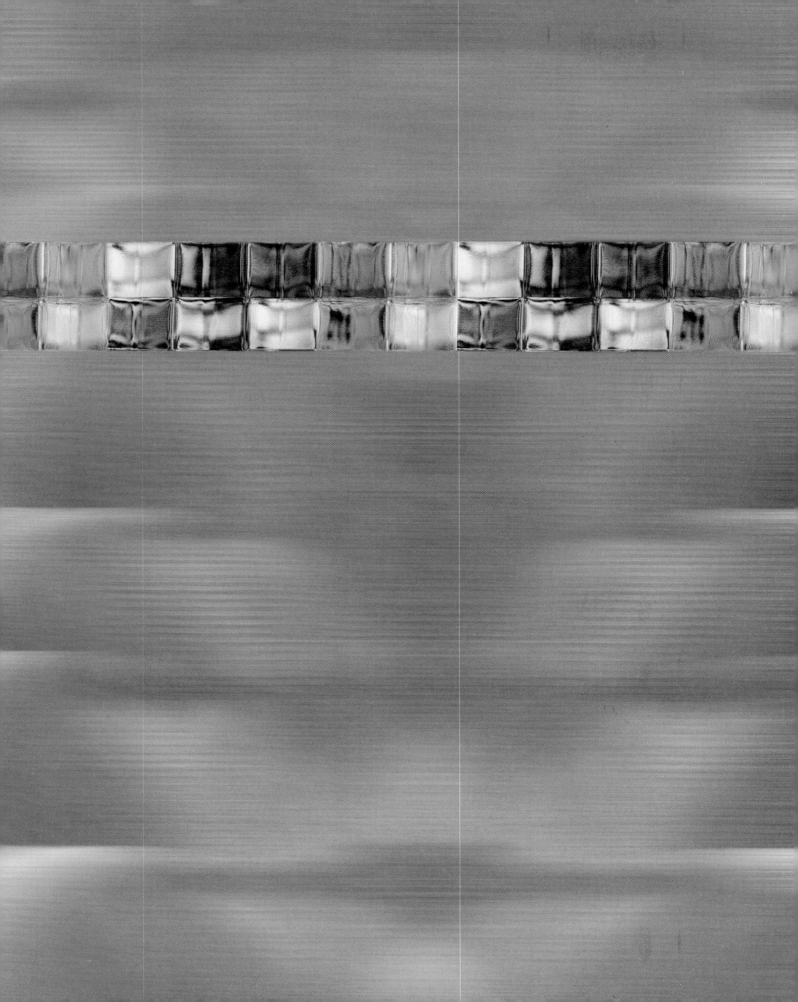

Unit
1

Review of Basic Mathematics Related to Dosage Computation

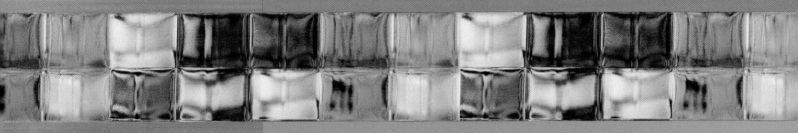

Chapter 1
Pretest in the Mathematics Involved in Dosage Computation

Chapter 2
Roman Numerals

Chapter 3
Fractions

Chapter 4
Decimals

Chapter 5
Percents

Chapter 6
Ratio

Chapter 7
Proportion

Chapter 8
Posttest in the Mathematics Involved in Dosage Computation

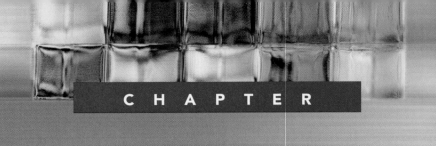

CHAPTER

1

Pretest in the Mathematics Involved in Dosage Computation

To safely administer medications, the nurse must master the ability to add, subtract, multiply, and divide whole numbers, fractions, and decimals. If you have a strong background in these basic skills, you should be able to compute proper dosage with relative ease.

Even though the pretest is time-consuming, it is vital for evaluating your knowledge of basic mathematics, so do not skip this process. Remember, we have used numbers here solely to demonstrate and review principles without regard to nursing situations. We recognize that the nurse would not encounter these numbers in patient-care settings. Aside from Unit 1, all the examples, questions, and problems relate to real-world situations that you might encounter during patient care.

Answer the five questions in each set. If, after scoring your paper, you find you have missed two or more questions in any set, work through the chapter that applies to that set. If you have four correct answers in each set, you can feel confident of your basic knowledge and move directly to Chapter 9.

Set 1.1

Write the following as Roman or Arabic numerals.

1. 29   _____

2. 63   _____

3. 92   _____

4. LIV   _____

5. XVIII   _____

Set 1.2

Add the following fractions and reduce to lowest terms.

1. $\frac{1}{2} + \frac{1}{4} + \frac{1}{16}$ _____

2. $\frac{1}{6} + \frac{4}{7} + \frac{5}{42}$ _____

3. $\dfrac{1}{3} + \dfrac{5}{12} + \dfrac{7}{36}$ _____

4. $2\dfrac{1}{4} + \dfrac{3}{8} + 1\dfrac{2}{9}$ _____

5. $3\dfrac{1}{7} + 24 + 10\dfrac{5}{21}$ _____

Set 1.3

Subtract the following fractions and reduce to lowest terms.

1. $\dfrac{7}{10} - \dfrac{3}{5}$ _____

2. $35 - 3\dfrac{3}{8}$ _____

3. $11\dfrac{5}{6} - 2\dfrac{1}{3}$ _____

4. $25\dfrac{1}{9} - 10\dfrac{4}{5}$ _____

5. $50\dfrac{1}{500} - 43\dfrac{2}{125}$ _____

Set 1.4

Multiply the following fractions and reduce to lowest terms.

1. $\dfrac{1}{2} \times \dfrac{1}{8}$ _____

2. $\dfrac{1}{16} \times \dfrac{1}{32}$ _____

3. $4\dfrac{3}{8} \times \dfrac{1}{10}$ _____

4. $7\dfrac{1}{2} \times 2 \times \dfrac{2}{3}$ _____

5. $12\dfrac{1}{2} \times 5\dfrac{7}{9} \times 2$ _____

Set 1.5

Divide the following fractions and reduce to lowest terms.

1. $\dfrac{1}{2} \div \dfrac{1}{4}$ _____

2. $7\dfrac{1}{2} \div 2$ _____

3. $2\dfrac{1}{2} \div \dfrac{3}{4}$ _____

4. $\dfrac{1}{64} \div \dfrac{1}{16}$ _____

5. $\dfrac{1}{100} \div \dfrac{1}{150}$ _____

Set 1.6

Change the following fractions to ratios.

1. $\dfrac{5}{7}$ _____

2. $\dfrac{1}{50}$ _____

3. $\dfrac{1}{120}$ _____

4. $\dfrac{3}{500}$ _____

5. $\dfrac{1}{9000}$ _____

Set 1.7

Arrange the following fractions in order from smallest to largest.

1. $\dfrac{3}{5}$; $\dfrac{1}{3}$; $\dfrac{3}{8}$; $\dfrac{3}{4}$; $\dfrac{5}{6}$ _____

2. $\dfrac{1}{10}$; $\dfrac{1}{2}$; $\dfrac{1}{12}$; $\dfrac{1}{3}$; $\dfrac{1}{9}$ _____

3. $\dfrac{1}{10}$; $\dfrac{3}{20}$; $\dfrac{5}{6}$; $\dfrac{7}{8}$; $\dfrac{1}{40}$ _____

4. $\dfrac{1}{8}$; $\dfrac{3}{16}$; $\dfrac{3}{4}$; $\dfrac{5}{64}$; $\dfrac{17}{32}$ _____

5. $\dfrac{1}{600}$; $\dfrac{1}{150}$; $\dfrac{1}{200}$; $\dfrac{1}{100}$; $\dfrac{1}{450}$ _____

Set 1.8

Change the following mixed numbers to improper fractions.

1. $12\dfrac{2}{5}$ _____

4. $42\dfrac{7}{9}$ _____

2. $33\dfrac{1}{3}$ _____

5. $5\dfrac{1}{150}$ _____

3. $16\dfrac{2}{3}$ _____

Set 1.9

Add the following decimals.

1. $1.5 + 2.7$ _____

4. $0.125 + 0.25$ _____

2. $0.75 + 0.66$ _____

5. $0.001 + 0.0101$ _____

3. $6.33 + 3.77$ _____

Set 1.10

Subtract the following decimals.

1. $1.6 - 0.35$ _____

4. $8.46 - 6.54$ _____

2. $1.5 - 0.75$ _____

5. $25.592 - 7.32$ _____

3. $0.5 - 0.125$ _____

Set 1.11

Multiply the following decimals.

1. 0.7×0.1 _____

4. 1.92×8.77 _____

2. 10.78×10 _____

5. 0.006×37.1 _____

3. 0.4×0.125 _____

Set 1.12

Divide the following decimals.

1. 0.4 ÷ 0.3 _____

2. 0.3 ÷ 0.15 _____

3. 6.42 ÷ 2.4 _____

4. 0.5 ÷ 0.125 _____

5. 0.006 ÷ 0.18 _____

Set 1.13

Arrange the following decimals in order from largest to smallest.

1. 0.9; 0.099; 0.1; 0.101; 0.17 _____

2. 0.125; 0.39; 0.6; 0.01; 0.015 _____

3. 0.4; 0.08; 0.014; 0.15; 0.375 _____

4. 0.01; 0.12; 0.2; 0.504; 0.102 _____

5. 0.006; 0.065; 0.6; 0.65; 0.0006 _____

Set 1.14

Convert the following fractions to decimals. Carry out to the fourth decimal place, if necessary.

1. $\dfrac{3}{8}$ _____

2. $\dfrac{1}{10}$ _____

3. $\dfrac{1}{64}$ _____

4. $\dfrac{1}{500}$ _____

5. $\dfrac{1}{9000}$ _____

Set 1.15

Convert the following decimals to fractions and reduce to lowest terms.

1. 0.7 _____

2. 0.25 _____

3. 0.05 _____

4. 0.50 _____

5. 0.004 _____

Set 1.16

Change the following fractions to percents.

1. $\dfrac{1}{2}$ _____

2. $\dfrac{3}{8}$ _____

3. $\dfrac{1}{125}$ _____

4. $\dfrac{1}{600}$ _____

5. $\dfrac{1}{1000}$ _____

Set 1.17

Change the following ratios to percents.

1. 1:4 _____
2. 1:20 _____
3. 1:300 _____

4. 1:5000 _____
5. 1:1500 _____

Set 1.18

Change the following decimals to percents.

1. 0.75 _____
2. 0.03 _____
3. 0.125 _____

4. 0.001 _____
5. 0.0006 _____

Set 1.19

Express the following percents as decimals.

1. 6% _____
2. 35% _____
3. 0.3% _____

4. 0.01% _____
5. 0.004% _____

Set 1.20

Express the following percents as fractions and reduce the answers to lowest terms.

1. 5% _____
2. 20% _____
3. 0.3% _____

4. $\frac{1}{4}$% _____
5. 0.05% _____

Set 1.21

Express the following percents as ratios.

1. 1% _____
2. 50% _____
3. 12.5% _____

4. 0.25% _____
5. 0.33% _____

Set 1.22

Express the following as ratios.

1. $\frac{1}{3}$ _____

2. $\frac{1}{500}$ _____

3. $\frac{\frac{2}{3}}{\frac{3}{4}}$ _____

4. $\dfrac{\frac{1}{2}}{150}$ _____

5. $\dfrac{\frac{1}{500}}{\frac{1}{1000}}$ _____

Set 1.23

Solve for x in the following proportions.

1. $1 : 5 = x : 20$ _____

2. $x : 3 = 7 : 21$ _____

3. $\dfrac{1}{2} : x = 3 : 12$ _____

4. $\dfrac{1}{3} : \dfrac{2}{3} = \dfrac{1}{6} : x$ _____

5. $25 : x = 75 : 1500$ _____

Set 1.24

Solve for x in the following proportions.

1. $\dfrac{1}{6} : \dfrac{1}{8} = x : 3$ _____

2. $0.3 : 0.4 = x : 0.5$ _____

3. $0.5 : 0.125 = 2 : x$ _____

4. $0.25 : 3 = 0.75 : x$ _____

5. $\dfrac{1}{150} : \dfrac{1}{100} = x : 1$ _____

Set 1.25

Make all of the following proportions "true" by changing one term in the ratio following the equal sign when necessary.

1. $1 : 4 = 25 : 100$ _____

2. $12 : 16 = \dfrac{3}{4} : \dfrac{2}{3}$ _____

3. $1 : \dfrac{1}{150} = 2 : \dfrac{1}{75}$ _____

4. $0.5 : 0.125 = 2 : 0.5$ _____

5. $\dfrac{1}{200} : 1 = \dfrac{1}{100} : \dfrac{1}{2}$ _____

ANSWERS TO PRETEST

Set 1.1   **1.** XXIX **2.** LXIII **3.** XCII **4.** 54 **5.** 18

Set 1.2   **1.** $\dfrac{13}{16}$ **2.** $\dfrac{6}{7}$ **3.** $\dfrac{17}{18}$ **4.** $3\dfrac{61}{72}$ **5.** $37\dfrac{8}{21}$

Set 1.3   **1.** $\dfrac{1}{10}$ **2.** $31\dfrac{5}{8}$ **3.** $9\dfrac{1}{2}$ **4.** $14\dfrac{14}{45}$ **5.** $6\dfrac{493}{500}$

Set 1.4   **1.** $\dfrac{1}{16}$ **2.** $\dfrac{1}{512}$ **3.** $\dfrac{7}{16}$ **4.** 10 **5.** $144\dfrac{4}{9}$

Set 1.5   **1.** 2 **2.** $3\dfrac{3}{4}$ **3.** $3\dfrac{1}{3}$ **4.** $\dfrac{1}{4}$ **5.** $1\dfrac{1}{2}$

Set 1.6   **1.** $5 : 7$ **2.** $1 : 50$ **3.** $1 : 120$ **4.** $3 : 500$ **5.** $1 : 9000$

Set 1.7   **1.** $\dfrac{1}{3} ; \dfrac{3}{8} ; \dfrac{3}{5} ; \dfrac{3}{4} ; \dfrac{5}{6}$ **2.** $\dfrac{1}{12} ; \dfrac{1}{10} ; \dfrac{1}{9} ; \dfrac{1}{3} ; \dfrac{1}{2}$ **3.** $\dfrac{1}{40} ; \dfrac{1}{10} ; \dfrac{3}{20} ; \dfrac{5}{6} ; \dfrac{7}{8}$ **4.** $\dfrac{5}{64} ; \dfrac{1}{8} ; \dfrac{3}{16} ; \dfrac{17}{32} ; \dfrac{3}{4}$ **5.** $\dfrac{1}{600} ; \dfrac{1}{450} ; \dfrac{1}{200} ; \dfrac{1}{150} ; \dfrac{1}{100}$

Set 1.8   1. $\dfrac{62}{5}$ 2. $\dfrac{100}{3}$ 3. $\dfrac{50}{3}$ 4. $\dfrac{385}{9}$ 5. $\dfrac{751}{150}$

Set 1.9   1. 4.2   2. 1.41   3. 10.1   4. 0.375   5. 0.0111

Set 1.10   1. 1.25   2. 0.75   3. 0.375   4. 1.92   5. 18.272

Set 1.11   1. 0.07   2. 107.8   3. 0.05   4. 16.8384   5. 0.2226

Set 1.12   1. 1.3333   2. 2   3. 2.675   4. 4   5. 0.0333

Set 1.13   1. 0.9; 0.17; 0.101; 0.1; 0.099   2. 0.6; 0.39; 0.125; 0.015; 0.01   3. 0.4; 0.375; 0.15; 0.08; 0.014   4. 0.504; 0.2; 0.12; 0.102; 0.01   5. 0.65; 0.6; 0.065; 0.006; 0.0006

Set 1.14   1. 0.375   2. 0.1   3. 0.0156   4. 0.002   5. 0.0001

Set 1.15   1. $\dfrac{7}{10}$ 2. $\dfrac{1}{4}$ 3. $\dfrac{1}{20}$ 4. $\dfrac{1}{2}$ 5. $\dfrac{1}{250}$

Set 1.16   1. 50%   2. 37.5%   3. 0.8%   4. $16\dfrac{2}{3}\%$ 5. 0.1%

Set 1.17   1. 25%   2. 5%   3. 0.33%   4. 0.02%   5. 0.06%

Set 1.18   1. 75%   2. 3%   3. 12.5%   4. 0.1%   5. 0.06%

Set 1.19   1. 0.06   2. 0.35   3. 0.003   4. 0.0001   5. 0.00004

Set 1.20   1. $\dfrac{1}{20}$ 2. $\dfrac{1}{5}$ 3. $\dfrac{3}{1000}$ 4. $\dfrac{1}{400}$ 5. $\dfrac{1}{2000}$

Set 1.21   1. 1 : 100   2. 1 : 2   3. 1 : 8   4. 1 : 400   5. 1 : 300

Set 1.22   1. 1 : 3   2. 1 : 500   3. $\dfrac{2}{3}:\dfrac{3}{4}$ 4. $\dfrac{1}{2}:150$ 5. $\dfrac{1}{500}:\dfrac{1}{1000}$

Set 1.23   1. x = 4   2. x = 1   3. x = 2   4. x = $\dfrac{1}{3}$ 5. x = 500

Set 1.24   1. x = 4   2. x = 0.375   3. x = 0.5   4. x = 9   5. x = $\dfrac{2}{3}$

Set 1.25   1. True proportion: 1 : 4 = 25 : 100   100 = 100   2. Change $\dfrac{2}{3}$ to 1

$$12:16 = \dfrac{3}{4}:1$$

$$12 = 12$$

3. True proportion: $1:\dfrac{1}{150} = 2:\dfrac{1}{75}$

$$\dfrac{1}{75} = \dfrac{1}{75}$$

4. True proportion: 0.5 : 0.125 = 2 : 0.5

0.25 = 0.25   5. Change $\dfrac{1}{2}$ to 2

$$\dfrac{1}{200}:1 = \dfrac{1}{100}:2$$

$$\dfrac{1}{100} = \dfrac{1}{100}$$

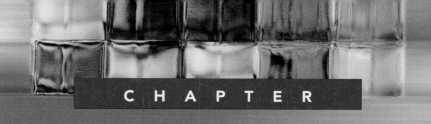

2

Roman Numerals

Learning Outcomes

After successfully completing this chapter, the learner should be able to:

- *Recognize the symbols used to represent numbers in the Roman system of numeration.*
- *Correctly write Arabic numerals as Roman numerals and Roman numerals as Arabic numerals.*

GENERAL INFORMATION

The numbers used throughout the world today are Arabic numerals. However, students in the health fields must also be able to interpret Roman numerals because they are still sometimes used.

VIP

Of these symbols, the I for 1, the V for 5, and the X for 10 are the most commonly encountered in the health fields. If an equal or smaller Roman numeral appears after a larger numeral, the value of the equal or smaller numeral is added to the value of the larger numeral. If the same Roman numeral is repeated, its value is added. For example, VIII = 8 (V = 5, III = 1 + 1 + 1 = 3) and 37 = XXXVII (XXX = 10 + 10 + 10 = 30; V = 5; II = 1 + 1 = 2).

Roman numerals are usually written as capital letters; however, in prescriptions they are frequently written as lowercase letters. In the Roman system of numeration, only seven symbols are needed to represent whole numbers, and these should be memorized:

I = 1	L = 50	D = 500
V = 5	C = 100	M = 1000
X = 10		

Problem Set 2.1

Convert the following:

1. VII _____
2. XVI _____
3. XXVIII _____
4. 22 _____
5. 6 _____

6. 33 _____
7. LXV _____
8. CCL _____
9. 70 _____
10. 125 _____

Answers 1. 7 2. 16 3. 28 4. XXII 5. VI 6. XXXIII 7. 65 8. 250 9. LXX 10. CXXV

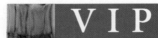

VIP

If a smaller Roman numeral appears before a larger numeral, the value of the smaller numeral is subtracted from the value of the larger numeral. Thus, IV = 4; IX = 9; and XIX = 19. Only one smaller numeral may precede a larger one, making expressions such as IIX, IVX, and XXXL unacceptable. When a smaller numeral is between two larger numerals, the rules for subtraction apply. Therefore, XXIX = 29, and XIV = 14.

Problem Set 2.2

Convert the following:

1. XIX _____
2. XXXIV _____
3. 43 _____
4. 64 _____
5. 92 _____

6. XCV _____
7. XLIX _____
8. XXXIX _____
9. 44 _____
10. 26 _____

Answers 1. 19 2. 34 3. XLIII 4. LXIV 5. XCII 6. 95 7. 49 8. 39 9. XLIV 10. XXVI

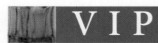

VIP

If there seem to be two ways of writing a numeral, the shorter form should be used. Because of this rule, a numeral should not be repeated more than three consecutive times in a given sequence. Thus, XVVI and XXXXII are incorrect, and XXI and XLII are correct.

Problem Set 2.3

Change the following to the correct form.

1. XVIIII   _____
2. XXXXV   _____
3. LXXXXIX   _____
4. CVVI   _____
5. XXXXXIIII   _____

6. XXLI   _____
7. CLXXXX   _____
8. XXCIIII   _____
9. XXVIIII   _____
10. CCCC   _____

Answers 1. XIX 2. XLV 3. IC 4. CXI 5. LIV 6. XXXI 7. CXC 8. LXXXIV 9. XXIX 10. CD

V I P

- If an equal or smaller Roman numeral appears after a larger numeral, the value of the equal or smaller numeral is added to the value of the larger numeral.
- If a smaller Roman numeral appears before a larger numeral, the value of the smaller numeral is subtracted from the value of the larger numeral.
- If there seem to be two ways of writing a numeral, the shorter form should be used.

Self-Evaluation Test 2.1
Roman Numerals

1. XXIV   _____
2. 32   _____
3. IX   _____
4. 48   _____
5. XVI   _____

6. 14   _____
7. 3   _____
8. LXXX   _____
9. XXIX   _____
10. 4   _____

Answers 1. 24 2. XXXII 3. 9 4. XLVIII 5. 16 6. XIV 7. III 8. 80 9. 29 10. IV

If you had fewer than three errors on Self-Evaluation Test 2.1, move on to Chapter 3, Fractions. If you had four or more errors, review the material on Roman numerals and complete Self-Evaluation Test 2.2 before continuing.

Self-Evaluation Test 2.2
Roman Numerals

1. LXIX   _____
2. 23   _____
3. XIX   _____

4. 2   _____
5. XXXVI   _____
6. 72   _____

7. XIV   _____

8. XLI   _____

9. XCII   _____

10. 1776 _____

Answers   **1.** 69   **2.** XXIII   **3.** 19   **4.** II   **5.** 36   **6.** LXXII   **7.** 14   **8.** 41   **9.** 92   **10.** MDCCLXXVI

The Self-Evaluation Tests on Roman numerals should be repeated until fewer than three errors occur.

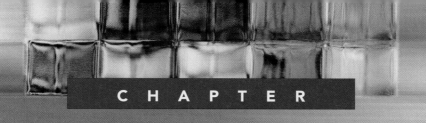

3

Fractions

Learning Outcomes

After successfully completing this chapter, the learner should be able to:

- *Define the parts of a fraction.*
- *Recognize the types of fractions.*
- *Identify the value of fractions.*
- *Find the least common denominator for fractions.*
- *Perform addition, subtraction, multiplication, and division of fractions.*

GENERAL INFORMATION

A fraction may be simply defined as a part of a whole. For example, one pie may be divided into four equal parts, each part being one fourth of the pie, with the four parts representing the whole pie (Figure 3-1).

One fourth can be written as $\frac{1}{4}$, 1/4, 1 ÷ 4, or 0.25, and one half can be written as $\frac{1}{2}$, 1/2, 1 ÷ 2, or 0.5 without any change in value. (Decimals are discussed in Chapter 4.)

A fraction is composed of two parts, a numerator and a denominator.

The denominator of a fraction is the number below the line, after the slash, or after the division sign. The denominator represents the number of parts into which the whole is divided. In the fraction $\frac{1}{4}$, the denominator is 4.

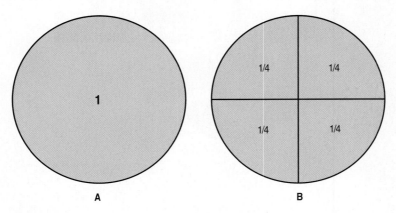

Figure 3-1   A. The whole   B. The whole divided into four equal parts

Problem Set 3.1

Identify the denominators of the following fractions.

1. $\dfrac{1}{3}$ _____

2. $\dfrac{1}{6}$ _____

3. $\dfrac{4}{11}$ _____

4. $\dfrac{33}{70}$ _____

5. $\dfrac{57}{61}$ _____

Answers   **1.** 3   **2.** 6   **3.** 11   **4.** 70   **5.** 61

The numerator is the number above the line, before the slash, or before the division sign. The numerator represents the number of parts taken from the whole. In the fraction $\frac{2}{7}$, the numerator is 2.

Problem Set 3.2

Identify the numerators of the following fractions.

1. $\dfrac{3}{4}$ _____

2. $\dfrac{5}{8}$ _____

3. $\dfrac{1}{5}$ _____

4. $\dfrac{19}{31}$ _____

5. $\dfrac{16}{57}$ _____

Answers   **1.** 3   **2.** 5   **3.** 1   **4.** 19   **5.** 16

A whole number may be expressed as a fraction by simply putting the whole number over a denominator of 1, producing the fraction $\frac{1}{1}$. This is true for any whole number.

Problem Set 3.3

Express the following whole numbers as fractions.

1. 5 _____
2. 23 _____
3. 567 _____

4. 1000 _____
5. 15,000 _____

Answers 1. $\frac{5}{1}$ 2. $\frac{23}{1}$ 3. $\frac{567}{1}$ 4. $\frac{1000}{1}$ 5. $\frac{15,000}{1}$

Changing a whole number to a fraction with a denominator of 1 does not change the value of the whole number, because dividing any number by 1 does not change its value.

For example, 20 can be written as $\frac{20}{1}$ or $20 \div 1$ without any change in value.

Problem Set 3.4

Divide the following whole numbers by 1.

1. $6 \div 1$ _____
2. $64 \div 1$ _____
3. $207 \div 1$ _____

4. $598 \div 1$ _____
5. $5424 \div 1$ _____

Answers 1. 6 2. 64 3. 207 4. 598 5. 5424

When a whole is divided into fractional parts, the smaller the denominator, the larger the portion it represents. If one pie is divided into four equal parts and a second pie is divided into eight equal parts, the larger portions would be in the pie divided into four equal parts; the smaller portions would be in the pie divided into eight equal parts.

Problem Set 3.5

Determine which fraction has the largest value.

1. $\frac{1}{2}$; $\frac{1}{6}$; or $\frac{1}{4}$ _____

2. $\frac{1}{32}$; $\frac{1}{60}$; or $\frac{1}{64}$ _____

3. $\frac{1}{100}$; $\frac{1}{175}$; or $\frac{1}{150}$ _____

4. $\frac{1}{1000}$; $\frac{1}{800}$; or $\frac{1}{500}$ _____

5. $\frac{1}{1500}$; $\frac{1}{5000}$; or $\frac{1}{10,000}$ _____

Answers 1. $\frac{1}{2}$ 2. $\frac{1}{32}$ 3. $\frac{1}{100}$ 4. $\frac{1}{500}$ 5. $\frac{1}{1500}$

If the denominators of two or more fractions are equal: the larger the numerator, the larger the amount it represents; and the smaller the numerator, the smaller the amount it represents. Given the fractions $\frac{1}{4}$, $\frac{2}{4}$, and $\frac{3}{4}$, the largest amount is represented by the fraction $\frac{3}{4}$ and the smallest amount is represented by the fraction $\frac{1}{4}$.

Problem Set 3.6

Determine which fraction has the smaller value.

1. $\frac{2}{3}$ or $\frac{1}{3}$ _____

2. $\frac{1}{8}$ or $\frac{3}{8}$ _____

3. $\frac{5}{64}$ or $\frac{7}{64}$ _____

4. $\frac{3}{1000}$ or $\frac{9}{1000}$ _____

5. $\frac{7}{10,000}$ or $\frac{31}{10,000}$ _____

Answers 1. $\frac{1}{3}$ 2. $\frac{1}{8}$ 3. $\frac{5}{64}$ 4. $\frac{3}{1000}$ 5. $\frac{7}{10,000}$

VIP

- The value of a number does not change when it is placed over a denominator of 1 or is divided by 1.
- If the numerators of the fractions are the same: the smaller the denominator, the larger the amount it represents.
- If the denominators of the fraction are the same: the larger the numerator, the larger the amount it represents.

Self-Evaluation Test 3.1
Assessing Fractions

Determine which fraction has the largest value.

1. $\frac{5}{8}$; $\frac{3}{8}$; or $\frac{7}{8}$ _____

2. $\frac{5}{12}$, $\frac{5}{32}$; or $\frac{5}{16}$ _____

3. $\frac{61}{64}$; $\frac{33}{64}$; or $\frac{1}{64}$ _____

4. $\frac{7}{150}$; $\frac{7}{300}$; or $\frac{7}{200}$ _____

5. $\frac{3}{1000}$; $\frac{33}{1000}$; or $\frac{1}{1000}$ _____

Express the following whole numbers as fractions.

6. 1 _____

7. 12 _____

8. 25 _____

9. 500 _____

10. 1000 _____

Arrange the following fractions in order from the largest to the smallest.

11. $\dfrac{1}{8}$; $\dfrac{1}{2}$; $\dfrac{1}{3}$; $\dfrac{1}{12}$; $\dfrac{1}{6}$ _____

12. $\dfrac{5}{16}$; $\dfrac{5}{32}$; $\dfrac{5}{8}$; $\dfrac{5}{6}$; $\dfrac{5}{64}$ _____

13. $\dfrac{3}{16}$; $\dfrac{1}{16}$; $\dfrac{5}{16}$; $\dfrac{13}{16}$; $\dfrac{7}{16}$ _____

14. $\dfrac{3}{350}$; $\dfrac{3}{200}$; $\dfrac{3}{500}$; $\dfrac{3}{150}$; $\dfrac{3}{100}$ _____

15. $\dfrac{3}{1000}$; $\dfrac{1}{1000}$; $\dfrac{99}{1000}$; $\dfrac{999}{1000}$; $\dfrac{7}{1000}$ _____

Answers   1. $\dfrac{7}{8}$ 2. $\dfrac{5}{12}$ 3. $\dfrac{61}{64}$ 4. $\dfrac{7}{150}$ 5. $\dfrac{33}{1000}$ 6. $\dfrac{1}{1}$ 7. $\dfrac{12}{1}$ 8. $\dfrac{25}{1}$ 9. $\dfrac{500}{1}$ 10. $\dfrac{1000}{1}$ 11. $\dfrac{1}{2}, \dfrac{1}{3}, \dfrac{1}{6}, \dfrac{1}{8}, \dfrac{1}{12}$
12. $\dfrac{5}{6}, \dfrac{5}{8}, \dfrac{5}{16}, \dfrac{5}{32}, \dfrac{5}{64}$ 13. $\dfrac{13}{16}, \dfrac{7}{16}, \dfrac{5}{16}, \dfrac{3}{16}, \dfrac{1}{16}$ 14. $\dfrac{3}{100}, \dfrac{3}{150}, \dfrac{3}{200}, \dfrac{3}{350}, \dfrac{3}{500}$ 15. $\dfrac{999}{1000}, \dfrac{99}{1000}, \dfrac{7}{1000}, \dfrac{3}{1000}, \dfrac{1}{1000}$

If you had fewer than three errors on Self-Evaluation Test 3.1, move on to the next section. If you had four or more errors, review the material just covered and complete Self-Evaluation Test 3.2 before continuing.

Self-Evaluation Test 3.2
Assessing Fractions

Determine which fraction has the largest value.

1. $\dfrac{2}{9}$; $\dfrac{7}{9}$; $\dfrac{5}{9}$ _____

4. $\dfrac{3}{125}$; $\dfrac{1}{125}$; $\dfrac{22}{125}$ _____

2. $\dfrac{5}{6}$; $\dfrac{5}{8}$; $\dfrac{5}{12}$ _____

5. $\dfrac{3}{1000}$; $\dfrac{3}{10,000}$; $\dfrac{3}{100}$ _____

3. $\dfrac{7}{500}$; $\dfrac{3}{500}$; $\dfrac{49}{500}$ _____

Express the following whole numbers as fractions.

6. 2   _____

9. 150   _____

7. 32   _____

10. 1500   _____

8. 75   _____

Arrange the following fractions in order from the smallest to the largest.

11. $\dfrac{1}{6}$; $\dfrac{1}{5}$; $\dfrac{1}{8}$; $\dfrac{1}{4}$; $\dfrac{1}{3}$ _____

12. $\dfrac{7}{10}$; $\dfrac{7}{9}$; $\dfrac{7}{12}$; $\dfrac{7}{8}$; $\dfrac{7}{16}$ _____

13. $\dfrac{1}{65}$; $\dfrac{1}{62}$; $\dfrac{1}{60}$; $\dfrac{1}{32}$; $\dfrac{1}{64}$ _____

14. $\dfrac{3}{150}$; $\dfrac{3}{200}$; $\dfrac{3}{100}$; $\dfrac{3}{250}$; $\dfrac{3}{300}$ _____

15. $\dfrac{1}{1000}$; $\dfrac{1}{10,000}$; $\dfrac{1}{100}$; $\dfrac{1}{150}$; $\dfrac{1}{1500}$ _____

Answers 1. $\dfrac{7}{9}$ 2. $\dfrac{5}{6}$ 3. $\dfrac{49}{500}$ 4. $\dfrac{22}{125}$ 5. $\dfrac{3}{100}$ 6. $\dfrac{2}{1}$ 7. $\dfrac{32}{1}$ 8. $\dfrac{75}{1}$ 9. $\dfrac{150}{1}$ 10. $\dfrac{1500}{1}$ 11. $\dfrac{1}{8}$, $\dfrac{1}{6}$, $\dfrac{1}{5}$, $\dfrac{1}{4}$, $\dfrac{1}{3}$
12. $\dfrac{7}{16}$, $\dfrac{7}{12}$, $\dfrac{7}{10}$, $\dfrac{7}{9}$, $\dfrac{7}{8}$ 13. $\dfrac{1}{65}$, $\dfrac{1}{64}$, $\dfrac{1}{62}$, $\dfrac{1}{60}$, $\dfrac{1}{32}$ 14. $\dfrac{3}{300}$, $\dfrac{3}{250}$, $\dfrac{3}{200}$, $\dfrac{3}{150}$, $\dfrac{3}{100}$ 15. $\dfrac{1}{10,000}$, $\dfrac{1}{1500}$, $\dfrac{1}{1000}$, $\dfrac{1}{150}$, $\dfrac{1}{100}$

The Self-Evaluation Tests on assessing fractions should be repeated until fewer than three errors occur.

PROPER AND IMPROPER FRACTIONS AND MIXED NUMBERS

When the numerator of a fraction is smaller than the denominator, it is called a proper fraction and has a value of less than 1. For example, $\dfrac{4}{9}$ is less than 1 and is a proper fraction. The fraction $\dfrac{2}{5}$ is classified as a proper fraction.

When the numerator of a fraction is equal to or greater than the denominator, it is called an improper fraction and has a value of 1 or greater than 1. For example, $\dfrac{9}{9}$ is equal to 1 and $\dfrac{13}{9}$ is greater than 1; both are improper fractions. The fraction $\dfrac{7}{3}$ is classified as an improper fraction.

Problem Set 3.7

Identify whether the following fractions are proper or improper fractions.

1. $\dfrac{15}{2}$ _____

2. $\dfrac{64}{65}$ _____

3. $\dfrac{9}{1000}$ _____

4. $\dfrac{201}{200}$ _____

5. $\dfrac{199}{200}$ _____

Answers 1. Improper 2. Proper 3. Proper 4. Improper 5. Proper

Changing Improper Fractions and Mixed Numbers

Every improper fraction may be written as a whole number or a mixed number (a whole number with a proper fraction) or a whole number and an improper fraction without any change in value. For example, $\dfrac{19}{6}$ can be written as $3\dfrac{1}{6}$, $2\dfrac{7}{6}$, $1\dfrac{13}{6}$ without any change in value. $\dfrac{5}{3}$ can be written as $1\dfrac{2}{3}$.

An improper fraction can be changed to a whole number or a mixed number by dividing the numerator of the fraction by the denominator of the fraction.

Example: Change $\dfrac{18}{9}$ to a whole number.

Solution: $\dfrac{18}{9} = 9\overline{)18}^{\,2}$

If there is a remainder as a result of the division, the remainder becomes the numerator of the fractional part of the mixed number, and the denominator of the improper fraction is used as the denominator of this fractional part.

Example: Change $\dfrac{13}{4}$ to a mixed number.

Solution: $\dfrac{13}{4} = 4\overline{)13}$ $\quad \dfrac{3}{}= 3\dfrac{1}{4}$

$$4\overline{)13}$$
$$\underline{12}$$
$$1$$

To review, $\dfrac{23}{7}$ can be changed to a mixed number by dividing the numerator 23 by the denominator 7. The whole-number part of the answer will be 3 and the fractional part will be $\dfrac{2}{7}$.

Problem Set 3.8

Change the following improper fractions to whole or mixed numbers.

1. $\dfrac{15}{2}$ _____

2. $\dfrac{100}{3}$ _____

3. $\dfrac{193}{64}$ _____

4. $\dfrac{325}{16}$ _____

5. $\dfrac{1500}{100}$ _____

Answers 1. $7\dfrac{1}{2}$ 2. $33\dfrac{1}{3}$ 3. $3\dfrac{1}{64}$ 4. $20\dfrac{5}{16}$ 5. 15

A mixed number can be changed to an improper fraction.

Example: Change $2\dfrac{3}{4}$ to an improper fraction.

Solution: Multiply the whole-number part of the mixed number by the denominator of the fraction part.

$2 \times 4 = 8$

Then add the numerator of the fraction part of the mixed number to this answer.

$3 + 8 = 11$

This answer becomes the numerator of the improper fraction, and the denominator of the fraction part of the mixed number becomes the denominator of the improper fraction.

$2\dfrac{3}{4} = \dfrac{11}{4}$

To review, $5\dfrac{3}{8}$ can be changed to an improper fraction by first multiplying 5 by 8 and adding 3, obtaining 43. The 43 becomes the numerator of the improper fraction. The denominator of the improper fraction will be 8. Therefore, $5\dfrac{3}{8}$ is equal to $\dfrac{43}{8}$.

Problem Set 3.9

Convert the following mixed numbers to improper fractions.

1. $33\dfrac{1}{3}$ _____

2. $37\dfrac{1}{8}$ _____

3. $83\dfrac{2}{3}$ _____

4. $120\dfrac{3}{5}$ _____

5. $100\dfrac{3}{64}$ _____

Answers 1. $\dfrac{100}{3}$ 2. $\dfrac{297}{8}$ 3. $\dfrac{251}{3}$ 4. $\dfrac{603}{5}$ 5. $\dfrac{6403}{64}$

Self-Evaluation Test 3.3
Improper Fractions and Mixed Numbers

Change the following improper fractions to whole or mixed numbers.

1. $\dfrac{23}{8}$ _____

2. $\dfrac{19}{4}$ _____

3. $\dfrac{89}{16}$ _____

4. $\dfrac{100}{33}$ _____

5. $\dfrac{128}{64}$ _____

6. $\dfrac{307}{150}$ _____

7. $\dfrac{451}{300}$ _____

Change the following mixed numbers to improper fractions.

8. $1\dfrac{1}{2}$ _____

9. $3\dfrac{3}{4}$ _____

10. $7\dfrac{1}{2}$ _____

11. $25\dfrac{3}{4}$ _____

12. $29\dfrac{2}{3}$ _____

13. $12\dfrac{1}{8}$ _____

14. $16\dfrac{2}{3}$ _____

15. $2\dfrac{49}{50}$ _____

Answers   1. $2\dfrac{7}{8}$ 2. $4\dfrac{3}{4}$ 3. $5\dfrac{9}{16}$ 4. $3\dfrac{1}{33}$ 5. 2 6. $2\dfrac{7}{150}$ 7. $1\dfrac{151}{300}$ 8. $\dfrac{3}{2}$ 9. $\dfrac{15}{4}$ 10. $\dfrac{15}{2}$ 11. $\dfrac{103}{4}$ 12. $\dfrac{89}{3}$ 13. $\dfrac{97}{8}$

14. $\dfrac{50}{3}$ 15. $\dfrac{149}{50}$

If you had fewer than three errors on Self-Evaluation Test 3.3, move on to the next section. If you had four or more errors, review the material just covered and complete Self-Evaluation Test 3.4 before continuing.

Self-Evaluation Test 3.4
Improper Fractions and Mixed Numbers

Change the following improper fractions to whole or mixed numbers.

1. $\dfrac{5}{2}$ _____

2. $\dfrac{9}{7}$ _____

3. $\dfrac{53}{5}$ _____

4. $\dfrac{32}{9}$ _____

5. $\dfrac{47}{6}$ _____

6. $\dfrac{52}{15}$ _____

7. $\dfrac{90}{45}$ _____

Change the following mixed numbers to improper fractions.

8. $1\dfrac{1}{4}$ _____

9. $2\dfrac{3}{8}$ _____

10. $1\frac{1}{32}$ _____   13. $12\frac{3}{8}$ _____

11. $2\frac{3}{64}$ _____   14. $2\frac{1}{150}$ _____

12. $66\frac{2}{3}$ _____   15. $50\frac{3}{64}$ _____

Answers   1. $2\frac{1}{2}$ 2. $1\frac{2}{7}$ 3. $10\frac{3}{5}$ 4. $3\frac{5}{9}$ 5. $7\frac{5}{6}$ 6. $3\frac{7}{15}$ 7. 2   8. $\frac{5}{4}$ 9. $\frac{19}{8}$ 10. $\frac{33}{32}$ 11. $\frac{131}{64}$ 12. $\frac{200}{3}$ 13. $\frac{99}{8}$

14. $\frac{301}{150}$ 15. $\frac{3203}{64}$

The Self-Evaluation Tests on improper fractions and mixed numbers should be repeated until fewer than three errors occur.

CHANGING THE FORM OF FRACTIONS

You can change the form of a fraction without changing its value. This can be accomplished by either multiplying or dividing both the numerator and the denominator by the same number.

The fraction $\frac{2}{3}$ can be changed to $\frac{8}{12}$ by multiplying both the numerator, 2, and the denominator, 3, by the number 4. This changes the form of the fraction but not the value.

The fraction $\frac{18}{20}$ can be changed to $\frac{9}{10}$ by dividing both the numerator, 18, and the denominator, 20, by the number 2. Again, this changes the form but not the value of the fraction. This is called reducing the fraction to its lowest terms.

The fraction $\frac{6}{8}$ is equal to $\frac{3}{4}$ (dividing both the numerator and the denominator by 2), $\frac{12}{16}$ (multiplying both the numerator and denominator by 2), $\frac{18}{24}$ (multiplying both the numerator and the denominator by 3), and so on. Consider the following set of fractions: $\frac{3}{21}$, $\frac{1}{7}$, $\frac{10}{28}$, and $\frac{6}{42}$. The one fraction in this set not equal to the others is $\frac{10}{28}$.

Calculation Alert

Multiplying or dividing both the numerator and the denominator of a fraction by the same number does not change the value of a fraction.

Problem Set 3.10

Identify the fraction in each set that is not equal in value to the other fractions in the set.

1. $\frac{1}{8}$; $\frac{3}{16}$; $\frac{4}{32}$; $\frac{5}{40}$ _____

2. $\frac{1}{12}$; $\frac{2}{36}$; $\frac{4}{48}$; $\frac{5}{60}$ _____

3. $\frac{1}{50}$; $\frac{2}{100}$; $\frac{3}{150}$; $\frac{5}{200}$ _____

4. $\dfrac{1}{100}$; $\dfrac{2}{200}$; $\dfrac{3}{400}$; $\dfrac{5}{500}$ _____

5. $\dfrac{1}{500}$; $\dfrac{2}{1000}$; $\dfrac{3}{1500}$; $\dfrac{5}{2000}$ _____

Answers   1. $\dfrac{3}{16}$ 2. $\dfrac{2}{36}$ 3. $\dfrac{5}{200}$ 4. $\dfrac{3}{400}$ 5. $\dfrac{5}{2000}$

Reducing fractions to their lowest terms minimizes confusion and simplifies the determination of the true value of the fraction. Therefore, in most instances, it is easier to work with fractions that are reduced to their lowest terms.

A fraction is in its lowest terms if no whole number other than 1 will divide equally into both the numerator and denominator. Thus, $\dfrac{3}{8}$ is in its lowest terms, but $\dfrac{3}{12}$ is not, because both the numerator and denominator are divisible by 3. Consider the following fractions: $\dfrac{3}{4}$, $\dfrac{5}{7}$, $\dfrac{7}{150}$, and $\dfrac{2}{300}$. The fraction not in lowest terms is $\dfrac{2}{300}$, which can be reduced to $\dfrac{1}{150}$.

To reduce a fraction to its lowest terms, divide both the numerator and the denominator by the largest number possible that divides exactly into both. Continue this process until no further division is possible. When no number will divide exactly into both the numerator and the denominator, the fraction is in its lowest terms.

In the fraction $\dfrac{56}{64}$, both the numerator 56 and the denominator 64 are divisible by 2. However, in the resulting fraction, both the numerator 28 and the denominator 32 are also divisible by 4, producing the fraction $\dfrac{7}{8}$, which is its lowest terms. A step could have been saved and the same results obtained if the original numerator and denominator had been divided by 8.

Calculation Alert

- A fraction is in its lowest terms if no whole number other than 1 will divide equally into both the numerator and the denominator.

- To reduce a fraction to its lowest terms, divide both the numerator and the denominator by the largest number possible that divides exactly into both.

Problem Set 3.11

Reduce the following fractions to their lowest terms.

1. $\dfrac{48}{72}$ _____ 5. $\dfrac{80}{96}$ _____

2. $\dfrac{18}{63}$ _____ 6. $\dfrac{54}{81}$ _____

3. $\dfrac{18}{24}$ _____ 7. $\dfrac{280}{630}$ _____

4. $\dfrac{39}{65}$ _____ 8. $\dfrac{105}{135}$ _____

9. $\dfrac{375}{1200}$ _____   10. $\dfrac{510}{1890}$ _____

Answers　1. $\frac{2}{3}$　2. $\frac{2}{7}$　3. $\frac{3}{4}$　4. $\frac{3}{5}$　5. $\frac{5}{6}$　6. $\frac{2}{3}$　7. $\frac{4}{9}$　8. $\frac{7}{9}$　9. $\frac{5}{16}$　10. $\frac{17}{63}$

A given fraction can be expressed as an equal fraction with a different denominator. For example, $\frac{1}{2}$ can be written as $\frac{5}{10}$, $\frac{25}{50}$, or $\frac{50}{100}$. Such a change is accomplished by multiplying both the numerator and denominator by the same number.

To change the form of a fraction when only the denominator of the new form is known, it is necessary to divide the new denominator by the denominator of the original fraction. The original numerator is then multiplied by this result. Thus, to express $\frac{2}{3}$ as a fraction with 12 as the new denominator, divide 12 by 3 (the original denominator) which equals 4; then multiply the original numerator, 2, by the 4 to obtain the new numerator, producing the fraction $\frac{8}{12}$. To change $\frac{1}{2}$ to a new fraction with a denominator of 12, divide 12 by 2, then multiply the numerator, 1, by 6. Thus, $\frac{1}{2}$ can be changed to $\frac{6}{12}$ without any change in value.

Problem Set 3.12

Change the following fractions to the forms shown.

1. $\dfrac{1}{2}$ _____ /10　　6. $\dfrac{5}{12}$ _____ /36

2. $\dfrac{3}{8}$ _____ /64　　7. $\dfrac{3}{50}$ _____ /200

3. $\dfrac{5}{6}$ _____ /96　　8. $\dfrac{1}{65}$ _____ /325

4. $\dfrac{3}{4}$ _____ /120　　9. $\dfrac{7}{16}$ _____ /48

5. $\dfrac{5}{9}$ _____ /99　　10. $\dfrac{1}{150}$ _____ /300

Answers　1. $\frac{5}{10}$　2. $\frac{24}{64}$　3. $\frac{80}{96}$　4. $\frac{90}{120}$　5. $\frac{55}{99}$　6. $\frac{15}{36}$　7. $\frac{12}{200}$　8. $\frac{5}{325}$　9. $\frac{21}{48}$　10. $\frac{2}{300}$

FINDING THE LEAST COMMON DENOMINATOR

It is frequently necessary to find a least common denominator (LCD) for a group of fractions. The least common denominator is the smallest number into which each of the denominators of each of the fractions in the group will divide exactly.

For example, 12 is the least common denominator for the fractions $\frac{1}{4}$, and $\frac{1}{3}$, because it is the smallest number that both 4 and 3 divide into exactly. For the fractions $\frac{1}{4}$, $\frac{1}{6}$, and $\frac{1}{8}$, the least common denominator is 24.

The number 48 could have been selected because 4, 6, and 8 also divide exactly into this number, but the LCD is the *smallest* number that all the denominators divide into exactly.

If the least common denominator for a group of fractions cannot be determined by looking, use the following procedure:

Example: Find the least common denominator of $\frac{1}{5}$, $\frac{1}{6}$, $\frac{2}{9}$, $\frac{5}{12}$, and $\frac{3}{24}$

Solution: Write all the denominators in a horizontal row: 5 6 9 12 24

Starting with the number 2, find the smallest whole number that divides exactly into two or more of the denominators. (If two or more of the denominators cannot be exactly divided by the number 2, try the number 3, and so on.)

Write the results of the division directly under the denominators, and bring down all the denominators that cannot be divided, thus completing a totally new row of numbers.

2	5	6	9	12	24
	5	3	9	6	12

Repeat the process until the final row of numbers contains no numbers that can be exactly divided by any whole number other than 1.

2	5	6	9	12	24
2	5	3	9	6	12
3	5	3	9	3	6
	5	1	3	1	2

The least common denominator can then be determined by multiplying each divisor (vertical numbers) and each number in the last row (horizontal numbers).

LCD = $2 \times 2 \times 3 \times 5 \times 1 \times 3 \times 1 \times 2$

LCD = $2 \times 2 \times 3 \times 5 \times 3 \times 2$ (the 1s can be dropped)

LCD = 360

When the least common denominator is obvious, this procedure is unnecessary.

Example: Find the least common denominator of $\frac{1}{4}$, $\frac{3}{12}$, $\frac{3}{20}$, and $\frac{7}{40}$

Solution: Write the row of denominators:

	4	12	20	40	divide this row by 2
2	2	6	10	20	divide this row by 2
2	1	3	5	10	divide this row by 5
5	1	3	1	2	which is only divisible by 1
	1	3	1	2	

Therefore, the LCD is determined by multiplying $2 \times 2 \times 5 \times 1 \times 3 \times 1 \times 2 = 120$

VIP

The least common denominator is the smallest number into which all of the denominators will divide equally.

Problem Set 3.13

Find the common denominator for the following fractions.

1. $\frac{1}{4}$, $\frac{1}{2}$, $\frac{3}{4}$ _____

2. $\frac{1}{6}$, $\frac{1}{8}$, $\frac{1}{4}$ _____

3. $\frac{9}{10}$, $\frac{1}{4}$, $\frac{1}{12}$ _____

4. $\frac{1}{3}$, $\frac{1}{12}$, $\frac{2}{9}$ _____

5. $\frac{1}{16}$, $\frac{1}{32}$, $\frac{1}{64}$ _____

6. $\frac{1}{15}$, $\frac{2}{5}$, $\frac{4}{45}$ _____

7. $\dfrac{3}{8}, \dfrac{1}{32}, \dfrac{1}{40}$ _____

8. $\dfrac{1}{16}, \dfrac{3}{48}, \dfrac{5}{8}$ _____

9. $\dfrac{1}{75}, \dfrac{1}{150}, \dfrac{3}{100}$ _____

10. $\dfrac{1}{200}, \dfrac{1}{150}, \dfrac{1}{100}$ _____

Answers **1.** 4 **2.** 24 **3.** 60 **4.** 36 **5.** 64 **6.** 45 **7.** 160 **8.** 48 **9.** 300 **10.** 600

Self-Evaluation Test 3.5
Changing the Form of Fractions

Reduce the following fractions to their lowest terms.

1. $\dfrac{84}{168}$ _____

2. $\dfrac{50}{175}$ _____

3. $\dfrac{84}{108}$ _____

4. $\dfrac{135}{675}$ _____

5. $\dfrac{217}{441}$ _____

Change the following fractions to the forms shown.

6. $\dfrac{3}{25}$ _____ /150

7. $\dfrac{3}{10}$ _____ /1000

8. $\dfrac{1}{8}$ _____ /96

9. $\dfrac{3}{8}$ _____ /64

10. $\dfrac{1}{100}$ _____ /300

Find the least common denominator for the following fractions.

11. $\dfrac{1}{4}, \dfrac{1}{16}, \dfrac{1}{8}$ _____

12. $\dfrac{1}{3}, \dfrac{1}{15}, \dfrac{1}{45}$ _____

13. $\dfrac{1}{7}, \dfrac{2}{35}, \dfrac{5}{14}$ _____

14. $\dfrac{1}{8}, \dfrac{1}{16}, \dfrac{1}{32}$ _____

15. $\dfrac{3}{16}, \dfrac{3}{32}, \dfrac{1}{96}$ _____

Answers **1.** $\dfrac{1}{2}$ **2.** $\dfrac{2}{7}$ **3.** $\dfrac{7}{9}$ **4.** $\dfrac{1}{5}$ **5.** $\dfrac{31}{63}$ **6.** $\dfrac{18}{150}$ **7.** $\dfrac{300}{1000}$ **8.** $\dfrac{12}{96}$ **9.** $\dfrac{24}{64}$ **10.** $\dfrac{3}{300}$ **11.** 16 **12.** 45 **13.** 70 **14.** 32 **15.** 96

  If you had fewer than three errors on Self-Evaluation Test 3.5, move on to the next section. If you had four or more errors, review the material just covered and complete Self-Evaluation Test 3.6 before continuing.

Self-Evaluation Test 3.6
Changing the Form of Fractions

Reduce the following fractions to their lowest terms.

1. $\dfrac{3}{150}$ _____

2. $\dfrac{16}{64}$ _____

3. $\dfrac{27}{108}$ _____

4. $\dfrac{60}{325}$ _____

5. $\dfrac{100}{125}$ _____

Change the following fractions to the forms shown.

6. $\dfrac{1}{65}$ _____ /325

7. $\dfrac{1}{16}$ _____ /64

8. $\dfrac{3}{64}$ _____ /320

9. $\dfrac{1}{75}$ _____ /150

10. $\dfrac{1}{200}$ _____ /600

Find the least common denominator for the following fractions.

11. $\dfrac{1}{2}, \dfrac{1}{6}, \dfrac{1}{8}$ _____

12. $\dfrac{1}{5}, \dfrac{1}{10}, \dfrac{1}{15}$ _____

13. $\dfrac{1}{25}, \dfrac{1}{150}, \dfrac{1}{300}$ _____

14. $\dfrac{1}{65}, \dfrac{1}{195}, \dfrac{1}{130}$ _____

15. $\dfrac{3}{200}, \dfrac{1}{100}, \dfrac{1}{300}$ _____

Answers   1. $\dfrac{1}{50}$ 2. $\dfrac{1}{4}$ 3. $\dfrac{1}{4}$ 4. $\dfrac{12}{65}$ 5. $\dfrac{4}{5}$ 6. $\dfrac{5}{325}$ 7. $\dfrac{4}{64}$ 8. $\dfrac{15}{320}$ 9. $\dfrac{2}{150}$ 10. $\dfrac{3}{600}$ **11.** 24   **12.** 30   **13.** 300   **14.** 390   **15.** 600

The Self-Evaluation Tests on changing the form of fractions should be repeated until fewer than three errors occur.

ADDING AND SUBTRACTING FRACTIONS

It is simple to combine fractions that have the same denominator. Just as three dimes plus four dimes equals seven dimes, three tenths plus four tenths equals seven tenths ($\frac{3}{10} + \frac{4}{10} = \frac{7}{10}$). In the same way, four fifths minus one fifth equals three fifths ($\frac{4}{5} + \frac{1}{5} = \frac{3}{5}$). These problems may also be written as:

$$\begin{array}{r} \dfrac{3}{10} \\ + \dfrac{4}{10} \\ \hline \dfrac{7}{10} \end{array} \quad 3 \atop 4 \qquad \text{and} \qquad \begin{array}{r} \dfrac{4}{5} \\ - \dfrac{1}{5} \\ \hline \dfrac{3}{5} \end{array} \quad 4 \atop 1$$

Adding or Subtracting Fractions That Have the Same Denominators

Example: Add $\dfrac{3}{4}$ and $\dfrac{5}{4}$

Solution: Add the numerators as indicated: 3 + 5 = 8

Place the result over the common denominator, which in this instance is 4

Reduce the result to lowest terms $\dfrac{3}{4} + \dfrac{5}{4} = \dfrac{8}{4}$, which can be reduced to 2

Example: Subtract $\dfrac{7}{6}$ from $\dfrac{17}{6}$

Solution: Subtract the numerators as indicated: 17 − 7 = 10

Place the result over the common denominator, which in this instance is 6

Reduce the result to lowest terms: $\frac{17}{6} - \frac{7}{6} = \frac{10}{6}$, which can be reduced to $\frac{5}{3}$, which can be further reduced to $1\frac{2}{3}$

Problem Set 3.14

Solve the following problems. Reduce to lowest terms.

1. $\frac{6}{4} + \frac{2}{4}$ _____

6. $\frac{5}{64} + \frac{7}{64} - \frac{1}{64}$ _____

2. $\frac{36}{8} - \frac{16}{8}$ _____

7. $\frac{31}{32} - \frac{3}{32} - \frac{1}{32}$ _____

3. $\frac{5}{6} - \frac{1}{6}$ _____

8. $\frac{6}{100} - \frac{2}{100} - \frac{3}{100}$ _____

4. $\frac{8}{10} + \frac{7}{10} + \frac{3}{10}$ _____

9. $\frac{9}{1000} - \frac{1}{1000} - \frac{3}{1000}$ _____

5. $\frac{1}{12} + \frac{6}{12} + \frac{5}{12}$ _____

10. $\frac{1}{1500} + \frac{17}{1500} + \frac{1483}{1500}$ _____

Answers   1. 2   2. $2\frac{1}{2}$ 3. $\frac{2}{3}$ 4. $1\frac{4}{5}$ 5. 1   6. $\frac{11}{64}$ 7. $\frac{27}{32}$ 8. $\frac{1}{100}$ 9. $\frac{1}{200}$ 10. $1\frac{1}{1500}$

Adding or Subtracting Fractions That Have Different Denominators

Example: Add $\frac{1}{4} + \frac{1}{6}$

Solution: Find the least common denominator: the LCD = 12

Write each fraction with this new denominator:

$\frac{1}{4}$ becomes $\frac{3}{12}$ and $\frac{1}{6}$ becomes $\frac{2}{12}$

Follow the procedure for fractions that have the same denominators and reduce the result to lowest terms:

$\frac{3}{12} + \frac{2}{12} = \frac{5}{12}$

Example: Subtract $\frac{1}{3}$ from $\frac{3}{8}$

Solution: Find the least common denominator: the LCD = 24

Write each fraction with this new denominator:

$\frac{3}{8}$ becomes $\frac{9}{24}$ and $\frac{1}{3}$ becomes $\frac{8}{24}$

Follow the procedure for fractions that have the same denominators and reduce the result to lowest terms:

$\frac{9}{24} - \frac{8}{24} = \frac{1}{24}$

These problems may also be written as:

$$
\begin{array}{c|c}
\frac{1}{4} & 3 \\
+ \ \frac{1}{6} & 2 \\
\hline
& 5 \\
& 12
\end{array}
\qquad
\begin{array}{c|c}
\frac{3}{8} & 9 \\
- \ \frac{1}{3} & 8 \\
\hline
& 1 \\
& 24
\end{array}
$$

To add $\frac{1}{6} + \frac{3}{9}$: find the least common denominator for these fractions, which is 18. Change $\frac{1}{6}$ to $\frac{3}{18}$, and $\frac{3}{9}$ to $\frac{6}{18}$. The sum of these two fractions is $\frac{9}{18}$, which should be reduced to $\frac{1}{2}$.

To subtract $\frac{3}{4} - \frac{1}{8}$: find the least common denominator for these fractions, which is 8. Change $\frac{3}{4}$ to $\frac{6}{8}$, and $\frac{1}{8}$ to $\frac{1}{8}$. The difference between these fractions is $\frac{5}{8}$.

Problem Set 3.15

Solve the following problems. Reduce to lowest terms.

1. $\frac{3}{7} + \frac{2}{9}$ _____

2. $\frac{1}{32} + \frac{1}{16}$ _____

3. $\frac{1}{12} - \frac{1}{60}$ _____

4. $\frac{3}{50} - \frac{1}{100}$ _____

5. $\frac{1}{6} + \frac{1}{8} + \frac{1}{3}$ _____

6. $\frac{2}{5} - \frac{1}{6} - \frac{1}{8}$ _____

7. $\frac{3}{100} + \frac{1}{150} + \frac{1}{75}$ _____

8. $\frac{1}{50} - \frac{1}{200} - \frac{1}{300}$ _____

9. $\frac{1}{500} + \frac{3}{100} + \frac{7}{250}$ _____

10. $\frac{1}{100} - \frac{1}{200} - \frac{1}{250}$ _____

Answers 1. $\frac{41}{63}$ 2. $\frac{3}{32}$ 3. $\frac{1}{15}$ 4. $\frac{1}{20}$ 5. $\frac{5}{8}$ 6. $\frac{13}{120}$ 7. $\frac{1}{20}$ 8. $\frac{7}{600}$ 9. $\frac{3}{50}$ 10. $\frac{1}{1000}$

Calculation Alert

- When adding or subtracting fractions that have the same denominators, simply add or subtract the numerators and place the results over the denominator.

- In adding or subtracting fractions that have different denominators, first find the least common denominator, then change each fraction to a new form using this common denominator. Then add or subtract the numerators and place the results over the common denominator.

- Always reduce the results to the lowest terms possible.

Self-Evaluation Test 3.7
Adding and Subtracting Fractions

1. $\dfrac{3}{8} + \dfrac{5}{8}$ _____

2. $\dfrac{1}{4} + \dfrac{1}{2}$ _____

3. $\dfrac{1}{6} + \dfrac{1}{8}$ _____

4. $\dfrac{7}{8} - \dfrac{3}{8}$ _____

5. $\dfrac{3}{4} - \dfrac{1}{2}$ _____

6. $\dfrac{1}{3} - \dfrac{1}{6}$ _____

7. $\dfrac{11}{12} - \dfrac{5}{6}$ _____

8. $\dfrac{3}{64} - \dfrac{1}{32}$ _____

9. $\dfrac{5}{8} - \dfrac{1}{4} - \dfrac{1}{6}$ _____

10. $\dfrac{1}{150} - \dfrac{1}{200}$ _____

11. $\dfrac{4}{7} + \dfrac{1}{6} - \dfrac{3}{21}$ _____

12. $\dfrac{3}{8} + \dfrac{1}{32} + \dfrac{3}{64}$ _____

13. $\dfrac{3}{5} + \dfrac{1}{10} + \dfrac{1}{30}$ _____

14. $\dfrac{1}{64} + \dfrac{1}{16} + \dfrac{1}{8}$ _____

15. $\dfrac{1}{150} + \dfrac{1}{200} + \dfrac{1}{100}$ _____

Answers 1. 1 2. $\dfrac{3}{4}$ 3. $\dfrac{7}{24}$ 4. $\dfrac{1}{2}$ 5. $\dfrac{1}{4}$ 6. $\dfrac{1}{6}$ 7. $\dfrac{1}{12}$ 8. $\dfrac{1}{64}$ 9. $\dfrac{5}{24}$ 10. $\dfrac{1}{600}$ 11. $\dfrac{25}{42}$ 12. $\dfrac{29}{64}$ 13. $\dfrac{11}{15}$ 14. $\dfrac{13}{64}$ 15. $\dfrac{13}{600}$

If you had fewer than three errors on Self-Evaluation Test 3.7, move on to the next section. If you had four or more errors, review the material just covered and complete Self-Evaluation test 3.8 before continuing.

Self-Evaluation Test 3.8
Adding and Subtracting Fractions

1. $\dfrac{3}{7} + \dfrac{1}{7}$ _____

2. $\dfrac{3}{4} + \dfrac{1}{8}$ _____

3. $\dfrac{1}{3} + \dfrac{1}{6}$ _____

4. $\dfrac{5}{9} - \dfrac{1}{9}$ _____

5. $\dfrac{1}{2} - \dfrac{1}{8}$ _____

6. $\dfrac{1}{15} + \dfrac{2}{45}$ _____

7. $\dfrac{14}{15} - \dfrac{4}{5}$ _____

8. $\dfrac{1}{100} + \dfrac{1}{150}$ _____

9. $\dfrac{1}{200} - \dfrac{1}{300}$ _____

10. $\dfrac{1}{6} + \dfrac{1}{8} + \dfrac{2}{3}$ _____

11. $\dfrac{1}{4} + \dfrac{5}{8} + \dfrac{1}{16}$ _____

12. $\dfrac{3}{4} - \dfrac{1}{6} - \dfrac{1}{8}$ _____

13. $\dfrac{1}{8} + \dfrac{1}{12} + \dfrac{1}{24}$ _____

14. $\dfrac{2}{5} + \dfrac{3}{10} - \dfrac{9}{20}$ _____

15. $\dfrac{3}{16} - \dfrac{1}{64} - \dfrac{1}{8}$ _____

Answers 1. $\dfrac{4}{7}$ 2. $\dfrac{7}{8}$ 3. $\dfrac{1}{2}$ 4. $\dfrac{4}{9}$ 5. $\dfrac{3}{8}$ 6. $\dfrac{1}{9}$ 7. $\dfrac{2}{15}$ 8. $\dfrac{1}{60}$ 9. $\dfrac{1}{600}$ 10. $\dfrac{23}{24}$ 11. $\dfrac{15}{16}$ 12. $\dfrac{11}{24}$ 13. $\dfrac{1}{4}$ 14. $\dfrac{1}{4}$ 15. $\dfrac{3}{64}$

The Self-Evaluation Tests on adding and subtracting fractions should be repeated until fewer than three errors occur.

ADDING AND SUBTRACTING MIXED NUMBERS

When adding mixed numbers, add the fractions by following the rules for adding fractions. When the sum of the fractions is a proper fraction, simply add the sum of the whole numbers to the fraction.

Example: Determine the sum of $2\frac{1}{3} + 6\frac{1}{3}$

Solution: First, add $\frac{1}{3} + \frac{1}{3} = \frac{2}{3}$, then add $2 + 6 = 8$

Therefore, $2\frac{1}{3} + 6\frac{1}{3} = 8\frac{2}{3}$

Example: Determine the sum of $9\frac{1}{4} + 6\frac{1}{2}$

Solution: First, add $\frac{1}{4} + \frac{1}{2} = \frac{3}{4}$, then add $9 + 6 = 15$

Therefore, $9\frac{1}{4} + 6\frac{1}{2} = 15\frac{3}{4}$

Example: Determine the sum of $8\frac{1}{4} + 4\frac{1}{6}$

Solution: First, add $\frac{1}{4} + \frac{1}{6} = \frac{5}{12}$, then add $8 + 4 = 12$

Therefore, $8\frac{1}{4} + 4\frac{1}{6} = 12\frac{5}{12}$

To add mixed numbers when the sum of the fractions is an improper fraction, change the improper fraction to a mixed number, then add the whole-number portion of this mixed number to the sum of the whole numbers.

Example: Determine the sum of $6\frac{3}{4} + 4\frac{1}{2}$

Solution: First, add the fractions $\frac{3}{4} + \frac{1}{2}$. The resulting answer is $\frac{5}{4}$, which is an improper fraction that should be

changed to $1\frac{1}{4}$.

Then, add $1\frac{1}{4} + 6 + 4$.

Therefore, $6\frac{3}{4} + 4\frac{1}{2} = 11\frac{1}{4}$

Example: Determine the sum of $7\frac{2}{8} + 3\frac{3}{4}$

Solution: First, add $\frac{2}{8} + \frac{3}{4} = \frac{8}{8}$ or 1

Then, add $7 + 3 + 1 = 11$

Therefore, $7\frac{2}{8} + 3\frac{3}{4} = 11$

Example: Determine the sum of $21\frac{5}{6} + 13\frac{5}{6}$

Solution: First, add $\frac{5}{6} + \frac{5}{6} = \frac{10}{6}$ or $1\frac{2}{3}$

Then, add $21 + 13 + 1\frac{2}{3}$

Therefore, $21\frac{5}{6} + 13\frac{5}{6} = 35\frac{2}{3}$

Problem Set 3.16

1. $1\frac{1}{8} + 3\frac{3}{4}$ _____

2. $3\frac{1}{12} + 4\frac{7}{8}$ _____

3. $24 + 1\frac{1}{4} + \frac{1}{30}$ _____

4. $1\frac{15}{16} + 25\frac{3}{32}$ _____

5. $9\frac{1}{100} + 3\frac{1}{150}$ _____

6. $15\frac{3}{16} + 10\frac{9}{10}$ _____

7. $7\frac{1}{2} + 3\frac{3}{4} + 15$ _____

8. $3\frac{4}{5} + 12\frac{5}{6} + 1\frac{7}{8}$ _____

9. $4\frac{3}{64} + 3\frac{1}{8} + 10\frac{1}{16}$ _____

10. $5\frac{1}{16} + 10\frac{3}{4} + 33\frac{6}{32}$ _____

Answers   1. $4\frac{7}{8}$ 2. $7\frac{23}{24}$ 3. $25\frac{17}{60}$ 4. $27\frac{1}{32}$ 5. $12\frac{1}{60}$ 6. $26\frac{7}{80}$ 7. $26\frac{1}{4}$ 8. $18\frac{61}{120}$ 9. $17\frac{15}{64}$ 10. 49

When subtracting mixed numbers, first subtract the fractions, following the rules for subtracting fractions. When the result of subtracting the fractions is a proper fraction, simply subtract the whole numbers and put the fractional results with this figure.

Example: Find the remainder of $6\frac{3}{4} - 4\frac{1}{4}$

Solution: First, subtract the fraction portions $\frac{3}{4} - \frac{1}{4} = \frac{2}{4}$

Then, subtract the whole number portions $6 - 4 = 2$

Therefore, $6\frac{3}{4} - 4\frac{1}{4} = 2\frac{2}{4} = 2\frac{1}{2}$

Example: Find the remainder of $9\frac{4}{5} - 7\frac{2}{3}$

Solution: First, subtract $\frac{2}{3}$ from $\frac{4}{5} = \frac{2}{15}$

Then, subtract 7 from $9 = 2$

Therefore, $9\frac{4}{5} - 7\frac{2}{3} = 2\frac{2}{15}$

Example: Find the remainder of $15\frac{2}{3} - 11\frac{1}{2}$

Solution: First, subtract $\frac{1}{2}$ from $\frac{2}{3} = \frac{1}{6}$

Then, subtract 11 from $15 = 4$

Therefore, $15\frac{2}{3} - 11\frac{1}{2} = 4\frac{1}{6}$

When subtracting mixed numbers in which the fraction portion of the number being subtracted is greater than the fraction portion of the number from which it is being subtracted, the smaller fraction must be increased before the subtraction can be done.

Example: Subtract $1\frac{1}{2}$ from $3\frac{1}{4}$

Solution: The fraction portion of $3\frac{1}{4}$ must be increased before the fraction portion of $1\frac{1}{2}$ can be subtracted from it.

Change the mixed number $3\frac{1}{4}$ to a whole number with an improper fraction. $3\frac{1}{4}$ can be expressed as $2\frac{5}{4}$

without changing its value by borrowing $1\left(\frac{4}{4}\right)$ from the whole-number portion.

Restate the problem as $2\frac{5}{4} - 1\frac{1}{2}$

Find the LCD, which is 4

Subtract the fraction $\left(\frac{5}{4} - \frac{2}{4} = \frac{3}{4}\right)$ and whole numbers (2 – 1 = 1)

Therefore, $3\frac{1}{4} - 1\frac{1}{2} = 1\frac{3}{4}$

Example: Subtract $2\frac{2}{3}$ from $15\frac{1}{6}$

Solution: Change the mixed number, $15\frac{1}{6}$, to $14\frac{7}{6}$

Then, change $2\frac{2}{3}$ to $2\frac{4}{6}$

Subtract $\frac{4}{6}$ from $\frac{7}{6}$ leaving a fractional portion of $\frac{3}{6}$, which reduces to $\frac{1}{2}$

Then subtract 2 from 14 = 12

Therefore, $15\frac{1}{6} - 2\frac{2}{3} = 12\frac{1}{2}$

Example: Subtract $1\frac{13}{18}$ from $4\frac{5}{36}$

Solution: First, change $4\frac{5}{36}$ to $3\frac{41}{36}$ and change $1\frac{13}{18}$ to $1\frac{26}{36}$

Then subtract $\frac{26}{36}$ from $\frac{41}{36}$ leaving a fractional portion of $\frac{15}{36}$, which reduces to $\frac{5}{12}$

Then subtract 1 from 3 leaving a whole-number portion of 2

Therefore, $4\frac{5}{36} - 1\frac{13}{18} = 2\frac{5}{12}$

Problem Set 3.17

1. $3\frac{1}{2} - 2\frac{1}{4}$ _____

2. $7\frac{1}{2} - 3\frac{3}{4}$ _____

3. $8\frac{1}{16} - 4\frac{1}{4}$ _____

4. $15\frac{5}{8} - 10\frac{1}{6}$ _____

5. $1\frac{1}{12} - \frac{3}{4} - \frac{1}{8}$ _____

6. $13\frac{1}{150} - 1\frac{1}{100}$ _____

7. $7\frac{1}{2} - 5\frac{3}{4} - 1\frac{1}{8}$ _____

8. $9\frac{3}{8} - 1\frac{1}{3} - 7\frac{3}{4}$ _____

9. $325\frac{1}{16} - 100\frac{1}{8} - 212$ _____

10. $21\frac{11}{12} - 5\frac{1}{2} - 16\frac{5}{12}$ _____

Answers 1. $1\frac{1}{4}$ 2. $3\frac{3}{4}$ 3. $3\frac{13}{16}$ 4. $5\frac{11}{24}$ 5. $\frac{5}{24}$ 6. $11\frac{299}{300}$ 7. $\frac{5}{8}$ 8. $\frac{7}{24}$ 9. $12\frac{15}{16}$ 10. 0

V I P

When subtracting mixed numbers in which the fraction portion of the number being subtracted is greater than the fraction portion of the number from which it is being subtracted, the smaller fraction must be increased before the subtraction can be done.

Self-Evaluation Test 3.9
Adding and Subtracting Mixed Numbers

1. $4\frac{1}{6} + 1\frac{1}{3}$ _____

2. $5\frac{1}{5} + 1\frac{1}{2}$ _____

3. $7\frac{1}{2} - 1\frac{3}{4}$ _____

4. $2\frac{1}{8} - 1\frac{1}{6}$ _____

5. $8\frac{7}{10} + 1\frac{3}{5}$ _____

6. $2\frac{1}{8} = 4\frac{1}{16}$ _____

7. $3\frac{1}{64} - \frac{1}{32}$ _____

8. $15\frac{2}{5} - \frac{3}{15}$ _____

9. $3\frac{1}{4} - \frac{1}{100}$ _____

10. $15\frac{3}{5} - 6\frac{7}{8}$ _____

11. $3\frac{1}{64} + 2\frac{1}{32}$ _____

12. $16\frac{2}{3} + 11\frac{1}{6}$ _____

13. $33\frac{1}{3} + 66\frac{2}{3}$ _____

14. $30\frac{1}{12} - 4\frac{1}{4}$ _____

15. $32\frac{1}{64} - 12\frac{1}{32}$ _____

Answers **1.** $5\frac{1}{2}$ **2.** $6\frac{7}{10}$ **3.** $5\frac{3}{4}$ **4.** $\frac{23}{24}$ **5.** $10\frac{3}{10}$ **6.** $6\frac{3}{16}$ **7.** $2\frac{63}{64}$ **8.** $15\frac{1}{5}$ **9.** $3\frac{6}{25}$ **10.** $8\frac{29}{40}$ **11.** $5\frac{3}{64}$ **12.** $27\frac{5}{6}$ **13.** 100

14. $25\frac{5}{6}$ **15.** $19\frac{63}{64}$

If you had fewer than three errors on Self-Evaluation Test 3.9, move on to the next section. If you had four or more errors, review the material just covered and complete Self-Evaluation Test 3.10 before continuing.

Self-Evaluation Test 3.10
Adding and Subtracting Mixed Numbers

1. $5\frac{1}{2} - \frac{3}{8}$ _____

2. $1\frac{1}{6} - \frac{3}{4}$ _____

3. $1\frac{1}{8} + 2\frac{1}{2}$ _____

4. $3\frac{4}{5} + 1\frac{1}{2}$ _____

5. $2\frac{1}{16} + \frac{3}{32}$ _____

6. $8\frac{1}{12} + 7\frac{1}{2}$ _____

7. $45\frac{1}{9} + 9\frac{1}{4}$ _____

8. $10\frac{1}{7} + 3\frac{1}{3}$ _____

9. $1\frac{1}{64} + 2\frac{1}{32}$ _____

10. $12\frac{1}{2} - 10\frac{3}{4}$ _____

11. $125\frac{3}{4} - 23\frac{1}{3}$ _____

12. $2\frac{1}{75} - 1\frac{1}{150}$ _____

13. $43\frac{1}{5} - 30\frac{3}{10}$ _____

14. $15\frac{1}{100} - \frac{1}{150}$ _____

15. $5\frac{1}{150} - 2\frac{1}{100}$ _____

The Self-Evaluation Tests on adding and subtracting mixed numbers should be repeated until fewer than three errors occur.

MULTIPLYING AND DIVIDING FRACTIONS

To multiply two or more fractions, the original numerators are multiplied to obtain a new numerator, and the original denominators are multiplied to obtain a new denominator. (There is no need to find a least common denominator.) Results should be reduced if possible.

Example: Multiply $\frac{2}{3}$ by $\frac{3}{4}$

Solution $\frac{2}{3} \times \frac{3}{4} = \frac{2 \times 3}{3 \times 4} = \frac{6}{12} = \frac{1}{2}$

Example: Multiply $\frac{5}{8}$ by $\frac{1}{3}$

Solution: $\frac{5}{8} \times \frac{1}{3} = \frac{5 \times 1}{8 \times 3} = \frac{5}{24}$

Example: Multiply $\frac{1}{8}$ by $\frac{1}{6}$ by $\frac{1}{4}$

Solution: $\frac{1}{8} \times \frac{1}{6} \times \frac{1}{4} = \frac{1 \times 1 \times 1}{8 \times 6 \times 4} = \frac{1}{192}$

When multiplying $\frac{3}{8} \times \frac{5}{6}$, the new numerator is 15, and the new denominator is 48. The product of the two fractions is $\frac{15}{48}$, which can be reduced to $\frac{5}{16}$.

Knowing that fractions can be reduced by dividing both the numerator and denominator by the same number without changing the value of the fraction assists in shortening the process of multiplication and division of fractions. The reduction or cancellation of terms of a fraction (the numerators and denominators) can be extended to any of the denominators or numerators involved in multiplication.

Example: Multiply $\frac{4}{5}$ by $\frac{5}{16}$

Solution: $\frac{4 \times 5}{5 \times 16} = \frac{20}{80} = \frac{1}{4}$

or by using **cancellation of terms.**

$$\frac{\overset{1}{\cancel{4}} \times \overset{1}{\cancel{5}}}{\underset{1}{\cancel{5}} \times \underset{4}{\cancel{16}}} = \frac{1}{4}$$

This example demonstrates the rule of reducing fractions by cancellation of terms, which means dividing both the numerator and the denominator by the same number.

Problem Set 3.18

1. $\frac{3}{8} \times \frac{1}{5}$ _____

2. $\frac{2}{3} \times \frac{3}{5}$ _____

3. $\frac{1}{6} \times \frac{3}{4}$ _____

4. $\frac{5}{6} \times \frac{3}{25}$ _____

5. $\dfrac{1}{12} \times \dfrac{1}{5}$ _____

6. $\dfrac{1}{64} \times \dfrac{1}{2}$ _____

7. $\dfrac{1}{64} \times \dfrac{4}{5}$ _____

8. $\dfrac{1}{100} \times \dfrac{1}{2}$ _____

9. $\dfrac{5}{6} \times \dfrac{1}{100}$ _____

10. $\dfrac{1}{150} \times \dfrac{1}{2}$ _____

Answers   1. $\dfrac{3}{40}$ 2. $\dfrac{2}{5}$ 3. $\dfrac{1}{8}$ 4. $\dfrac{1}{10}$ 5. $\dfrac{1}{60}$ 6. $\dfrac{1}{128}$ 7. $\dfrac{1}{80}$ 8. $\dfrac{1}{200}$ 9. $\dfrac{1}{120}$ 10. $\dfrac{1}{300}$

To divide one fraction by another fraction or by a whole number, the numerator and denominator of the fraction used for dividing (the fraction or whole number following the division sign or the word "by") must be interchanged. This is called inverting the fraction. The division sign is then changed to a multiplication sign and the rules for multiplication are then followed.

Example: Divide $\dfrac{5}{6} \div \dfrac{1}{4}$

Solution: Invert the fraction $\dfrac{1}{4}$, rewriting it as $\dfrac{4}{1}$ and change the "÷" to "×."

$$\dfrac{5}{6} \times \dfrac{4}{1} =$$

$$\dfrac{20}{6} = 3\dfrac{2}{6} = 3\dfrac{1}{3}$$

Example: Divide $\dfrac{1}{2} \div \dfrac{4}{5}$

Solution: Invert the fraction $\dfrac{4}{5}$, rewriting it as $\dfrac{5}{4}$ and change the "÷" to "×."

$$\dfrac{1}{2} \times \dfrac{5}{4} = \dfrac{5}{8}$$

Example: Divide $\dfrac{1}{8} \div 2$

Solution: The whole number (2) must first be expressed as a fraction with a numerator of 2 and a denominator of 1 $\left(\dfrac{2}{1}\right)$. Invert the fraction $\dfrac{2}{1}$, rewrite it as $\dfrac{1}{2}$ and change the "÷" to "×."

$$\dfrac{1}{8} \div \dfrac{2}{1} =$$

$$\dfrac{1}{8} \times \dfrac{1}{2} = \dfrac{1}{16}$$

Example: Divide $\dfrac{2}{5}$ by 5

Solution: $\dfrac{2}{5} \div \dfrac{5}{1} =$

$$\dfrac{2}{5} \times \dfrac{1}{5} = \dfrac{2}{25}$$

Problem Set 3.19

1. $\dfrac{1}{2} \div 8$ _____

2. $\dfrac{1}{16} \div 4$ _____

3. $\dfrac{1}{8} \div \dfrac{1}{6}$ _____

4. $\dfrac{2}{3} \div \dfrac{1}{3}$ _____

5. $\dfrac{3}{4} \div \dfrac{1}{2}$ _____

6. $\dfrac{1}{4} \div \dfrac{2}{3}$ _____

7. $\dfrac{1}{150} \div 2$ _____

8. $\dfrac{1}{64} \div \dfrac{1}{32}$ _____

9. $\dfrac{1}{100} \div \dfrac{1}{150}$ _____

10. $\dfrac{1}{100} \div \dfrac{1}{200}$ _____

Answers 1. $\dfrac{1}{16}$ 2. $\dfrac{1}{64}$ 3. $\dfrac{3}{4}$ 4. 2 5. $1\dfrac{1}{2}$ 6. $\dfrac{3}{8}$ 7. $\dfrac{1}{300}$ 8. $\dfrac{1}{2}$ 9. $1\dfrac{1}{2}$ 10. 2

Calculation Alert

- When multiplying fractions, the numerators are multiplied to form a new numerator, and the denominators are multiplied to form a new denominator.
- When dividing fractions, the number after the division sign is always inverted, the division sign is changed to a multiplication sign, and the rule for multiplication of fractions is used.
- When multiplying and dividing fractions, there is no need to find a common denominator.

Self-Evaluation Test 3.11
Multiplying and Dividing Fractions

1. $\dfrac{1}{2} \times \dfrac{1}{3}$ _____

2. $\dfrac{1}{7} \times \dfrac{3}{5}$ _____

3. $\dfrac{5}{12} \times \dfrac{1}{15}$ _____

4. $\dfrac{1}{100} \times \dfrac{1}{4}$ _____

5. $\dfrac{1}{200} \times \dfrac{1}{2}$ _____

6. $\dfrac{1}{150} \times \dfrac{3}{5}$ _____

7. $\dfrac{1}{100} \times \dfrac{1}{150}$ _____

8. $\dfrac{1}{3} \times \dfrac{2}{7} \times \dfrac{1}{5}$ _____

9. $\dfrac{1}{6} \div 2$ _____

10. $\dfrac{5}{8} \div \dfrac{3}{4}$ _____

11. $\dfrac{1}{2} \div \dfrac{1}{6}$ _____

12. $\dfrac{1}{8} \div \dfrac{3}{4}$ _____

13. $\dfrac{1}{100} \div 3$ _____

14. $\dfrac{1}{300} \div \dfrac{1}{2}$ _____

15. $\dfrac{1}{200} \div \dfrac{1}{100}$ _____

Answers 1. $\dfrac{1}{6}$ 2. $\dfrac{3}{35}$ 3. $\dfrac{1}{36}$ 4. $\dfrac{1}{400}$ 5. $\dfrac{1}{400}$ 6. $\dfrac{1}{250}$ 7. $\dfrac{1}{15,000}$ 8. $\dfrac{2}{105}$ 9. $\dfrac{1}{12}$ 10. $\dfrac{5}{6}$ 11. 3 **12.** $\dfrac{1}{6}$ 13. $\dfrac{1}{300}$

14. $\dfrac{1}{150}$ 15. $\dfrac{1}{2}$

If you had fewer than three errors on Self-Evaluation Test 3.11, move on to the next section. If you had four or more errors, review the material just covered and complete Self-Evaluation Test 3.14 before continuing.

Self-Evaluation Test 3.12
Multiplying and Dividing Fractions

1. $\dfrac{1}{4} \times \dfrac{1}{2}$ _____

2. $\dfrac{1}{6} \times \dfrac{7}{8}$ _____

3. $\dfrac{2}{3} \times \dfrac{3}{5}$ _____

4. $\dfrac{1}{32} \times \dfrac{1}{2}$ _____

5. $\dfrac{1}{150} \times \dfrac{3}{4}$ _____

6. $\dfrac{2}{3} \times \dfrac{1}{200}$ _____

7. $\dfrac{2}{5} \times \dfrac{1}{8} \times \dfrac{1}{2}$ _____

8. $\dfrac{1}{3} \times \dfrac{3}{10} \times \dfrac{5}{6}$ _____

9. $\dfrac{3}{8} \div \dfrac{1}{2}$ _____

10. $\dfrac{1}{32} \div 2$ _____

11. $\dfrac{1}{6} \div \dfrac{1}{8}$ _____

12. $\dfrac{1}{100} \div 3$ _____

13. $\dfrac{1}{300} \div \dfrac{1}{2}$ _____

14. $\dfrac{1}{100} \div \dfrac{1}{200}$ _____

15. $\dfrac{1}{150} \div \dfrac{1}{100}$ _____

Answers   1. $\frac{1}{8}$ 2. $\frac{7}{48}$ 3. $\frac{2}{5}$ 4. $\frac{1}{64}$ 5. $\frac{1}{200}$ 6. $\frac{1}{300}$ 7. $\frac{1}{40}$ 8. $\frac{1}{12}$ 9. $\frac{3}{4}$ 10. $\frac{1}{64}$ 11. $1\frac{1}{3}$ 12. $\frac{1}{300}$ 13. $\frac{1}{150}$ 14. 2 15. $\frac{2}{3}$

The Self-Evaluation Tests on multiplying and dividing fractions should be repeated until fewer than three errors occur.

MULTIPLYING AND DIVIDING MIXED NUMBERS

To multiply mixed numbers, first convert the mixed number to an improper fraction and then follow the rules for multiplying fractions.

Example: $4\dfrac{2}{5} \times 7\dfrac{1}{2}$

Solution: First change the mixed number $4\dfrac{2}{5}$ to the improper fraction $\dfrac{22}{5}$ and the mixed number $7\dfrac{1}{2}$ to the improper fraction $\dfrac{15}{2}$; then rewrite as:

$$\dfrac{22}{5} \times \dfrac{15}{2} =$$

$$\dfrac{22}{5} \times \dfrac{15}{2} = \dfrac{\overset{11}{22} \times \overset{3}{15}}{\underset{1}{5} \times \underset{1}{2}} = 33$$

Therefore, $4\dfrac{2}{5} \times 7\dfrac{1}{2} = 33$

Example: $3\dfrac{3}{4} \times 1\dfrac{1}{3}$

Solution: First change the mixed numbers to fractions, rewriting as $\dfrac{15}{4} \times \dfrac{4}{3}$

$$\dfrac{\overset{5}{15} \times \overset{1}{4}}{\underset{1}{4} \times \underset{1}{3}} = 5$$

Therefore, $3\dfrac{3}{4} \times 1\dfrac{1}{3} = 5$

Problem Set 3.20

1. $5 \times \dfrac{3}{4}$ _____

2. $1\dfrac{1}{2} \times 4$ _____

3. $2 \times 1\dfrac{1}{2}$ _____

4. $7\dfrac{1}{2} \times 6$ _____

5. $3\dfrac{3}{4} \times \dfrac{1}{2}$ _____

6. $7\dfrac{1}{2} \times 3\dfrac{3}{4}$ _____

7. $1\dfrac{1}{2} \times \dfrac{1}{150}$ _____

8. $2\dfrac{1}{4} \times \dfrac{1}{300}$ _____

9. $1\dfrac{1}{2} \times \dfrac{3}{4} \times 16$ _____

10. $3\dfrac{3}{4} \times 7\dfrac{1}{2} \times \dfrac{1}{15}$ _____

Answers 1. $3\dfrac{3}{4}$ 2. 6 3. 3 4. 45 5. $1\dfrac{7}{8}$ 6. $28\dfrac{1}{8}$ 7. $\dfrac{1}{100}$ 8. $\dfrac{3}{400}$ 9. 18 10. $1\dfrac{7}{8}$

To divide mixed numbers, first convert the mixed number to an improper fraction and then follow the rule for dividing fractions.

Example: $9\dfrac{3}{8} \div 6\dfrac{1}{4}$

Solution: Change the mixed number $9\dfrac{3}{8}$ to the improper fraction $\dfrac{75}{8}$, and the mixed number $6\dfrac{1}{4}$ to the improper

fraction $\dfrac{25}{4}$; rewrite as $\dfrac{75}{8} \div \dfrac{25}{4}$

Following the rules for division of fractions (inverting the term following the division sign) this can be rewritten as:

$$\dfrac{\overset{3}{\cancel{75}}}{\underset{2}{\cancel{8}}} \times \dfrac{\overset{1}{\cancel{4}}}{\underset{1}{\cancel{25}}} = \dfrac{3}{2} = 1\dfrac{1}{2}$$

Therefore, $9\dfrac{3}{8} \div 6\dfrac{1}{4} = 1\dfrac{1}{2}$

Example: $7\dfrac{1}{2} \div 15$

Solution: Change the mixed number to a fraction, make the whole number a fraction, and rewrite as

$$\dfrac{15}{2} \div \dfrac{15}{1}$$

$$\dfrac{\overset{1}{\cancel{15}}}{2} \times \dfrac{1}{\underset{1}{\cancel{15}}} = \dfrac{1}{2}$$

Therefore, $7\dfrac{1}{2} \div 15 = \dfrac{1}{2}$

Problem Set 3.21

1. $3\dfrac{1}{3} \div 5$ _____

2. $3\dfrac{3}{4} \div 3$ _____

3. $1\dfrac{2}{3} \div \dfrac{1}{4}$ _____

4. $\dfrac{5}{9} \div 7\dfrac{1}{2}$ _____

5. $15 \div 2\dfrac{1}{2}$ _____

6. $1\dfrac{1}{2} \div \dfrac{1}{100}$ _____

7. $\dfrac{1}{200} \div 2\dfrac{1}{2}$ _____

8. $2\dfrac{1}{2} \div \dfrac{1}{200}$ _____

9. $2\dfrac{1}{2} \div \dfrac{3}{4} \div 7\dfrac{1}{2}$ _____

10. $7\dfrac{1}{2} \div 3\dfrac{3}{4} \div 1\dfrac{1}{2}$ _____

Answers   1. $\dfrac{2}{3}$ 2. $1\dfrac{1}{4}$ 3. $6\dfrac{2}{3}$ 4. $\dfrac{2}{27}$ 5. 6   6. 150   7. $\dfrac{1}{500}$ 8. 500   9. $\dfrac{4}{9}$ 10. $1\dfrac{1}{3}$

V I P

- When multiplying mixed numbers, convert the mixed numbers to improper fractions and follow the rules for multiplying fractions.
- When dividing mixed numbers, convert the mixed numbers to improper fractions and follow the rule for dividing fractions.

Self-Evaluation Test 3.13
Multiplying and Dividing Mixed Numbers

1. $1\dfrac{1}{2} \times 2$ _____

2. $8\dfrac{3}{4} \times 16$ _____

3. $1\dfrac{1}{5} \times \dfrac{2}{3}$ _____

4. $\dfrac{1}{15} \times 3\dfrac{3}{4}$ _____

5. $3\dfrac{5}{9} \times 6\dfrac{3}{4}$ _____

6. $12\dfrac{1}{2} \times \dfrac{1}{200}$ _____

7. $1 \times \dfrac{1}{15} \times 2\dfrac{1}{7}$ _____

8. $\dfrac{1}{200} \times \dfrac{1}{150} \times 2$ _____

9. $15 \div 7\dfrac{1}{2}$ _____

10. $\dfrac{1}{16} \div 3\dfrac{3}{4}$ _____

11. $7\dfrac{1}{2} \div 3\dfrac{3}{4}$ _____

12. $11\dfrac{1}{5} \div 2\dfrac{2}{3}$ _____

13. $36\dfrac{3}{5} \div 5\dfrac{1}{12}$ _____

14. $2\dfrac{1}{2} \div 1\dfrac{1}{4} \div 1\dfrac{3}{8}$ _____

15. $\dfrac{3}{200} \div \dfrac{1}{150} \div 3\dfrac{3}{4}$ _____

Answers   1. 3   2. 140   3. $\dfrac{4}{5}$ 4. $\dfrac{1}{4}$ 5. 24   6. $\dfrac{1}{16}$ 7. $1\dfrac{1}{7}$ 8. $\dfrac{1}{15,000}$ 9. 2   10. $\dfrac{1}{60}$ 11. 2   12. $4\dfrac{1}{5}$ 13. $7\dfrac{1}{5}$ 14. $1\dfrac{5}{11}$

15. $\dfrac{3}{5}$

If you had fewer than three errors on Self-Evaluation Test 3.13, move on to the next chapter. If you had four or more errors, review the material just covered and complete Self-Evaluation Test 3.14 before continuing.

Self-Evaluation Test 3.14
Multiplying and Dividing Mixed Numbers

1. $5 \times \frac{3}{4}$ _____

2. $16 \times 1\frac{1}{2}$ _____

3. $1\frac{1}{2} \times \frac{3}{4}$ _____

4. $7\frac{1}{2} \times 5\frac{2}{3}$ _____

5. $\frac{1}{100} \times 2\frac{1}{2}$ _____

6. $10\frac{1}{8} \times 1\frac{1}{3}$ _____

7. $3 \times \frac{1}{100} \times \frac{1}{150}$ _____

8. $2\frac{1}{2} \times 1\frac{1}{4} \times 1\frac{3}{5}$ _____

9. $7\frac{1}{2} \div 15$ _____

10. $1\frac{1}{2} \div \frac{3}{4}$ _____

11. $2\frac{2}{3} \div 3\frac{5}{9}$ _____

12. $10\frac{7}{8} \div 1\frac{1}{2}$ _____

13. $1\frac{1}{64} \div 2\frac{1}{32}$ _____

14. $3\frac{3}{4} \div \frac{1}{150} \div 5\frac{1}{4}$ _____

15. $\frac{1}{300} \div \frac{3}{100} \div 3\frac{1}{3}$ _____

Answers 1. $3\frac{3}{4}$ 2. 24 3. $1\frac{1}{8}$ 4. $42\frac{1}{2}$ 5. $\frac{1}{40}$ 6. $13\frac{1}{2}$ 7. $\frac{1}{5000}$ 8. 5 9. $\frac{1}{2}$ 10. 2 11. $\frac{3}{4}$ 12. $7\frac{1}{4}$ 13. $\frac{1}{2}$ 14. $107\frac{1}{7}$ 15. $\frac{1}{30}$

The Self-Evaluation Tests on multiplying and dividing mixed numbers should be repeated until fewer than three errors occur.

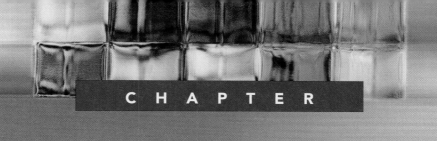

4

Decimals

Learning Outcomes

After successfully completing this chapter, the learner should be able to:

- *Recognize the numerical value of decimals.*
- *Understand the relationship between decimals and fractions.*
- *Perform the arithmetic skills of addition, subtraction, multiplication, and division with decimals.*
- *Convert decimals to fractions and fractions to decimals.*

GENERAL INFORMATION

The Arabic system of numeration is positional. This means that the value of any numeral is affected by the position it occupies in a number. Starting at the right and moving to the left, the value assigned to the numerical place is 10 times greater than the value of the place that preceded it. The number 7,213,456 is thus assigned the following places:

7	2	1	3	4	5	6
millions	hundred thousands	ten thousands	thousands	hundreds	tens	ones

This number is read as seven million, two hundred thirteen thousand, four hundred fifty-six.

Every whole number ends with a period called a decimal point, although it is usually not written. When this period is placed to the right of a number's last whole digit, any digit to the right of this decimal point becomes a decimal fraction, occupying a decimal place representing tenths, hundredths, thousandths, and so on, as shown by the number 26.43275:

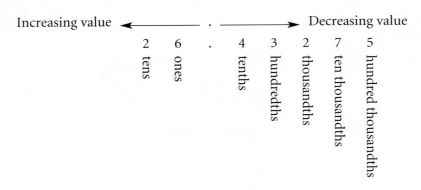

In a decimal fraction, the first digit to the right of the decimal point represents tenths and the digit three places to the right of the decimal point represents thousandths. Thus, the number 47.63 is read as 47 and 63 hundredths. Therefore, 5.6 represents 5 and 6 tenths ($5\frac{6}{10}$), and 0.33 stands for 33 hundredths ($\frac{33}{100}$).

When there is no whole-number part, a zero is placed to the left of the decimal point to avoid an error in interpreting the value. For example, .5 should be written as 0.5 and stated as "zero point five." A zero at the end of a decimal number does not change the value of the number. However, any zeros following the decimal number should be removed from the final answer to avoid errors in interpretation. For example, 0.5 ($\frac{5}{10} = \frac{1}{2}$) may be written as 0.50 and its value is unchanged ($\frac{50}{100} = \frac{5}{10} = \frac{1}{2}$).

In evaluating decimals, remember that the larger the whole-number portion of a decimal, the greater the value of the decimal. If the whole-number portion of the decimals are equal or no whole-number portions are present, the decimal fraction with the larger number in the tenth position has the greater value. This evaluation continues down the decimal places until a difference can be evaluated. For example, 3.5 is greater than 2.9; 5.8 is greater than 5.6; and 0.53 is greater than 0.51.

The evaluation of decimal fractions can be made easier by applying the rules for evaluating fractions:

- If the denominators of the fraction are the same: the larger the numerator, the greater the value
- If the numerators of the fraction are the same: the smaller the denominator, the greater the value

Problem Set 4.1

Determine which decimal has the greater value.

1. 0.2; 0.5; 0.1 _____
2. 0.7; 0.67; 0.86 _____
3. 1.3; 1.05; 1.25 _____
4. 0.01; 0.75; 0.9 _____
5. 7.5; 7.87; 7.19 _____

6. 0.33; 0.6; 0.25 _____
7. 0.3; 0.03; 0.003 _____
8. 32.5; 33.1; 32.97 _____
9. 2.25; 2.167; 2.125 _____
10. 0.125; 0.25; 0.025 _____

Answers 1. 0.5 2. 0.86 3. 1.3 4. 0.9 5. 7.87 6. 0.6 7. 0.3 8. 33.1 9. 2.25 10. 0.25

V I P

- Every whole number ends with a decimal point, although it is usually not written.
- Numbers to the right of the decimal point have a value less than 1, and numbers to the left have a value greater than 1.
- A zero may be added to the end of a decimal number without changing the value of the decimal. Any zeros following the decimal number should be removed from the final answer to avoid errors in interpretation.
- A zero should be placed in front of the decimal point when there is no whole-number part of a decimal.

CHANGING THE FORM OF DECIMALS

In general, if a decimal is to be written as a fraction, the numerator of the fraction will be the decimal number without the decimal point, and the denominator will be the number 1 followed by as many zeros as there are digits or decimal places to the right of the decimal point.

Example Write 0.518 as a fraction.

Solution: Use 518 as the numerator and 1000 (1 followed by three zeros) as the denominator

Therefore, 0.518 can be written as $\frac{518}{1000}$ (518 thousandths)

Example: Write 0.3 as a fraction.

Solution: Use 3 as the numerator and 10 (1 followed by one zero) as the denominator

Therefore, 0.3 can be written as $\frac{3}{10}$ (3 tenths)

Example: Write 6.291 as a fraction.

Solution: Use 291 as the numerator and 1000 (1 followed by three zeros) as the denominator; this fraction follows the whole number, 6

Therefore, 6.291 can be written as $6\frac{291}{1000}$ (6 and 291 thousandths)

Problem Set 4.2

Convert these decimals to fractions or mixed numbers. Reduce if necessary.

1. 0.04 _____
2. 0.16 _____
3. 0.002 _____
4. 7.025 _____
5. 8.125 _____

6. 0.0001 _____
7. 0.0002 _____
8. 0.0025 _____
9. 0.0375 _____
10. 1.0005 _____

Answers 1. $\frac{1}{25}$ 2. $\frac{4}{25}$ 3. $\frac{1}{500}$ 4. $7\frac{1}{40}$ 5. $8\frac{1}{8}$ 6. $\frac{1}{10,000}$ 7. $\frac{1}{5000}$ 8. $\frac{1}{400}$ 9. $\frac{3}{80}$ 10. $1\frac{1}{2000}$

Self-Evaluation Test 4.1
Evaluating and Changing the Form of Decimals

Identify the decimal with the greatest value.

1. 0.3; 0.33; 0.033   _____

2. 9.9; 9.09; 9.099   _____

3. 0.001; 0.01; 0.09   _____

4. 5.01; 5.0125; 5.125   _____

5. 0.125; 0.025; 0.375   _____

Convert these decimals to fractions or mixed numbers. Reduce if necessary.

6. 0.2   _____   11. 0.125   _____

7. 0.5   _____   12. 0.009   _____

8. 2.75   _____   13. 1.005   _____

9. 0.25   _____   14. 9.075   _____

10. 0.01   _____   15. 12.001   _____

Answers   1. 0.33   2. 9.9   3. 0.09   4. 5.125   5. 0.375   6. $\frac{1}{5}$ 7. $\frac{1}{2}$ 8. $2\frac{3}{4}$ 9. $\frac{1}{4}$ 10. $\frac{1}{100}$ 11. $\frac{1}{8}$ 12. $\frac{9}{1000}$ 13. $1\frac{1}{200}$ 14. $9\frac{3}{40}$ 15. $12\frac{1}{1000}$

If you had fewer than three errors on Self-Evaluation Test 4.1, move on to the next section. If you had four or more errors, review the material just covered and complete Self-Evaluation Test 4.2 before continuing.

Self-Evaluation Test 4.2
Evaluating and Changing the Form of Decimals

Identify the decimal with the greatest value.

1. 0.3; 0.6; 0.125   _____   4. 0.125; 0.25; 0.025   _____

2. 7.5; 7.75; 7.52   _____   5. 15.1; 15.001; 15.111   _____

3. 0.01; 0.005; 0.05   _____

Convert these decimals to fractions or mixed numbers. Reduce if necessary.

6. 0.1   _____   11. 0.002   _____

7. 0.4   _____   12. 0.075   _____

8. 0.01   _____   13. 5.125   _____

9. 0.75   _____   14. 3.001   _____

10. 0.05   _____   15. 0.009   _____

Answers   1. 0.6   2. 7.75   3. 0.05   4. 0.25   5. 15.111   6. $\frac{1}{10}$ 7. $\frac{2}{5}$ 8. $\frac{1}{100}$ 9. $\frac{3}{4}$ 10. $\frac{1}{20}$ 11. $\frac{1}{500}$ 12. $\frac{3}{40}$ 13. $5\frac{1}{8}$ 14. $3\frac{1}{1000}$ 15. $\frac{9}{1000}$

The Self-Evaluation Tests on multiplying and dividing mixed numbers should be repeated until fewer than three errors occur.

ADDING AND SUBTRACTING DECIMALS

When adding decimals, it is necessary to align the decimal points before the decimals are added, including those unwritten ones at the end of whole numbers, before beginning addition. In other words, tenths must be added to tenths, hundredths must be added to hundredths, and so on. When adding decimals with different numbers of places following the decimal point, zeros may be added to the end of the shorter decimals to assist in alignment, without changing the value of the decimals.

Example: 0.6 + 1.23

Solution: Align decimal points and add the columns:

```
0.60
1.23
----
1.83
```

Example: 4 + 22.4 + 16.181

Solution: Align decimal points and add the columns:

```
 4.000
22.400
16.181
------
42.581
```

Problem Set 4.3

1. 15.1 + 7.5 + 3.75 _____
2. 7.5 + 3.75 + 1.00 _____
3. 0.1 + 0.01 + 0.12 _____
4. 0.1 + 0.25 + 0.375 _____
5. 1.5 + 8.375 + 5.67 _____
6. 33.3 + 6.67 + 0.03 _____
7. 0.2 + 0.25 + 0.251 _____
8. 3.7 + 2.35 + 3.375 _____
9. 0.07 + 0.71 + 0.075 _____
10. 64.1 + 60.01 + 0.009 _____

Answers   **1.** 26.35 **2.** 12.25 **3.** 0.23 **4.** 0.725 **5.** 15.545 **6.** 40 **7.** 0.701 **8.** 9.425 **9.** 0.855 **10.** 124.119

When subtracting decimals, it is necessary to align the decimal points before the decimals are subtracted, including those unwritten ones at the end of whole numbers, before beginning subtraction. In other words, tenths must be subtracted from tenths, hundredths must be subtracted from hundredths, and so on. When subtracting decimals with different numbers of places following the decimal point, zeros may be added to the end of the shorter decimals to assist in alignment, without changing the value.

Example: 8.67 – 0.23

Solution: Align decimal points and subtract, adding zeros to align the columns:

$$
\begin{array}{r}
8.67 \\
-0.23 \\
\hline
8.44
\end{array}
$$

Therefore, 8.67 – 0.23 = 8.44

Example: 0.534 – 0.32

Solution: Align decimal points and subtract, adding zeros to align the columns:

$$
\begin{array}{r}
0.534 \\
-0.320 \\
\hline
0.214
\end{array}
$$

Therefore, 0.534 – 0.32 = 0.214

Example: 5 – 2.73

Solution: Align decimal points and subtract, adding zeros to align the columns:

$$
\begin{array}{r}
5.00 \\
-2.73 \\
\hline
2.27
\end{array}
$$

Therefore, 5 – 2.73 = 2.27

Problem Set 4.4

1. 7.35 – 1.5 _____
2. 15.75 – 3.5 _____
3. 0.25 – 0.125 _____
4. 0.32 – 0.016 _____
5. 1.575 – 0.25 _____

6. 64.1 – 0.009 _____
7. 15.545 – 8.375 _____
8. 325 – 0.25 – 4.75 _____
9. 1.5 – 0.125 – 0.25 _____
10. 33.3 – 6.67 – 0.03 _____

Answers   **1.** 5.85   **2.** 12.25   **3.** 0.125   **4.** 0.304   **5.** 1.325   **6.** 64.091   **7.** 7.17   **8.** 320   **9.** 1.125   **10.** 26.6

V I P

- Always align decimal points before adding or subtracting decimals.
- Zeros placed after shorter decimals assist in correct alignment.

Self-Evaluation Test 4.3
Adding and Subtracting Decimals

1. 0.5 + 0.3 _____
2. 1.23 + 0.7 _____

3. 0.02 + 0.09 _____
4. 15 + 7.5 + 3.75 _____

5. $20.1 + 1.001 + 0.03$ _____

6. $8.001 + 6.334 + 1.667$ _____

7. $0.375 - 0.1$ _____

8. $0.06 - 0.004$ _____

9. $5.758 - 2.321$ _____

10. $0.001 - 0.0005$ _____

11. $5.35 - 2.0 - 0.01$ _____

12. $0.35 - 0.025 - 0.125$ _____

13. $14.97 + 0.62 - 0.4$ _____

14. $7.297 - 6.725 + 5.21$ _____

15. $2.005 + 0.01 - 0.995$ _____

Answers **1.** 0.8 **2.** 1.93 **3.** 0.11 **4.** 26.25 **5.** 21.131 **6.** 16.002 **7.** 0.275 **8.** 0.056 **9.** 3.437 **10.** 0.0005 **11.** 3.34 **12.** 0.2 **13.** 15.19 **14.** 5.782 **15.** 1.02

If you had fewer than three errors on Self-Evaluation Test 4.3, move on to the next section. If you had four or more errors, review the material just covered and complete Self-Evaluation Test 4.4 before continuing.

Self-Evaluation Test 4.4
Adding and Subtracting Decimals

1. $0.6 + 0.7$ _____

2. $0.123 + 0.4$ _____

3. $12.3 + 0.07$ _____

4. $1.0154 + 5.02 + 12.34$ _____

5. $5.005 + 1.375 + 0.001$ _____

6. $0.375 + 0.025 + 0.125$ _____

7. $2.5 - 1.375$ _____

8. $0.016 - 0.0153$ _____

9. $0.1666 - 0.125$ _____

10. $3.03125 - 0.01562$ _____

11. $15 - 7.5 - 3.75$ _____

12. $7.5 - 3.75 - 0.001$ _____

13. $8.001 - 6.334 - 1.667$ _____

14. $0.009 + 4 - 3.50$ _____

15. $5.01 - 0.009 + 0.999$ _____

Answers **1.** 1.3 **2.** 0.523 **3.** 12.37 **4.** 18.3754 **5.** 6.381 **6.** 0.525 **7.** 1.125 **8.** 0.0007 **9.** 0.0416 **10.** 3.01563 **11.** 3.75 **12.** 3.749 **13.** 0 **14.** 0.509 **15.** 6

The Self-Evaluation Tests on adding and subtracting decimals should be repeated until fewer than three errors occur.

MULTIPLYING AND DIVIDING DECIMALS

When multiplying decimals, follow the procedure for regular multiplication, temporarily disregarding the decimal points. After multiplication is completed, the decimal points must be considered and the decimal places marked off, starting from the last number in the answer. The number of places to mark off—that is, where to place the decimal point—in the answer is determined by adding the number of decimal places to the right of the decimal point in each of the numbers being multiplied.

Example: Multiply 3.1 by 1.2

Solution:

$$\begin{array}{r} 3.1 \\ \times\ 1.2 \\ \hline 3.72 \end{array}$$

The answer is written as 3.72. Because there is one decimal place in each of the numbers being multiplied (1 + 1 = 2), two places are marked off in the answer.

Therefore, 3.1 × 1.2 = 3.72

Example: Multiply 2.3 × 1.5

Solution:

$$\begin{array}{r} 2.3 \\ \times\ 1.5 \\ \hline 3.45 \end{array}$$

Two decimal places are marked off in the answer.

Therefore, 2.3 × 1.5 = 3.45

Example: Multiply 3.5 × 0.009 × 50

Solution:

$$\begin{array}{r} 3.5 \\ \times\ 0.009 \\ \hline 0.0315 \\ \times\ \quad 50 \\ \hline 1.5750 \end{array}$$

Four decimal places are marked off in the answer.

Therefore, 3.5 × 0.009 × 50 = 1.5750

Problem Set 4.5

1. 7.5 × 2 _____
2. 0.125 × 2 _____
3. 1.5 × 0.25 _____
4. 0.06 × 2.5 _____
5. 0.008 × 7.5 _____

6. 3.75 × 0.25 _____
7. 0.125 × 0.25 _____
8. 750 × 0.005 _____
9. 0.02 × 15 × 1.5 _____
10. 0.0001 × 50 × 7.5 _____

Answers   **1.** 15   **2.** 0.25   **3.** 0.375   **4.** 0.15   **5.** 0.06   **6.** 0.9375   **7.** 0.0313   **8.** 3.75   **9.** 0.45   **10.** 0.0375

When dividing a decimal by a whole number, the decimal point in the answer (quotient) is positioned in the same place as it is in the number being divided (dividend). The procedure for division is then followed.

Example: Divide 2.4 by 8

Solution: Place the decimal point over the number being divided:

$$\begin{array}{r} 0.3 \\ 8\overline{)2.4} \end{array}$$

Therefore, 2.4 ÷ 8 = 0.3

Example: Divide 3.602 by 2

Solution: Place the decimal point over the number being divided:

$$\begin{array}{r} 1.801 \\ 2\overline{)3.602} \end{array}$$

Therefore, 3.602 ÷ 2 = 1.801

Example: Divide 224.14 by 7

Solution: Place the decimal point over the number being divided:

$$\begin{array}{r} 32.02 \\ 7\overline{)224.14} \end{array}$$

Therefore, 224.14 ÷ 7 = 32.02

When dividing a whole number or a decimal by a decimal, it is necessary to observe the following procedure before dividing. First, make the divisor (the number you are dividing by) a whole number by moving the decimal point to the end after the last digit on the right in the divisor. Then move the decimal point in the dividend (the number being divided) the same number of places to the right. Zeros may be added if they are necessary to complete the move. Then follow the preceding rule for dividing a decimal by a whole number.

Example: Divide 4.797 by 1.23

Solution: Move the decimal point in the divisor to the end after the last digit. Move decimal point in the dividend (the number being divided) the same number of places to the right.

$$\begin{array}{r} 3.9 \\ 1.23\,\overline{)4.79.7} \\ \underline{369} \\ 1107 \\ \underline{1107} \end{array}$$

Therefore, 4.797 ÷ 1.23 = 3.9

Example: Divide 130.4 by 0.16

Solution: Move the decimal point in the divisor to the end after the last digit. Move the decimal point in the dividend (the number being divided) the same number of places to the right.

$$\begin{array}{r} 8\;15. \\ 0.16\,\overline{)130.40.} \\ \underline{128} \\ 24 \\ \underline{16} \\ 80 \\ \underline{80} \end{array}$$

Therefore, 130.4 ÷ 0.16 = 815

Calculation Alert

When dividing decimals, carry the results out to four decimal places. If the digit in the fourth decimal place is equal to or greater than 5, add 1 to the digit in the third decimal place; if the digit in the fourth decimal place is 4 or less, drop it.

Problem Set 4.6

1. $0.25 \div 4$ _____
2. $0.006 \div 2$ _____
3. $0.009 \div 3$ _____
4. $0.375 \div 8$ _____
5. $0.05 \div 25$ _____

6. $325 \div 1.5$ _____
7. $7.5 \div 0.25$ _____
8. $250 \div 0.005$ _____
9. $0.125 \div 0.25$ _____
10. $0.006 \div 0.125$ _____

Answers   1. 0.063   2. 0.003   3. 0.003   4. 0.047   5. 0.002   6. 216.667   7. 30   8. 50,000   9. 0.5   10. 0.048

VIP

■ When multiplying decimals, first multiply the numbers; then count the total number of decimal places in the numbers being multiplied and, starting from behind the last digit in the answer, mark off the total number of decimal places.

■ When dividing decimals, first convert the decimal in the divisor (if a decimal is present) to a whole number by moving the decimal point of the divisor number to the end following the last digit in the divisor. Move the decimal point in the number being divided the same number of places to the right. The decimal point in the answer is always placed in the same position as it appears in the number being divided.

Self-Evaluation Test 4.5
Multiplying and Dividing Decimals

1. 9.2×3 _____
2. $18 \div 2.4$ _____
3. $15 \div 0.25$ _____
4. 0.8×0.4 _____
5. $0.75 \div 15$ _____
6. 7.5×3.75 _____
7. $0.1 \div 0.375$ _____
8. 0.001×0.2 _____

9. 64.5×0.375 _____
10. $2.003 \div 0.16$ _____
11. $0.166 \div 0.125$ _____
12. $0.125 \div 0.025$ _____
13. $0.325 \div 0.125$ _____
14. 1.066×0.0625 _____
15. 0.156×0.03215 _____

Answers   1. 27.6   2. 7.5   3. 60   4. 0.32   5. 0.05   6. 28.125   7. 0.267   8. 0.0002   9. 24.188   10. 12.519   11. 1.328   12. 5   13. 2.6   14. 0.067   15. 0.005

If you had fewer than three errors on Self-Evaluation Test 4.5, move on to the next section. If you had four or more errors, review the material just covered and complete Self-Evaluation Test 4.6 before continuing.

Self-Evaluation Test 4.6
Multiplying and Dividing Decimals

1. $0.8 \div 0.4$ _____

2. $15 \div 3.75$ _____

3. 3.125×4 _____

4. 10×0.001 _____

5. $0.0625 \div 3$ _____

6. $15 \div 0.125$ _____

7. $0.002 \div 0.2$ _____

8. 1.875×0.5 _____

9. 2.2×56.81 _____

10. $0.005 \div 0.01$ _____

11. $0.156 \div 0.18$ _____

12. 1.75×2.166 _____

13. 0.375×0.125 _____

14. 0.003×0.004 _____

15. $150.345 \div 2.2$ _____

Answers   **1.** 2   **2.** 4   **3.** 12.5   **4.** 0.01   **5.** 0.021   **6.** 120   **7.** 0.01   **8.** 0.938   **9.** 124.982   **10.** 0.5   **11.** 0.867   **12.** 3.791
13. 0.047   **14.** 0.000012   **15.** 68.339

The Self-Evaluation Tests on multiplying and dividing decimals should be repeated until fewer than three errors occur.

CONVERTING FRACTIONS TO DECIMALS AND DECIMALS TO FRACTIONS

Recognizing that there is a relationship between fractions and decimals is useful when it becomes necessary to convert a fraction to its decimal equivalent. To accomplish this task, simply divide the numerator of the fraction (the top number of the fraction) by the denominator of the fraction (the bottom number of the fraction: remember that the **d** in *denominator* denotes down).

Example: Convert $\frac{3}{4}$ to a decimal

Solution: Divide the numerator of the fraction by the denominator:

$$
\begin{array}{r}
0.75 \\
4\overline{)3.00} \\
\underline{2\ 8} \\
20 \\
\underline{20} \\
\end{array}
$$

Therefore, $\frac{3}{4} = 0.75$

Example: Convert $\frac{1}{100}$ to a decimal

Solution: Divide the numerator of the fraction by the denominator:

$$
\begin{array}{r}
0.01 \\
100\overline{)1.00} \\
\underline{1\ 00} \\
\end{array}
$$

Therefore, $\frac{1}{100} = 0.01$

Example: Convert 0.75 to a fraction

Solution: Make the decimal number without the decimal point the numerator of the fraction. The number 1 followed by as many zeros as there are digits to the right of the decimal point will be the denominator.

$$\frac{75}{100} = \frac{3}{4}$$

Therefore, $0.75 = \frac{3}{4}$

Problem Set 4.7

Convert to decimals or fractions. Reduce to lowest terms.

1. $\dfrac{3}{8}$ _____

2. $\dfrac{1}{4}$ _____

3. $\dfrac{1}{8}$ _____

4. $\dfrac{5}{6}$ _____

5. $\dfrac{1}{10}$ _____

6. $\dfrac{1}{100}$ _____

7. $\dfrac{1}{200}$ _____

8. 0.15 _____

9. 0.075 _____

10. 0.0002 _____

Answers 1. 0.375 2. 0.25 3. 0.125 4. 0.833 5. 0.1 6. 0.01 7. 0.005 8. $\dfrac{3}{20}$ 9. $\dfrac{3}{40}$ 10. $\dfrac{1}{5000}$

Self-Evaluation Test 4.7
Converting Fractions to Decimals and Decimals to Fractions

Convert to decimals or fractions. Reduce to lowest terms.

1. $\dfrac{1}{2}$ _____

2. $\dfrac{2}{5}$ _____

3. $\dfrac{1}{6}$ _____

4. $\dfrac{5}{8}$ _____

5. $\dfrac{2}{15}$ _____

6. $\dfrac{1}{150}$ _____

7. $\dfrac{3}{200}$ _____

8. $\dfrac{1}{120}$ _____

9. $\dfrac{1}{500}$ _____

10. $\dfrac{7}{100}$ _____

11. $\dfrac{1}{3000}$ _____

12. $\dfrac{9}{1000}$ _____

13. 0.005 _____

14. 0.009 _____

15. 0.0033 _____

Answers 1. 0.5 2. 0.4 3. 0.166 4. 0.625 5. 0.133 6. 0.007 7. 0.015 8. 0.008 9. 0.002 10. 0.07 11. 0.0003 12. 0.009

13. $\dfrac{1}{200}$ 14. $\dfrac{9}{1000}$ 15. $\dfrac{33}{10,000}$

If you had fewer than three errors on Self-Evaluation Test 4.7, move on to the next chapter. If you had four or more errors, review the material just covered and complete Self-Evaluation Test 4.8 before continuing.

Self-Evaluation Test 4.8
Converting Fractions to Decimals and Decimals to Fractions

Convert to decimals or fractions. Reduce to lowest terms.

1. $\dfrac{1}{4}$ _____

2. $\dfrac{1}{3}$ _____

3. $\dfrac{3}{10}$ _____

4. $\dfrac{1}{40}$ _____

5. $\dfrac{1}{60}$ _____

6. $\dfrac{1}{64}$ _____

7. $\dfrac{1}{32}$ _____

8. $\dfrac{3}{50}$ _____

9. $\dfrac{1}{100}$ _____

10. $\dfrac{1}{200}$ _____

11. $\dfrac{1}{1000}$ _____

12. $\dfrac{1}{1500}$ _____

13. 0.05 _____

14. 0.025 _____

15. 0.0002 _____

Answers **1.** 0.25 **2.** 0.333 **3.** 0.3 **4.** 0.025 **5.** 0.017 **6.** 0.016 **7.** 0.031 **8.** 0.06 **9.** 0.01 **10.** 0.005 **11.** 0.001 **12.** 0.00066

13. $\dfrac{1}{20}$ **14.** $\dfrac{1}{40}$ **15.** $\dfrac{1}{5000}$

The Self-Evaluation Tests on converting fractions to decimals and decimals to fractions should be repeated until fewer than three errors occur.

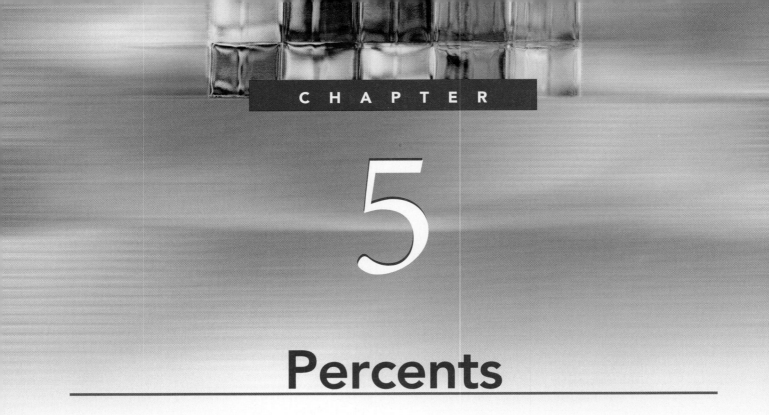

CHAPTER

5

Percents

Learning Outcomes

After successfully completing this chapter, the learner should be able to:

- ■ *Recognize the numerical value of percents.*
- ■ *Convert percents to decimals, and decimals to percents.*
- ■ *Convert percents to fractions, and fractions to percents.*
- ■ *Determine the percent of numbers.*

GENERAL INFORMATION

Percent, which is represented by the symbol %, means hundredths.
A percent can be expressed arithmetically in different forms without changing its value.

Example: 3% can be expressed as:

A fraction with a denominator of 100: $\frac{3}{100}$

A decimal with two decimal places: 0.03

A ratio (as covered in Chapter 6): 3 : 100

Example: 50% can be expressed as:

A fraction with a denominator of 100: $\frac{50}{100}$

A decimal with two decimal places: 0.50

A ratio (as covered in Chapter 6): 50 : 100

A percent can be:

A whole number, such as 20%

A mixed number, such as $3\frac{1}{2}$%

A decimal, such as 0.5%

A fraction, such as $\frac{1}{2}$%

The numbers can be expressed in various forms without changing the value of the percent.

Example: $\frac{1}{4}$% can be written as 0.25%

0.3% can be written as $\frac{3}{10}$%

$3\frac{1}{2}$% can be written as 3.5%

CONVERTING BETWEEN PERCENTS AND DECIMALS

To change a percent to a decimal, remove the percent sign and divide by 100. This division by 100 can be accomplished by moving the decimal point two places to the left of its current position, and adding zeros as necessary.

Example: Convert 15% to a decimal.

Solution: Remove the percent sign and divide by 100:

15% = 0.15. = 0.15
← x

To change a decimal to a percent, multiply by 100 and add a percent sign. The multiplication by 100 can be accomplished by moving the decimal point two places to the right of its current position, adding zeros as necessary, and adding a percent sign.

Example: Change 0.22 to a percent.

Solution: Multiply by 100 and add a percent sign:

0.22 = 0.22. = 22%
x →

Problem Set 5.1

Convert the following to percents or decimals.

1. 5% _____
2. 0.4 _____
3. 25% _____
4. 0.75 _____
5. 0.3% _____

6. 0.375 _____
7. 0.009 _____
8. 12.5% _____
9. 1.25% _____
10. 0.00125 _____

Answers   **1.** 0.05   **2.** 40%   **3.** 0.25   **4.** 75%   **5.** 0.003   **6.** 37.5%   **7.** 0.9%   **8.** 0.125   **9.** 0.0125   **10.** 0.125%

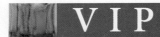

VIP

- When changing a percent to a decimal, move the decimal point two places to the left and remove the percent sign.
- When changing a decimal to a percent, move the decimal point two places to the right and add a percent sign.

Self-Evaluation Test 5.1
Converting Percents to Decimals and Decimals to Percents

Convert the following to percents or decimals.

1. 7% _____
2. 0.45 _____
3. 0.05 _____
4. 75% _____
5. 25% _____
6. 0.2% _____
7. 0.5% _____
8. 0.125 _____

9. 0.075 _____
10. 0.001 _____
11. 0.009 _____
12. 16.2% _____
13. 0.33% _____
14. 87.5% _____
15. 0.0002 _____

Answers   **1.** 0.07   **2.** 45%   **3.** 5%   **4.** 0.75   **5.** 0.25   **6.** 0.002   **7.** 0.005   **8.** 12.5%   **9.** 7.5%   **10.** 0.1%   **11.** 0.9%   **12.** 0.162   **13.** 0.0033   **14.** 0.875   **15.** 0.02%

If you had fewer than three errors on Self-Evaluation Test 5.1, move on to the next section. If you had four or more errors, review the material just covered and complete Self-Evaluation Test 5.2 before continuing.

Self-Evaluation Test 5.2
Converting Percents to Decimals and Decimals to Percents

Convert the following to percents or decimals.

1. 3% _____
2. 1% _____
3. 0.5 _____
4. 50% _____
5. 0.04 _____
6. 0.01 _____
7. 0.25 _____
8. 0.09 _____

9. 7.5% _____
10. 0.1% _____
11. 0.005 _____
12. 83.3% _____
13. 0.25% _____
14. 0.0001 _____
15. 0.0015 _____

Answers   **1.** 0.03   **2.** 0.01   **3.** 50%   **4.** 0.50   **5.** 4%   **6.** 1%   **7.** 25%   **8.** 9%   **9.** 0.075   **10.** 0.001   **11.** 0.5%   **12.** 0.833   **13.** 0.0025   **14.** 0.01%   **15.** 0.15%

The Self-Evaluation Tests on converting percents to decimals and decimals to percents should be repeated until fewer than three errors occur.

CONVERTING BETWEEN PERCENTS AND FRACTIONS

To change a percent to a fraction, first convert the percent to a decimal by dividing by 100 and removing the percent sign. Then, convert the decimal to a fraction by following the procedure discussed in Chapter 4. Always reduce the fraction to its lowest terms.

Example: Change 30% to a fraction.

Solution: Convert the percent to a decimal, then convert the decimal to a fraction:

$$30\% = 0.3 = \frac{3}{10}$$

Example: Change 0.1% to a fraction.

Solution: Convert the percent to a decimal, then convert the decimal to a fraction:

$$0.1\% \left(\frac{1}{10}\%\right) = 0.001 = \frac{1}{1000}$$

To change a fraction to a percent, first convert the fraction to a decimal by following the procedure discussed in Chapter 4. Then, convert the decimal to a percent by multiplying by 100, adding zeros if necessary, and add a percent sign.

Example: Convert $\frac{3}{5}$ to a percent.

Solution: Convert the fraction to a decimal, then convert the decimal to a percent:

$$\frac{3}{5} = 0.6 = 60\%$$

Example: Convert $\frac{1}{4}$ to a percent.

Solution: Convert the fraction to a decimal, then convert the decimal to a percent:

$$\frac{1}{4} = 0.25 = 25\%$$

Problem Set 5.2

Convert the following percents to fractions and fractions to percent. Reduce to lowest terms.

1. 4% _____

2. $\frac{1}{6}$ _____

3. $\frac{1}{8}$ _____

4. $\frac{1}{20}$ _____

5. 60% _____

6. 7.5% _____

7. $\frac{1}{300}$ _____

8. 37.5% _____

9. $\frac{1}{5000}$ _____

10. $33\frac{1}{3}\%$ _____

Answers 1. $\frac{1}{25}$ 2. 16.6%, $\left(16\frac{2}{3}\%\right)$ 3. 12.5%, $\left(12\frac{1}{2}\%\right)$ 4. 5% 5. $\frac{3}{5}$ 6. $\frac{3}{40}$ 7. $0.33\frac{1}{3}\%$, $\left(\frac{1}{3}\%\right)$ 8. $\frac{3}{8}$ 9. 0.02%, $\left(\frac{1}{50}\%\right)$
10. $\frac{1}{3}$

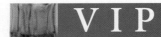

VIP

- When changing a percent to a fraction, convert the percent to a decimal and follow the rules for changing a decimal to a fraction.
- When changing a fraction to a percent, convert the fraction to a decimal and follow the rules for changing a decimal to a percent.

Self-Evaluation Test 5.3
Converting Percents to Fractions and Fractions to Percents

Change percents to fractions and fractions to percents. Reduce to lowest terms.

1. 1% _____

2. 0.5% _____

3. $\dfrac{1}{2}$ _____

4. $\dfrac{1}{5}$ _____

5. $\dfrac{1}{10}$ _____

6. $\dfrac{1}{25}$ _____

7. $\dfrac{1}{60}$ _____

8. 25% _____

9. 35% _____

10. $\dfrac{1}{3}$% _____

11. 0.9% _____

12. 0.07% _____

13. $\dfrac{1}{500}$ _____

14. $\dfrac{1}{1000}$ _____

15. $\dfrac{1}{2500}$ _____

Answers 1. $\dfrac{1}{100}$ 2. $\dfrac{1}{200}$ 3. 50% 4. 20% 5. 10% 6. 4% 7. $1.66\dfrac{2}{3}$%, $\left(1\dfrac{2}{3}\%\right)$ 8. $\dfrac{1}{4}$ 9. $\dfrac{7}{20}$ 10. $\dfrac{1}{300}$ 11. $\dfrac{9}{1000}$

12. $\dfrac{7}{10,000}$ 13. 0.2%, $\left(\dfrac{1}{5}\%\right)$ 14. 0.1%, $\left(\dfrac{1}{10}\%\right)$ 15. 0.04%, $\left(\dfrac{1}{25}\%\right)$

If you had fewer than three errors on Self-Evaluation Test 5.3, move on to the next section. If you had four or more errors, review the material just covered and complete Self-Evaluation Test 5.4 before continuing.

Self-Evaluation Test 5.4
Converting Percents to Fractions and Fractions to Percents

Convert percents to fractions and fractions to percents. Reduce to lowest terms.

1. 5% _____

2. $\dfrac{3}{4}$ _____

3. $\dfrac{9}{10}$ _____

4. $\dfrac{1}{12}$ _____

5. $\dfrac{1}{25}$ _____ 11. $\dfrac{1}{200}$ _____

6. 75% _____ 12. 0.02% _____

7. 20% _____ 13. $\dfrac{1}{100}$ % _____

8. 2.5% _____

9. 0.1% _____ 14. $\dfrac{9}{1000}$ _____

10. $\dfrac{1}{150}$ _____ 15. $\dfrac{1}{10,000}$ _____

Answers 1. $\dfrac{1}{20}$ 2. 75% 3. 90% 4. $8\dfrac{1}{3}$% 5. 4% 6. $\dfrac{3}{4}$ 7. $\dfrac{1}{5}$ 8. $\dfrac{1}{40}$ 9. $\dfrac{1}{1000}$ 10. $0.6\dfrac{2}{3}$% 11. 0.5%, $\left(\dfrac{1}{2}\%\right)$ 12. $\dfrac{1}{5000}$

13. $\dfrac{1}{10,000}$ 14. 0.9%, $\left(\dfrac{9}{10}\%\right)$ 15. 0.01%

The Self-Evaluation Tests on converting percents to fractions and fractions to percents should be repeated until fewer than three errors occur.

DETERMINING PERCENTS

Determining a Given Percent of a Number

When determining a given percent of a number, first change the percent to a decimal or fraction, then multiply the decimal or fraction by the number.

Example: Determine 25% of 60

Solution: Change the percent to a decimal:

25% = 0.25

Multiply the decimal by the number:

0.25 × 60 = 15

Therefore, 25% of 60 = 15

Example: Determine 40% of 90

Solution: Change the percent to a fraction:

$40\% = \dfrac{40}{100} = \dfrac{2}{5}$

Multiply the fraction by the number:

$\dfrac{2}{5} \times 90 = 36$

Therefore, 40% of 90 = 36

Determining What Percent One Number Is of Another Number

When determining what percent one number is of another number, it is necessary to create a fraction. The denominator of the fraction is the number following the word "of" in the problem statement and the numerator is the remaining number. This fraction is then converted to a decimal following the rules discussed previously. The decimal result is then converted to a percent.

Example: 15 is what % of 60? or, What % of 60 is 15?

Solution: Create a fraction using these two numbers.

The fraction created is $\frac{15}{60}$

Convert this fraction to a decimal:

$$\frac{15}{60} = 60\overline{)15.00}^{\,0.25}$$

Convert the resulting decimal to a percent:

0.25 = 25%

Therefore, 15 is 25% of 60 or 25% of 60 = 15

Problem Set 5.3

1. 5% of 1500 _____

2. 1% of 2500 _____

3. 25% of 500 _____

4. 2.5% of 750 _____

5. $\frac{9}{10}$ % of 2000 _____

6. 20 is what percent of 100 _____

7. 5 is what percent of 2500 _____

8. 1 is what percent of 1000 _____

9. 100 is what percent of 750 _____

10. 50 is what percent of 1000 _____

Answers **1.** 75 **2.** 25 **3.** 125 **4.** 18.75 **5.** 18 **6.** 20% **7.** 0.2% **8.** 0.1% **9.** 13.3% **10.** 5%

V I P

A percent can be a whole number, a mixed number, a decimal, or a fraction and can be expressed in any of these various forms without changing the value of the percent.

Self-Evaluation Test 5.5
Determining Percents

Solve the following problems on determining percents.

1. 80% of 30 _____

2. 20% of 75 _____

3. $\frac{1}{2}$ % of 7.5 _____

4. 0.06% of 40 _____

5. 50% of 1000 _____

6. $\frac{1}{4}$ % of 2000 _____

7. $\frac{9}{10}$ % of 1000 _____

8. 15 is what % of 75 _____

9. 25 is what % of 65 _____

10. 30 is what % of 45 _____

11. 3 is what % of 600 _____

12. $\frac{1}{2}$ is what % of 60 _____

13. 5 is what % of 2000 _____

14. 15 is what % of 1000 _____

15. 25 is what % of 1500 _____

Answers **1.** 24 **2.** 15 **3.** 0.0375 **4.** 0.024 **5.** 500 **6.** 5 **7.** 9 **8.** 20% **9.** 38% **10.** $66\frac{2}{3}$% **11.** 0.5% **12.** 0.83%

13. 0.25% **14.** 1.5% **15.** $1.6\frac{2}{3}$% (can be written as 1.67%)

If you had fewer than three errors on Self-Evaluation Test 5.5, move on to the next chapter. If you had four or more errors, review the material just covered and complete Self-Evaluation Test 5.6 before continuing.

Self-Evaluation Test 5.6
Determining Percents

1. 75% of 250 _____

2. $\frac{1}{2}$% of 500 _____

3. 2.5% of 750 _____

4. 0.3% of 500 _____

5. 5% of 1000 _____

6. 0.9% of 1500 _____

7. $\frac{1}{3}$% of 1200 _____

8. 2 is what % of 200 _____

9. 3 is what % of 150 _____

10. 50 is what % of 500 _____

11. 30 is what % of 120 _____

12. 60 is what % of 180 _____

13. 75 is what % of 500 _____

14. 1 is what % of 5000 _____

15. 35 is what % of 1000 _____

Answers **1.** 187.5 **2.** 2.5 **3.** 18.75 **4.** 1.5 **5.** 50 **6.** 13.5 **7.** 4 **8.** 1% **9.** 2% **10.** 10% **11.** 25% **12.** $33\frac{1}{3}$% **13.** 15% **14.** 0.02% **15.** 3.5%

The Self-Evaluation Tests on determining percents should be repeated until fewer than three errors occur.

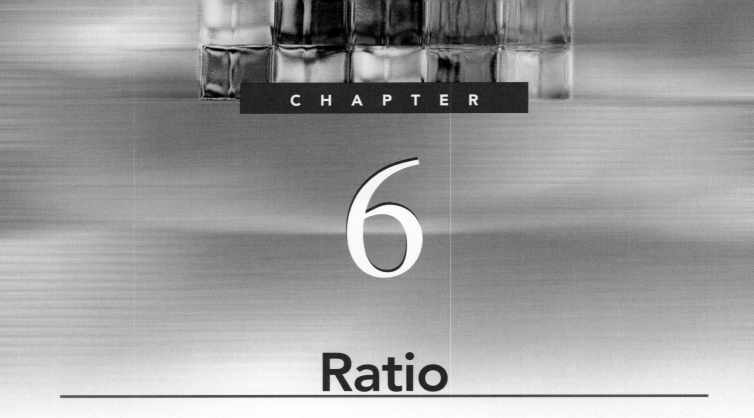

6

Ratio

Learning Outcomes

After successfully completing this chapter, the learner should be able to:

- *Recognize the numerical relationships represented by ratio.*
- *Convert ratios to fractions, and fractions to ratios.*
- *Convert ratios to decimals, and decimals to ratios.*
- *Convert ratios to percents, and percents to ratios.*

GENERAL INFORMATION

A ratio expresses the numerical relationship between two quantities. For example, if lemonade contained 1 oz of lemon juice to 8 oz of water, the ratio of lemon juice to water could be expressed as 1:8. (The ratio of lemon juice in the total mixture could be expressed as 1:9 (1 oz of lemon juice + 8 oz of water, or a total of 9 oz).

   If a cat had a litter of two white kittens and three gray kittens, the ratio of white kittens to gray kittens could be expressed as 2:3. The ratio of white kittens to the total litter could be expressed as 2:5.

Problem Set 6.1

Express as ratios.

1. 3 girls to 10 boys   _____

2. 5 mice to 200 squirrels   _____

3. 25 Pooh bears to 110 Piglets   _____

4.   45 blue cars to 1000 red cars   _____

5.   1000 6-year olds to 3000 8-year-olds   _____

A ratio is the result of the division of two numbers that can also be expressed as a fraction. The first number of the ratio becomes the numerator, and the second number becomes the denominator. The colon (:) represents the slash or the division sign. Once expressed as a fraction, a ratio can be reduced to its lowest terms.

Example: $3:12 = \dfrac{3}{12} = \dfrac{1}{4}$

Example: $2:6$ can be expressed as $\dfrac{2}{6}$ which can be reduced to $\dfrac{1}{3}$

Problem Set 6.2

Express as fractions; reduce to lowest terms.

1.   3:4   _____

2.   1:500   _____

3.   25:100   _____

4.   9:1000   _____

5.   1000:3000   _____

Because ratios are another way of expressing a fraction, multiplying or dividing both parts of the ratio by the same number does not change the value of the ratio.

Example: Multiplying:

4:12 multiplied by 3 produces the ratio 12:36

Dividing:

4:12 divided by 4 produces the ratio 1:3

Problem Set 6.3

1. $1:5 \times 4$ _____

2. $1:20 \times 5$ _____

3. $3:8 \times 10$ _____

4. $150:300 \div 150$ _____

5. $1000:3000 \div 1000$ _____

By processes previously explained (see Chapter 4), once a ratio is converted to a fraction, the fraction can be converted to a decimal, and the decimal can be converted to a percent.

Example: $5:10 = \dfrac{5}{10} = \dfrac{1}{2} = 0.5 = 50\%$

Example: $1:250 = \dfrac{1}{250} = 0.004 = 0.4\%$

Problem Set 6.4

Express as decimals and percents.

1. 1:8   _____
2. 1:10   _____
3. 1:200   _____

4. 1:5000   _____
5. 1:10,000   _____

Answers   **1.** 0.125, $12\frac{1}{2}$%   **2.** 0.1, 10%   **3.** 0.005, 0.5%   **4.** 0.0002, 0.02%   **5.** 0.0001, 0.01%

VIP

A ratio can be expressed as a fraction, a decimal, or a percent without any change in value.

Self-Evaluation Test 6.1
Converting Ratios, Fractions, Decimals, and Percents

Ratio	Fraction	Decimal	Percent
1:2			
	$\frac{1}{4}$		
		0.125	
			75%
1:50			
	$\frac{1}{100}$		
		0.005	
			0.9%

Answers

Ratio	Fraction	Decimal	Percent
1:2	$\frac{1}{2}$	0.5	50%
1:4	$\frac{1}{4}$	0.25	25%
1:8	$\frac{1}{8}$	**0.125**	$12\frac{1}{2}\%$
3:4	$\frac{3}{4}$	0.75	**75%**
1:50	$\frac{1}{50}$	0.02	2%
1:100	$\frac{1}{100}$	0.01	1%
1:200	$\frac{1}{200}$	**0.005**	0.5%
9:1000	$\frac{9}{1000}$	0.009	**0.9%**

If you had fewer than three errors on Self-Evaluation Test 6.1, move on to the next chapter. If you had four or more errors, review the material just covered and complete Self-Evaluation Test 6.2 before continuing.

Self-Evaluation Test 6.2
Converting Ratios, Fractions, Decimals, and Percents

Ratio	Fraction	Decimal	Percent
1:6			
	$\frac{1}{5}$		
		0.333	
			1.33%
1:100			
	$\frac{1}{300}$		
		0.0025	
			0.1%

Answers

Ratio	Fraction	Decimal	Percent
1:6	$\dfrac{1}{6}$	0.166	$16\dfrac{2}{3}\%$
1:5	$\dfrac{1}{5}$	0.2	20%
1:3	$\dfrac{1}{3}$	**0.333**	$33\dfrac{1}{3}\%$
1:75	$\dfrac{1}{75}$	0.0133	**1.33%**
1:100	$\dfrac{1}{100}$	0.01	1%
1:300	$\dfrac{1}{\mathbf{300}}$	0.0033	0.33%
1:400	$\dfrac{1}{400}$	**0.0025**	0.25%
1:1000	$\dfrac{1}{1000}$	0.001	**0.1%**

The Self-Evaluation Tests on converting ratios, fractions, decimals, and percents should be repeated until fewer than three errors occur.

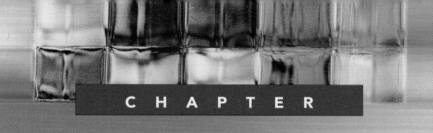

7

Proportion

Learning Outcomes

After successfully completing this chapter, the learner should be able to:

- ■ *Recognize the relationship of terms in a proportion.*
- ■ *Determine the value of an unknown quantity in a proportion.*

GENERAL INFORMATION

A proportion is an equation that contains two ratios of equal value. The proportion (equation) uses an equal sign **or** double colon to demonstrate that the ratios on both sides of the equal sign (or double colon) are equal.

Example: $4:12 = (::) \ 8:24$, or $\frac{4}{12} = (::) \frac{8}{24}$

(reducing these fractions to lowest terms demonstrates their equality): $\frac{1}{3} = \frac{1}{3}$

    Each of the numbers composing a proportion has a name. The first number in the first ratio (the numerator of the first fraction) is called Term 1. The second number in the first ratio (the denominator of the first fraction) is called Term 2. The first number of the second ratio (the numerator of the second fraction) is called Term 3. The second number of the second ratio (the denominator of the second fraction) is called Term 4.

Example: $4 \ : \ 12 \ = \ 8 \ : \ 24$

      1st 2nd   3rd 4th

           or

    1st $\dfrac{4}{12} = \dfrac{8}{24}$ 3rd

    2nd   4th

The 1st and 4th terms of the proportion (the outermost terms) are called the extremes. The 2nd and 3rd terms of the proportion (the innermost terms) are called the means.

Example:

```
            ┌──────── Extremes ────────┐
            │   ┌── Means ──┐          │
     4   :   12   =    8   :   24
    1st      2nd       3rd      4th
                    or
  Extreme 1st   4     8   3rd Mean
  Mean 2nd     ── = ──   4th Extreme
               12    24
```

The product of the means always equals the product of the extremes in a true proportion.

Example: In the proportion 2:4 = 6:12, the extremes are 2 and 12, and the means are 4 and 6.

2:4 = 6:12   the product of the means $4 \times 6 = 24$ equals the
product of the extremes $2 \times 12 = 24$ (24 = 24).

Therefore, 2:4 = 6:12 is a true proportion.

Example: In the proportion $\dfrac{6}{8} = \dfrac{12}{16}$, the extremes are 6 and 16, and the means are 8 and 12.

$\dfrac{6}{8} = \dfrac{12}{16}$ the product of the means $8 \times 12 = 96$, equals the
product of the extremes $6 \times 16 = 96$ (96 = 96).

Therefore, $\dfrac{6}{8} = \dfrac{12}{16}$ is a true proportion.

Problem Set 7.1

Identify the extremes:

1. 5:10 = 25:50 _____

2. 1:100 = 5:500 _____

3. $\dfrac{10}{100} = \dfrac{15}{150}$ _____

4. $\dfrac{1}{300} = \dfrac{10}{3000}$ _____

5. $\dfrac{\frac{1}{2}}{100} : \dfrac{\frac{3}{4}}{150}$ _____

Identify which of the following proportions are true:

6. 1:3 = 35:70 _____

7. $\dfrac{1}{8} : 1 = \dfrac{3}{4} : 6$ _____

8. $\dfrac{0.1}{0.2} = \dfrac{1}{0.02}$ _____

9. $\dfrac{\frac{1}{150}}{1} = \dfrac{\frac{1}{200}}{2}$ _____

10. 10%:30% = 30%:90% _____

Answers   1. 5 & 50   2. 1 & 500   3. 10 & 150   4. 1 & 3000   5. $\frac{1}{2}$ & 150   6. Not true   7. True   8. Not true   9. Not true
10. True

V I P

The equal sign or double colon in a proportion demonstrates that the values of the ratios on either side of the equal sign or double colon are equal to each other.

Self-Evaluation Test 7.1
Identifying True Proportions

1. $3:15 = 4:20$ _____

2. $16:32 = 20:40$ _____

3. $3:150 = 6:300$ _____

4. $\dfrac{1}{32}:\dfrac{1}{64} = 1:2$ _____

5. $0.125:1 = 0.5:4$ _____

6. $\dfrac{1}{6}:1 = \dfrac{1}{8}:1\dfrac{1}{2}$ _____

7. $0.325:1 = 0.65:2$ _____

8. $0.01:5 = 0.05:25$ _____

9. $25:0.005 = 100:2$ _____

10. $\dfrac{1}{1000} = \dfrac{0.5}{5000}$ _____

11. $\dfrac{1}{8}:\dfrac{1}{2} = \dfrac{3}{32}:\dfrac{3}{8}$ _____

12. $\dfrac{1}{200}:1 = \dfrac{1}{100}:2$ _____

13. $0.001:0.5 = 0.02:1$ _____

14. $0.25:0.5 = 0.125:1$ _____

15. $9:1000 = 27:3000$ _____

Answers   1. True   2. True   3. True   4. Not true   5. True   6. Not true   7. True   8. True   9. Not true   10. Not true   11. True
12. True   13. Not true   14. Not true   15. True

If you had fewer than three errors on Self-Evaluation Test 7.1, move on to the next section. If you had four or more errors, review the material just covered and complete Self-Evaluation test 7.2 before continuing.

Self-Evaluation Test 7.2
Identifying True Proportions

1. $1:10 = 2:20$ _____

2. $3:15 = 4:60$ _____

3. $\dfrac{1}{8}:1 = \dfrac{1}{6}:2$ _____

4. $\dfrac{0.25}{0.125} = \dfrac{2}{1}$ _____

5. $\dfrac{1}{16}:2 = \dfrac{1}{8}:4$ _____

6. $16:32 = 20:64$ _____

7. $3:350 = 4:450$ _____

8. $75:1.5 = 125:3$ _____

9. $\dfrac{9}{1000} = \dfrac{1}{9000}$ _____

10. $0.5:15 = 1.5:45$ _____

11. $0.01:5 = 0.5:25$ _____

12. $\dfrac{1}{150}:\dfrac{1}{75} = 2:1$ _____

13. $\dfrac{1}{8}:\dfrac{1}{2} = \dfrac{1}{16}:\dfrac{1}{4}$ _____

14. $\dfrac{1}{1000}:4 = \dfrac{1}{250}:16$ _____

15. $0.001:0.1 = 0.002:0.2$ _____

Answers   1. True   2. Not true   3. Not true   4. True   5. True   6. Not true   7. Not true   8. Not true   9. Not true   10. True
11. Not true   12. Not true   13. True   14. True   15. True

The Self-Evaluation Tests on identifying true proportions should be repeated until fewer than three errors occur.

SOLVING FOR AN UNKNOWN TERM

Before solving for an unknown term in a proportion (equation), it is important to recognize that certain principles influence this task.

In a true proportion, the product of the means equals the product of the extremes (or the product of the extremes equals the product of the means). When two ratios are set up as equal, both sides of the equation may be divided or multiplied by the same number without changing the relationship between the ratios.

Example: Both sides of the equation $2:4 = 6:12$ can be divided by the same number, such as 2, producing the equation $1:2 = 3:6$, without changing the relationship between the ratios.

Both sides of the equation $2:4 = 6:12$ can also be multiplied by the same number, such as 3, producing the equation $6:12 = 18:36$, without changing the relationship between the ratios.

The value of the new equations produced by dividing or multiplying both sides of a true proportion by the same number does not change the proportional relationship.

A true proportion can be set up in a variety of ways as long as the ratios on both sides of the equal sign are written in the same order or sequence.

Example: smaller number : larger number = smaller number : larger number

or

larger number : smaller number = larger number : smaller number

or

denominator : numerator = denominator : numerator

or

numerator : denominator = numerator : denominator

The fact that in a true proportion the product of the means equals the product of the extremes is an important principle that is used to determine the value of an unknown term, usually signified by the letter x.

Example: Determine the value of x in the proportion: $1:4 = x:12$

Solution: Because the product of the means equals the product of the extremes, and the letter x is usually placed on the left side, this equation can be rewritten as $4x = 12$.

Solving for x can now be accomplished by dividing both sides of the equation by the number preceding the x, in this instance 4, without changing the relationship. The number used for division should always be the number preceding the unknown (x), so that when this step is completed the unknown (x) will stand alone on the left side of the equation.

$$1:4 = x:12$$

$$\frac{\cancel{4}x}{\cancel{4}} = \frac{\cancel{12}^{\,3}}{\cancel{4}}$$

$$x = \frac{3}{1}$$

$$x = 3$$

A check of the accuracy of the computation can be accomplished by substituting the determined value of x (the answer) for the x in the original equation.

Example: Substitute the determined value of x (3) in the original equation:

$1:4 = x:12$ produces an equation that reads:

$1:4 = 3:12$

By multiplying the means and the extremes, the answer is proven correct because $12 = 12$.

Example: Determine the value of x in the equation 7:x = 21:48

Solution: Multiply the means and the extremes:

21x = 336

Divide both sides of the equation by the number preceding x (21):

x = 16

Check answer by substituting the determined value of x in the equation:

7:16 = 21:48

Multiplying the means and the extremes proves that 336 = 336.

Calculation Alert

■ The product of the means always equals the product of the extremes.

■ When solving for an unknown, always divide both sides of the equation by the number preceding the unknown.

Although the unknown quantity may be any of the four terms of an equation, after multiplying the means and the extremes, the unknown is usually placed on the left side of the equation.

Example:

9:x = 27:36	20:50 = 30:x
27x = 324	20x = 1500
x = 12	x = 75
Proof:	
9:12 = 27:36	20:50 = 30:75
324 = 324	1500 = 1500

Problem Set 7.2

1. 1:15 = x:60 _____

2. $16:\dfrac{1}{4} = x:1$ _____

3. $\dfrac{1}{12}:x = \dfrac{1}{8}:1$ _____

4. $7\dfrac{1}{2}:\dfrac{1}{2} = x:2$ _____

5. x:0.125 = 2:0.5 _____

6. 0.001:0.5 = x:2 _____

7. $\dfrac{1}{32}:\dfrac{1}{64} = 2:x$ _____

8. $\dfrac{1}{200}:\dfrac{1}{150} = x:1$ _____

9. 400,000:8 = x:1.5 _____

10. 1,000,000:10 = 400,000:x _____

Answers   1. x = 4   2. x = 64   3. $x = \dfrac{2}{3}$ 4. x = 30   5. x = 0.5   6. x = 0.004   7. x = 1   8. $x = \dfrac{3}{4}$ 9. x = 75,000   10. x = 4

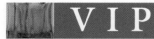 **V I P**

Regardless of which term of the equation is the unknown, after multiplying the means and extremes, the unknown value (the x) is usually placed on the left side of the equation.

Self-Evaluation Test 7.3
Solving for X

1. $1:60 = 5:x$ _____

2. $1:15 = x:45$ _____

3. $2.2:1 = 25:x$ _____

4. $0.1:x = 0.5:2$ _____

5. $15:20 = x:30$ _____

6. $0.125:1 = x:2$ _____

7. $2.2:1 = x:145$ _____

8. $\frac{1}{4}:16 = \frac{1}{8}:x$ _____

9. $0.25:2 = x:\frac{1}{2}$ _____

10. $1000:1 = 750:x$ _____

11. $x:0.5 = 0.125:1$ _____

12. $\frac{1}{150}:1 = x:\frac{3}{5}$ _____

13. $1:5000 = x:1000$ _____

14. $\frac{1}{200}:1 = \frac{1}{150}:x$ _____

15. $\frac{1}{150}:x = \frac{1}{300}:1$ _____

Answers   1. $x = 300$ 2. $x = 3$ 3. $x = 11.364$ 4. $x = 0.4$ 5. $x = 22.5$ 6. $x = 0.25$ 7. $x = 319$ 8. $x = 8$ 9. $x = 0.0625$

10. $x = 0.75$ 11. $x = 0.0625$ 12. $x = \frac{1}{250}$ 13. $x = 0.2$ 14. $x = 1\frac{1}{3}$ 15. $x = 2$

If you had fewer than three errors on Self-Evaluation Test 7.3, move on to the next chapter, the Posttest in Basic Mathematics. If you had four or more errors, review the material just covered and complete Self-Evaluation Test 7.4 before continuing.

Self-Evaluation Test 7.4
Solving for X

1. $1:3 = x:15$ _____

2. $1:64 = 3:x$ _____

3. $\frac{1}{6}:1 = 2:x$ _____

4. $1:2.2 = 60:x$ _____

5. $\frac{1}{8}:1 = \frac{1}{6}:x$ _____

6. $1\frac{1}{2}:2 = x:3$ _____

7. $10:15 = x:45$ _____

8. $2.2:1 = 135:x$ _____

9. $\frac{1}{200}:1 = x:2$ _____

10. $1:3.6 = x:170$ _____

11. $1:0.05 = x:0.1$ _____

12. $1:0.25 = x:0.125$ _____

13. $50:1000 = x:100$ _____

14. $\frac{1}{150}:\frac{1}{100} = x:1$ _____

15. $x:1000 = 1.5:3000$ _____

Answers   1. $x = 5$ 2. $x = 192$ 3. $x = 12$ 4. $x = 132$ 5. $x = 1\frac{1}{3}$ 6. $x = 2\frac{1}{4}$ 7. $x = 30$ 8. $x = 61.36$ 9. $x = \frac{1}{100}$ 10. $x = 47.2$

11. $x = 2$ 12. $x = 0.5$ 13. $x = 5$ 14. $x = \frac{2}{3}$ 15. $x = 0.5$

The Self-Evaluation Tests on solving for x should be repeated until fewer than three errors occur.

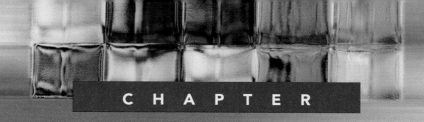

CHAPTER

8

Posttest in the Mathematics Involved in Dosage Computation

Set 8.1

Write the following as Roman or Arabic numerals.

1. 19 _____
2. 38 _____
3. 122 _____
4. XLIV _____
5. XCVI _____

Set 8.2

Add the following fractions and reduce to lowest terms.

1. $\dfrac{1}{8} + \dfrac{5}{6} + \dfrac{2}{3}$ _____

2. $\dfrac{1}{32} + \dfrac{1}{64} + \dfrac{3}{8}$ _____

3. $\dfrac{1}{10} + \dfrac{1}{15} + \dfrac{1}{50}$ _____

4. $2\dfrac{2}{3} + 1\dfrac{1}{4} + 7\dfrac{1}{2}$ _____

5. $\dfrac{1}{150} + \dfrac{1}{200} + \dfrac{1}{300}$ _____

Set 8.3

Subtract the following fractions and reduce to lowest terms.

1. $\dfrac{9}{10} - \dfrac{2}{5}$ _____

2. $65 - 4\dfrac{1}{5}$ _____

3. $7\dfrac{1}{2} - 1\dfrac{1}{8}$ _____

4. $33\dfrac{1}{3} - 3\dfrac{3}{8}$ _____

5. $25\dfrac{1}{300} - \dfrac{1}{60}$ _____

Set 8.4

Multiply the following fractions and reduce to lowest terms.

1. $\dfrac{1}{6} \times \dfrac{1}{8}$ _____

2. $\dfrac{1}{100} \times \dfrac{1}{3}$ _____

3. $7\dfrac{1}{2} \times 2\dfrac{2}{3}$ _____

4. $250 \times \dfrac{1}{2} \times \dfrac{3}{5}$ _____

5. $1\dfrac{1}{2} \times 1\dfrac{7}{8} \times \dfrac{1}{15}$ _____

Set 8.5

Divide the following fractions and reduce to lowest terms.

1. $\dfrac{1}{8} \div \dfrac{1}{6}$ _____

2. $\dfrac{1}{1000} \div 2$ _____

3. $\dfrac{1}{64} \div \dfrac{1}{32}$ _____

4. $7\dfrac{1}{2} \div 3\dfrac{3}{8}$ _____

5. $\dfrac{1}{150} \div \dfrac{1}{200}$ _____

Set 8.6

Change the following fractions to ratios.

1. $\dfrac{1}{2}$ _____

2. $\dfrac{3}{8}$ _____

3. $\dfrac{1}{64}$ _____

4. $\dfrac{3}{100}$ _____

5. $\dfrac{\frac{1}{2}}{\frac{1}{8}}$ _____

Set 8.7

Arrange the following fractions in order from smallest to largest.

1. $\dfrac{1}{2}; \dfrac{1}{3}; \dfrac{3}{8}; \dfrac{1}{12}; \dfrac{7}{16}$ _____

2. $\dfrac{3}{16}; \dfrac{3}{8}; \dfrac{3}{4}; \dfrac{29}{32}; \dfrac{1}{2}$

3. $\dfrac{3}{5}$; $\dfrac{4}{15}$; $\dfrac{9}{10}$; $\dfrac{1}{30}$; $\dfrac{1}{12}$ _____

4. $\dfrac{3}{200}$; $\dfrac{1}{150}$; $\dfrac{9}{100}$; $\dfrac{3}{50}$; $\dfrac{2}{75}$ _____

5. $\dfrac{1}{1000}$; $\dfrac{9}{1000}$; $\dfrac{7}{2000}$; $\dfrac{3}{500}$; $\dfrac{1}{250}$ _____

Set 8.8

Change the following mixed numbers to improper fractions.

1. $2\dfrac{3}{4}$ _____

2. $7\dfrac{1}{2}$ _____

3. $66\dfrac{2}{3}$ _____

4. $10\dfrac{2}{25}$ _____

5. $250\dfrac{3}{4}$ _____

Set 8.9

Add the following decimals.

1. $0.125 + 0.9$ _____

2. $1.75 + 0.25$ _____

3. $0.06 + 0.125$ _____

4. $0.006 + 0.325$ _____

5. $0.0101 + 0.001$ _____

Set 8.10

Subtract the following decimals.

1. $7.5 - 1.5$ _____

2. $1.7 - 0.9$ _____

3. $7.5 - 0.25$ _____

4. $64 - 0.064$ _____

5. $0.75 - 0.03$ _____

Set 8.11

Multiply the following decimals.

1. 0.5×0.3 _____

2. 3.75×1.5 _____

3. 7.5×1.25 _____

4. 0.0125×0.5 _____

5. 0.375×0.25 _____

Set 8.12

Divide the following decimals.

1. $7.5 \div 1.5$ _____

2. $0.6 \div 0.12$ _____

3. $0.75 \div 0.25$ _____

4. $1.25 \div 0.125$ _____

5. $0.065 \div 0.002$ _____

Set 8.13

Arrange the following decimals in order from the largest to the smallest.

1. 0.4; 0.5; 0.375; 0.001; 0.12 _____

2. 0.065; 0.06; 0.6; 0.003; 0.013 _____

3. 0.3; 0.025; 0.666; 0.75; 0.125 _____

4. 0.0101; 0.101; 0.001; 0.1; 1.01 _____

5. 2.125; 2.01; 2.51; 0.0125; 0.125 _____

Set 8.14

Convert the following fractions to decimals. Carry out to the fourth decimal place, if necessary.

1. $\dfrac{1}{4}$ _____   4. $\dfrac{1}{150}$ _____

2. $\dfrac{5}{6}$ _____   5. $\dfrac{9}{1000}$ _____

3. $\dfrac{1}{32}$ _____

Set 8.15

Convert the following decimals to fractions and reduce to lowest terms.

1. 0.04 _____   4. 0.015 _____

2. 0.50 _____   5. 0.009 _____

3. 0.125 _____

Set 8.16

Change the following fractions to percent.

1. $\dfrac{1}{8}$ _____   4. $\dfrac{1}{200}$ _____

2. $\dfrac{1}{12}$ _____   5. $\dfrac{1}{1000}$ _____

3. $\dfrac{1}{60}$ _____

Set 8.17

Change the following ratios to percents.

1. 1:6 _____   4. 5:1000 _____

2. $\dfrac{3}{4}$:1 _____   5. 1:2000 _____

3. 3:400 _____

Set 8.18

Change the following decimals to percents.

1. 0.1 _____
2. 0.03 _____
3. 0.75 _____

4. 0.001 _____
5. 0.0002 _____

Set 8.19

Express the following percents as decimals.

1. 3% _____
2. 40% _____
3. 0.7% _____

4. 0.9% _____
5. 0.03% _____

Set 8.20

Express the following percents as fractions and reduce to lowest terms.

1. 1% _____
2. 1.5% _____
3. $\frac{1}{2}$% _____

4. $\frac{9}{10}$% _____
5. 0.01% _____

Set 8.21

Express the following percents as ratios.

1. 5% _____
2. 75% _____
3. 0.4% _____

4. 37.5% _____
5. $\frac{9}{10}$% _____

Set 8.22

Determine the given percents.

1. 8% of 32 _____
2. $\frac{1}{2}$% of 5 _____
3. 60% of 462 _____

4. 300% of 200 _____
5. 20% of 20,000 _____

Set 8.23

Solve for x in the following proportions.

1. 1:5 = x:25 _____
2. x:4 = 15:60 _____
3. $\frac{3}{8}$:x = 1:24 _____

4. $\frac{1}{2}:\frac{1}{4}$ = x:2 _____
5. 1:100 = x:1000 _____

Set 8.24

Solve for x in the following proportions.

1. $1:50 = x:35$ _____
2. $1:80 = x:45$ _____
3. $0.5:1 = x:50$ _____

4. $0.2:0.3 = 1:x$ _____
5. $0.75:1 = 0.25:x$ _____

Set 8.25

Make all of the following proportions "true" by changing one term in the ratio following the equal sign when necessary.

1. $1:15 = 3:60$ _____
2. $16:\dfrac{1}{4} = 128:2$ _____
3. $\dfrac{1}{100}:3 = \dfrac{1}{300}:\dfrac{1}{3}$ _____

4. $\dfrac{1}{1000}:2 = \dfrac{1}{200}:10$ _____
5. $100,000:4 = 25,000:2.5$ _____

ANSWERS TO POSTTEST

Set 8.1

1. XIX
2. XXXVIII
3. CXXII

4. 44
5. 96

Set 8.2

1. $1\dfrac{5}{8}$
2. $\dfrac{27}{64}$
3. $\dfrac{14}{75}$

4. $11\dfrac{5}{12}$
5. $\dfrac{3}{200}$

Set 8.3

1. $\dfrac{1}{2}$
2. $60\dfrac{4}{5}$
3. $6\dfrac{3}{8}$

4. $29\dfrac{33}{24}$
5. $24\dfrac{74}{75}$

Set 8.4

1. $\dfrac{1}{48}$
2. $\dfrac{1}{300}$
3. 20

4. 75
5. $\dfrac{3}{16}$

Set 8.5

1. $\dfrac{3}{4}$
2. $\dfrac{1}{2000}$
3. $\dfrac{1}{2}$

4. $2\dfrac{2}{9}$
5. $1\dfrac{1}{3}$

Set 8.6

1. $1:2$
2. $3:8$
3. $1:64$

4. $3:100$
5. $\dfrac{1}{2}:\dfrac{1}{8}$

Set 8.7

1. $\dfrac{1}{12}$; $\dfrac{1}{3}$; $\dfrac{3}{8}$; $\dfrac{7}{16}$; $\dfrac{1}{2}$

2. $\dfrac{3}{16}$; $\dfrac{3}{8}$; $\dfrac{1}{2}$; $\dfrac{3}{4}$; $\dfrac{29}{32}$

3. $\dfrac{1}{30}$; $\dfrac{1}{12}$; $\dfrac{4}{15}$; $\dfrac{3}{5}$; $\dfrac{9}{10}$

4. $\dfrac{1}{150}$; $\dfrac{3}{200}$; $\dfrac{2}{75}$; $\dfrac{3}{50}$; $\dfrac{9}{100}$

5. $\dfrac{1}{1000}$; $\dfrac{7}{2000}$; $\dfrac{1}{250}$; $\dfrac{3}{500}$; $\dfrac{9}{1000}$

Set 8.8

1. $\dfrac{11}{4}$

2. $\dfrac{15}{2}$

3. $\dfrac{200}{3}$

4. $\dfrac{252}{25}$

5. $\dfrac{1003}{4}$

Set 8.9

1. 1.025
2. 2
3. 0.185
4. 0.331
5. 0.0111

Set 8.10

1. 6.0
2. 0.8
3. 7.25
4. 63.936
5. 0.72

Set 8.11

1. 0.15
2. 5.625
3. 9.375
4. 0.00625
5. 0.09375

Set 8.12

1. 5
2. 5
3. 3
4. 10
5. 32.5

Set 8.13

1. 0.5; 0.4; 0.375; 0.12; 0.001
2. 0.6; 0.065; 0.06; 0.013; 0.003
3. 0.75; 0.666; 0.3; 0.125; 0.025
4. 1.01; 0.101; 0.1; 0.0101; 0.001
5. 2.51; 2.125; 2.01; 0.125; 0.0125

Set 8.14

1. 0.25
2. 0.8333
3. 0.0312
4. 0.0066
5. 0.009

Set 8.15

1. $\dfrac{1}{25}$

2. $\dfrac{1}{2}$

3. $\dfrac{1}{8}$

4. $\dfrac{3}{200}$

5. $\dfrac{9}{1000}$

Set 8.16

1. $12\dfrac{1}{2}\%$ or 12.5%

2. $8\dfrac{1}{3}\%$ or 8.333%

3. $1\dfrac{2}{3}\%$ or 1.667%

4. $\dfrac{1}{2}\%$ or 0.5%

5. $\dfrac{1}{10}\%$ or 0.1%

Set 8.17

1. $16\dfrac{2}{3}\%$ or 16.67%

2. 75%

3. $\dfrac{3}{4}\%$ or 0.75%

4. $\dfrac{1}{2}\%$ or 0.5%

5. $\dfrac{1}{20}\%$ or 0.05%

Set 8.18

1. 10%
2. 3%
3. 75%
4. 0.1%
5. 0.02%

Set 8.19

1. 0.03
2. 0.4
3. 0.007
4. 0.009
5. 0.0003

Set 8.20

1. $\dfrac{1}{100}$
2. $\dfrac{3}{200}$
3. $\dfrac{1}{200}$
4. $\dfrac{9}{1000}$
5. $\dfrac{1}{10,000}$

Set 8.21

1. 1:20
2. 3:4
3. 1:250
4. 3:8
5. 9:1000

Set 8.22

1. 2.56
2. 0.025
3. 277.2
4. 600
5. 4000

Set 8.23

1. x = 5
2. x = 1
3. x = 9
4. x = 4
5. x = 10

Set 8.24

1. x = 0.7
2. x = 0.5625
3. x = 25
4. x = 1.5
5. x = 0.333

Set 8.25

1. Change 60 to 45
   $$1:15 = 3:45$$
   $$45 = 45$$

2. True proportion:
   $$16:\dfrac{1}{4} = 128:2$$
   $$32 = 32$$

3. Change $\dfrac{1}{3}$ to 1
   $$\dfrac{1}{100}:3 = \dfrac{1}{300}:1$$
   $$\dfrac{1}{100} = \dfrac{1}{100}$$

4. True proportion:
   $$\dfrac{1}{1000}:2 = \dfrac{1}{200}:10$$
   $$\dfrac{1}{100} = \dfrac{1}{100}$$

5. Change 2.5 to 1
   $$100,000:4 = 25,000:1$$
   $$100,000 = 100,000$$

Unit 2

Systems of Measurement

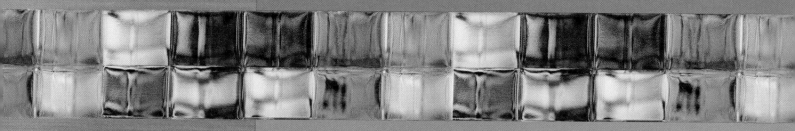

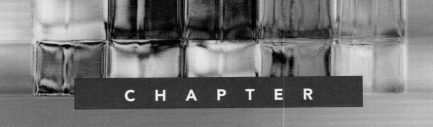

9

Celsius (Centigrade) and Fahrenheit Temperature Scales

Learning Outcomes

After successfully completing this chapter, the learner should be able to:

- *Recognize the relationship between the Celsius and Fahrenheit temperature scales.*
- *Convert a given temperature from one temperature scale to the other.*
- *Recognize how to set up and use the formula for conversion.*

GENERAL INFORMATION

Two temperature scales are in common use throughout the world. In the United States the Fahrenheit scale is still used, although the Celsius scale, which is used in most other parts of the world, is becoming fairly common. To indicate which scale is being used, a temperature measured on the Fahrenheit scale is followed by an F and a temperature measured on the Celsius scale is followed by a C.

Using Figure 9-1, it can be determined that water freezes at 32 degrees Fahrenheit and at 0 degrees Celsius. This 32-degree difference is used in converting temperature from one scale to the other. Using Figure 9-1, it can also be determined that water boils at 212 degrees Fahrenheit and at 100 degrees Celsius.

There is a 180-degree difference between the freezing and boiling points on the Fahrenheit scale and a 100-degree difference between these two points on the Celsius scale. The difference between the boiling point and freezing point on the Fahrenheit scale and the Celsius scale can be set as a ratio, 180:100. This ratio can be used to determine arithmetically that each Celsius degree is $\frac{9}{5}$ times greater than each Fahrenheit degree:

$$180:100 = \frac{180}{100} = \frac{9}{5}$$

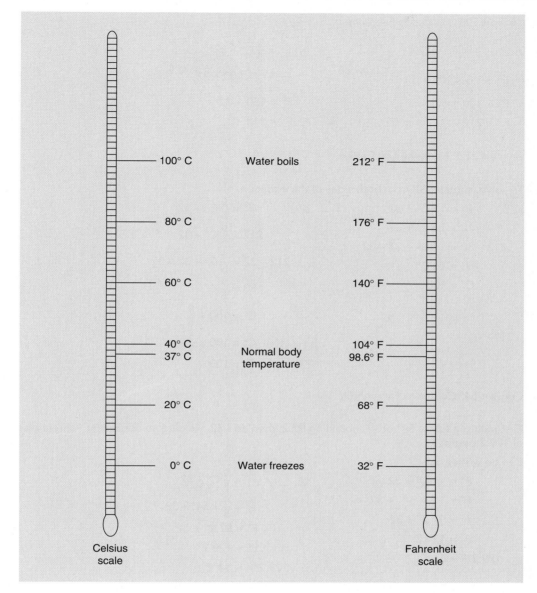

Figure 9-1   Celsius and Fahrenheit temperature scales and the relationship of significant temperatures

If the fraction $\frac{9}{5}$ is expressed as a decimal, it can be stated that each Celsius degree is 1.8 times greater than each Fahrenheit degree.

CONVERTING BETWEEN FAHRENHEIT AND CELSIUS TEMPERATURE SCALES

It may be necessary to convert a given temperature from one scale to the other, and two formulas are available to accomplish this. Either formula may be used, depending on whether you prefer to work with a decimal or a fraction. The formulas are:

a) $F° = 1.8C° + 32$ b) $F° = \frac{9}{5}C° + 32$

Example: Convert 100° Celsius to Fahrenheit:

Solution: a) $F° = 1.8C° + 32$

                 $F° = 1.8 \times 100 + 32$

                 $F° = 180 + 32$

                 $F° = 212$

b) $F° = \frac{9}{5}C° + 32$

     $F° = \frac{9}{5} \times 100 + 32$

     $F° = 180 + 32$

     $F° = 212$

Example: Convert 212° Fahrenheit to Celsius:

Solution: To solve, subtract 32 from both sides of the equation.

a) $F° = 1.8C° + 32$

           $212 = 1.8C° + 32$

      $212 - 32 = 1.8C° + 32 - 32$

             $180 = 1.8C°$

               $C° = 100$

b) $F° = \frac{9}{5}C° + 32$

        $212 = \frac{9}{5}C° + 32$

   $212 - 32 = \frac{9}{5}C° + 32 - 32$

         $180 = \frac{9}{5}C°$

          $C° = 180 \div \frac{9}{5}$

          $C° = 180 \times \frac{5}{9}$

          $C° = 100$

Example: Convert 54° Celsius to Fahrenheit:

Solution: First multiply 1.8 by 54° or $\frac{9}{5}$, obtaining 97.2; then add 32, yielding an equivalent Fahrenheit temperature of 129.2 degrees.

Can be written as:

a) $F° = 1.8C° + 32$

          $F° = 1.8 \times 54° + 32$

          $F° = 97.2° + 32$

          $F° = 129.2°$

       $129.2°F = 54°C$

b) $F° = \frac{9}{5}C° + 32$

      $F° = \frac{9}{5} \times 54° + 32$

      $F° = 97.2° + 32$

      $F° = 129.2°$

   $129.2°F = 54°C$

Example: Convert 100° Fahrenheit to Celsius:

Solution: First subtract 32 from 100°F to obtain 68, and 32 from the other side of the equation, leaving $\frac{9}{5}C°$ (1.8C°) to stand alone.

The equation now reads $68 = \frac{9}{5}C°$ (or 1.8C°).

By dividing both sides of the equation by $\frac{9}{5}$ (or 1.8),

we can determine that the equivalent Celsius temperature is 37.77 or, rounded to one decimal, 37.8 degrees.

Can be written as:

a) $F° = 1.8C° + 32$

         $100° = 1.8C° + 32$

     $100° - 32 = 1.8C° + 32 - 32$

           $68 = 1.8C°$

          $37.8° = C°$

       $100°F = 37.8°C$

b) $F° = \frac{9}{5}C° + 32$

      $100° = \frac{9}{5}C° + 32$

   $100° - 32 = \frac{9}{5}C° + 32 - 32$

       $68° = \frac{9}{5}C°$

      $37.8° = C°$

    $100°F = 37.8°C$

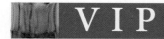

VIP

A way to remember the relationship between Celsius and Fahrenheit scales is to recall that 16°C is approximately 61°F and 28°C is approximately 82°F.

Some common Celsius and Fahrenheit body temperature equivalents are as follows:

Celsius	Fahrenheit
35°	95°
36°	96.8°
37°	98.6°
38°	100.4°
39°	102.2°
40°	104°
41°	105.8°

Problem Set 9.1

Convert to the Celsius or Fahrenheit scale.

1. 16°F _____
2. 68°F _____
3. 82°F _____
4. 104°F _____
5. 100.4°F _____

6. 36°C _____
7. 28°C _____
8. 63°C _____
9. 39°C _____
10. 106°C _____

Answers   **1.** –8.9°C **2.** 20°C **3.** 27.8°C **4.** 40°C **5.** 38°C **6.** 96.8°F **7.** 82.4°F **8.** 145.4°F **9.** 102.2°F **10.** 222.8°F

VIP

To convert temperature from one scale to the other, either of two formulas may be used:

$$F = 1.8\,C + 32 \quad \textit{or} \quad F = \frac{9}{5}C + 32$$

When the unknown temperature is Celsius, start by subtracting 32 from both sides of the equation before solving.

Self-Evaluation Test 9.1
Converting Celsius and Fahrenheit Temperatures

Convert to the Celsius or Fahrenheit scale.

1. 4°F   _____
2. 42°F   _____
3. 50°F   _____
4. 70°F   _____
5. 102°F   _____
6. 103°F   _____
7. 98.6°F   _____
8. 18°C   _____

9. 20°C   _____
10. 21°C   _____
11. 32°C   _____
12. 72°C   _____
13. 96°C   _____
14. 37.5°C   _____
15. 39.6°C   _____

Answers   **1.** −15.6°C   **2.** 5.6°C   **3.** 10°C   **4.** 21.1°C   **5.** 38.9°C   **6.** 39.4°C   **7.** 37°C   **8.** 64.4°F   **9.** 68°F   **10.** 69.8°F   **11.** 89.6°F
12. 161.6°F   **13.** 204.8°F   **14.** 99.5°F   **15.** 103.3°F

If you had fewer than three errors on Self-Evaluation Test 9.1, proceed to the next chapter. If you had four or more errors, review the material on converting temperatures and complete Self-Evaluation Test 9.2 before continuing.

Self-Evaluation Test 9.2
Converting Celsius and Fahrenheit Temperatures

Convert to the Celcius or Fahrenheit scale.

1. 40°F   _____
2. 60°F   _____
3. 81°F   _____
4. 97°F   _____
5. 101°F   _____
6. 99.8°F   _____
7. −12°F   _____
8. 15°C   _____

9. 19°C   _____
10. 29°C   _____
11. 36°C   _____
12. 39°C   _____
13. 64°C   _____
14. 22.2°C   _____
15. 37.6°C   _____

Answers   **1.** 4.4°C   **2.** 15.6°C   **3.** 27.2°C   **4.** 36.1°C   **5.** 38.3°C   **6.** 37.7°C   **7.** −24.4°C   **8.** 59°F   **9.** 66.2°F   **10.** 84.2°F
11. 96.8°F   **12.** 102.2°F   **13.** 147.2°F   **14.** 72°F   **15.** 99.7°F

The Self-Evaluation Tests on converting celsius and fahrenheit temperatures should be repeated until fewer than three errors occur.

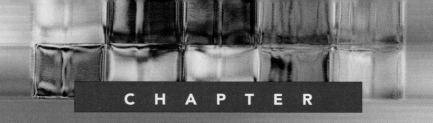

10

The Household System

Learning Outcomes

After successfully completing this chapter, the learner should be able to:

■ *Recognize the units of measure in the household system of measurement.*

■ *Convert units of measure to equivalent units of measure within the household system of measurement.*

■ *Use the proper form and abbreviations to write the amounts and the names of the various units of measure.*

GENERAL INFORMATION

The household system is rather inaccurate. It is perfectly safe to use in cooking, but should be avoided when administering medications, especially in health care settings. If it is necessary to use a household measure for medications, it should be used only until some other, more accurate instrument of measure is available. The household system is still the most commonly used system of measurement in the home.

The smallest unit of measure in the household system is the drop, and there are 75 drops in 1 teaspoon. There are 3 teaspoons in 1 tablespoon.

There are 2 tablespoons to 1 ounce, 6 ounces to an average teacup, and 8 ounces to an average cup or glass. Because spoons, cups, and glasses come in all sizes and shapes, you can understand why this system is considered totally inaccurate.

In writing, the following abbreviations are used: gtt for drop, small letter t or tsp for teaspoon, capital letter T or Tbs for tablespoon, and oz for ounce. The tsp and Tbs are the preferred abbreviations, because they avoid the possibility of error.

In writing, the amount given always precedes the unit name regardless of whether the full unit name or an abbreviation is used. The amount to be given is always written in Arabic numerals. Fractions are written as fractions and always precede the unit name.

Example: Three and one-half teaspoons = $3\frac{1}{2}$ teaspoons = $3\frac{1}{2}$ tsp

Five tablespoons = 5 tablespoons = 5 Tbs

Thirty-five drops = 35 drops = 35 gtts

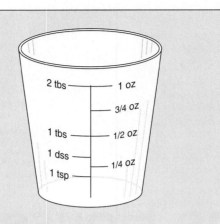

Equivalents in the Household System

75 drops = 1 teaspoon

3 teaspoons = 1 tablespoon

2 tablespoons = 1 ounce

6 ounces = 1 teacup

8 ounces = 1 average cup or glass

16 ounces = 1 pound

Problem Set 10.1

Convert the following:

1. 10 ounces _____ Tbs   4. 24 ounces _____ pounds

2. 45 drops _____ tsp   5. 1 tsp _____ gtt

3. 4 Tbs _____ tsp

Answers   1. 20 Tbs 2. $\frac{3}{5}$ tsp 3. 12 tsp 4. $1\frac{1}{2}$ pounds 5. 75 gtt

■ When household utensils are used, all of these measures are extremely variable and depend on the size of the drop, the size of the teaspoon, and the size of the tablespoon.

Self-Evaluation Test 10.1
The Household System

Convert the following to the equivalent unit indicated. (Make certain the answers to all the conversions are in the correct form.)

1. 75 drops _____ tsp   6. 8 tsp _____ oz

2. 8 tsp _____ Tbs   7. 4 cups _____ oz

3. 24 oz _____ cups   8. 8 Tbs _____ oz

4. 24 oz _____ teacups   9. $\frac{1}{2}$ tsp _____ gtt

5. 3 Tbs _____ oz   10. 4 Tbs _____ tsp

Answers   1. 1 tsp 2. $2\frac{2}{3}$ Tbs 3. 3 cups 4. 4 teacups 5. $1\frac{1}{2}$ oz 6. $1\frac{1}{3}$ oz 7. 32 oz 8. 4 oz 9. $37\frac{1}{2}$ gtt 10. 12 tsp

If you had fewer than two errors on Self-Evaluation Test 10.1, proceed to the next chapter. If you had three or more errors, review the material on the household system and complete Self-Evaluation Test 10.2 before continuing.

Self-Evaluation Test 10.2
The Household System

Convert the following to the equivalent unit indicated. (Make certain the answers to all the conversions are in the correct form.)

1. 2 pounds _____ oz
2. 8 teacups _____ oz
3. 48 oz _____ lb
4. 32 oz _____ cups
5. 10 oz _____ Tbs

6. 45 drops _____ tsp
7. 2 tsp _____ gtt
8. 16 oz _____ glasses
9. 3 cups _____ oz
10. 3 oz _____ Tbs

Answers   **1.** 32 oz   **2.** 48 oz   **3.** 3 lbs   **4.** 4 cups   **5.** 20 Tbs   **6.** $\frac{3}{5}$ tsp   **7.** 150 gtt   **8.** 2 glasses   **9.** 24 oz   **10.** 6 Tbs

The Self-Evaluation Tests on the household system should be repeated until fewer than two errors occur.

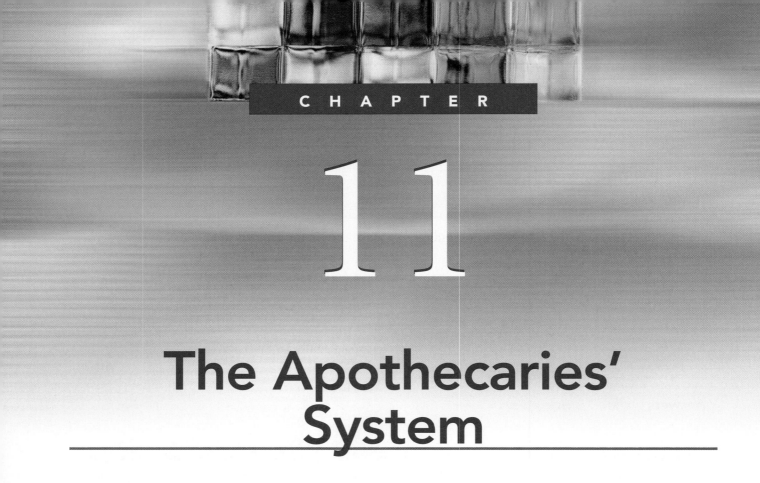

11

The Apothecaries' System

Learning Outcomes

After successfully completing this chapter, the learner should be able to:

- *Recognize the units of measure in the apothecaries' system of measurement.*
- *Convert units of measure to equivalent units of measure within the apothecaries' system of measurement.*
- *Use the proper form and abbreviations to write the amounts and the names for the various units of measure.*

GENERAL INFORMATION

The basic unit for measuring volume (liquid) in the apothecaries' system is the minim. The basic unit for measuring weight is the grain. The two basic units in the apothecaries' system are the minim and the grain.

Inasmuch as 1 minim is about the size of a drop of water, and a drop of water weighs about 1 grain, the liquid and weight units are approximately equal. Therefore, 1 minim equals 1 grain. It should be noted that although 1 minim is the size of a drop of water, drops may not be substituted for minims, because there is no way to accurately control their size.

The next larger unit in both the volume (liquid) and weight table is the dram. The word *fluid* is used with the dram to designate liquid measure, because the identical term is used in both the liquid and weight tables. There are 60 minims in 1 fluid dram, and there are 60 grains in 1 dram. It should be noted that although a dram is the approximate size of a teaspoon, teaspoons may not be substituted for drams, because the size of teaspoons may vary.

Changing minims to fluid drams or grains to drams:

Example: How many grains are there in 3 drams?

Solution: Using the equivalent 60 grains = 1 dram, multiply the 3 drams by 60.

Therefore, there are 180 grains in 3 drams.

The ounce is the next larger unit in both the volume (liquid) and weight tables. The word *fluid* is also used with the ounce to designate liquid measure, because the identical term is used in both the liquid and weight tables. Now we know 60 minims equals 1 fluid dram and 60 grains equals 1 dram, so we can move on to the next unit: 8 fluid drams equals 1 fluid ounce, and 8 drams equals 1 ounce.

Changing fluid ounces to fluid drams, and ounces to drams:

Example: How many fluid ounces are there in 32 fluid drams?

Solution: Using the equivalent 8 fluid drams = 1 fluid ounce, divide the 32 fluid drams by 8. Therefore, 32 fluid drams equals 4 fluid ounces.

To complete the volume (liquid) table, 16 fluid ounces equals 1 pint, 2 pints equals 1 quart, and 4 quarts equals 1 gallon.

A way to remember the symbols for drams and ounces is to recall that ounces are the larger unit and therefore have the larger symbol. To review, ɱ or M is the abbreviation for minim, ℥ is the symbol for ounce, ʒ is the symbol for dram, and pt or O is the abbreviation for pint.

In addition, remember when converting from a smaller unit or measure to a larger unit, divide. When converting from a larger unit to a smaller unit, multiply.

In writing, if an abbreviation or symbol is used, the amount to be given follows the unit abbreviation and is written in lowercase Roman numerals. If the full unit name is used, the amount to be given is written in Arabic numerals and precedes the unit name. Fractions are written as fractions and either follow or precede the unit name, depending on whether an abbreviation or symbol is used. The only deviation from this rule is with the fraction $\frac{1}{2}$. The symbol s̄s̄ is used to represent the fraction $\frac{1}{2}$ and follows the unit name when an abbreviation is used. For example, gr iii is 3 grains, ʒ v is 5 drams, and gr $\frac{1}{4}$ is $\frac{1}{4}$ grain. O viis̄s̄ is $7\frac{1}{2}$ pints, and ℥ ix or oz ix is 9 ounces.

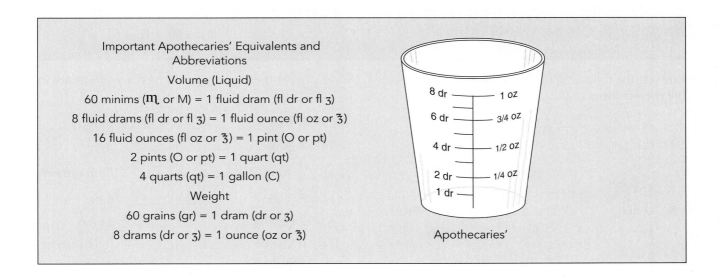

Important Apothecaries' Equivalents and Abbreviations

Volume (Liquid)

60 minims (ɱ or M) = 1 fluid dram (fl dr or fl ʒ)

8 fluid drams (fl dr or fl ʒ) = 1 fluid ounce (fl oz or ℥)

16 fluid ounces (fl oz or ℥) = 1 pint (O or pt)

2 pints (O or pt) = 1 quart (qt)

4 quarts (qt) = 1 gallon (C)

Weight

60 grains (gr) = 1 dram (dr or ʒ)

8 drams (dr or ʒ) = 1 ounce (oz or ℥)

8 dr — 1 oz
6 dr — 3/4 oz
4 dr — 1/2 oz
2 dr — 1/4 oz
1 dr —

Apothecaries'

Problem Set 11.1

Write the following amounts correctly:

1. 10 ʒ _____
2. $\frac{1}{2}$ gr _____
3. grains 3 _____

4. minim 60 _____
5. dram $7\frac{1}{2}$ _____

Convert:

6. ʒ 8 _____ drams
7. ʒ xxiv _____ ounces
8. fl ʒ x _____ minims
9. gr xxx _____ dram
10. 5 pints _____ fluid ounces

11. 8 pints _____ quarts
12. fl ʒ xxiv _____ pints
13. fl ʒ iss̄ _____ minims
14. 32 quarts _____ gallons
15. 300 grains _____ drams

Answers 1. 10 ounces or ʒ x 2. $\frac{1}{2}$ grain or gr ss̄ 3. 3 grains or gr iii 4. 60 minims or ♏ 60 5. $7\frac{1}{2}$ drams or ʒ viiss̄

6. 64 drams 7. 3 ounces 8. 600 minims 9. $\frac{1}{2}$ dram 10. 80 fluid ounces 11. 4 quarts 12. $1\frac{1}{2}$ pints 13. 90 minims 14. 8 gallons

15. 5 drams

V I P

In the apothecaries' system:

- Use the equivalent chart.
- When moving from a larger unit to a smaller unit, multiply by the equivalent value of the smaller unit.
- When moving from a smaller unit to a larger unit, divide by the equivalent value of the larger unit.

Self-Evaluation Test 11.1
The Apothecaries' System

Convert the following to the equivalent unit indicated. (Make certain the answers to all the conversions are in the correct form.)

1. ʒ x _____ drams
2. C v _____ quarts
3. ʒ x _____ grains
4. ʒ vi _____ ounce
5. O iii _____ fluid ounces
6. ʒ ss̄ _____ grains
7. ʒ iss̄ _____ grains
8. ʒ viii _____ grains

9. fl ʒ ii _____ minims
10. fl ʒ iv _____ fluid drams
11. $\frac{1}{2}$ pint _____ fluid ounces
12. fl ʒ xxiv _____ pints
13. 2 quarts _____ gallon
14. fl ʒ xxxii _____ fluid ounces
15. 120 grains _____ drams

If you had fewer than three errors on Self-Evaluation Test 11.1, move on to the next chapter. If you had four or more errors, review the material on the apothecaries' system and complete Self-Evaluation Test 11.2 before continuing.

Self-Evaluation Test 11.2
The Apothecaries' System

Convert the following to the equivalent unit indicated. (Make certain the answers to all the conversions are in the correct form.)

1. O v _____ fluid ounces

2. C vi _____ pints

3. oz v _____ drams

4. qt iii _____ fluid ounces

5. ʒ xx _____ ounces

6. qt xx _____ pints

7. O viii _____ quarts

8. ℳ xxx _____ fluid drams

9. O xxxii _____ quarts

10. fl ʒ xvi _____ fluid ounces

11. fl ʒ xxv _____ fluid drams

12. fl ʒ xxiv _____ fluid ounces

13. $\frac{3}{4}$ dram _____ grains

14. 5 gallons _____ quarts

15. 4 ounces _____ drams

The Self-Evaluation Tests on the apothecaries' system should be repeated until fewer than three errors occur.

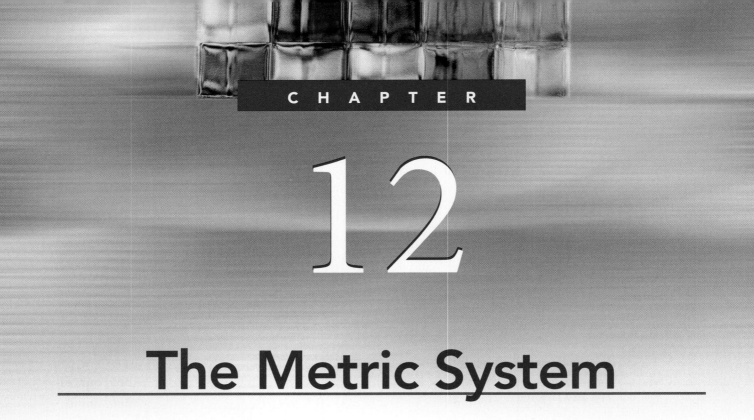

12

The Metric System

Learning Outcomes

After successfully completing this chapter, the learner should be able to:

- *Recognize the units of measure in the metric system of measurement.*
- *Convert units of measure to equivalent units of measure within the metric system of measurement.*
- *Use the proper form and abbreviations to write the amounts and the names for the various units of measure.*

GENERAL INFORMATION

Two systems of measurement have been used in the preparation and administration of medications: the apothecaries' system and the metric system. With the health care system in the United States moving toward the use of the international metric system, the use of the apothecaries' system in the prescription of medications has greatly diminished.

In the metric system, the basic unit for measuring volume (liquid) is the liter, the basic unit for measuring weight is the gram, and the basic unit for measuring length is the meter. The three basic units in the metric system are the liter, the gram, and the meter.

The metric system is a decimal system that is based on multiples or powers of the number 10. In the metric system, Latin prefixes are used to denote which multiples or powers of the basic unit are being considered. For example, the prefix *kilo* means 1000 times the basic unit. Therefore, a kilogram contains 1000 grams and a kiloliter contains 1000 liters. The prefix *milli* means 0.001 times the basic unit. Therefore, a milligram is 0.001 (one thousandth) of a gram and a milliliter is 0.001 (one thousandth) of a liter.

The prefixes used with the basic units in the metric system and their meanings are:

kilo = one thousand times   (1000)

hecto = one hundred times   (100)

deka = ten times   (10)

Basic unit = liter, gram, meter   (whole units)

deci = one tenth   (0.1)

centi = one hundredth   (0.01)

milli = one thousandth   (0.001)

micro = one millionth   (0.000001)

A mnemonic that may help in improving recall of these prefixes is:

kilo	hecto	deka	basic	deci	centi	milli	micro
K	H	D	B	D	C	M	M
King	Henry	Dates	Beth's	Darling	Cousin	Mary	May

VIP

To reduce the size of the decimal and to minimize errors, the *micro* prefix is the most commonly used with milliunits (milliliter, milligram, or millimeter), where it represents one thousandth of the milliunit, rather than with the basic unit (liter, gram, or meter) where it represents one millionth of the basic unit.

In the metric system, the following rules apply when changing a basic unit to a smaller or larger unit or when changing a smaller or larger unit to a basic unit:

■ To change a basic unit (liter, gram, or meter) to a smaller unit (deci-, centi-, or milli-), multiply by 10, 100, or 1000. For example: 1 gram = 1000 milligrams

■ To change a basic unit (liter, gram, or meter) to a larger unit (deka-, hecto-, or kilo-), divide by 10, 100, or 1000. For example: 1 gram = 0.001 kilograms

■ To change a smaller unit (deci-, centi-, or milli-) to a basic unit (liter, gram, or meter), divide by 10, 100, or 1000. For example: 1 milligram = 0.001 gram

■ To change a larger unit (deka-, hecto-, or kilo-) to a basic unit (liter, gram, or meter), multiply by 10, 100, or 1000. For example: 1 kilogram = 1000 grams

In the metric system, the terms most commonly used in the health care field are the gram, liter, microgram, milligram, milliliter, millimeter, centimeter, and kilogram.

Because 1 milliliter of water weighs about 1 gram, the liquid and the weight units are approximately equal. Therefore, 1000 milliliters of water weighs about 1000 grams. The term *cubic centimeter* is sometimes encountered. A cubic centimeter is the amount of space occupied by a milliliter of water and is therefore considered the equivalent of 1 milliliter. See Figure 12-1 for an illustration of these relationships.

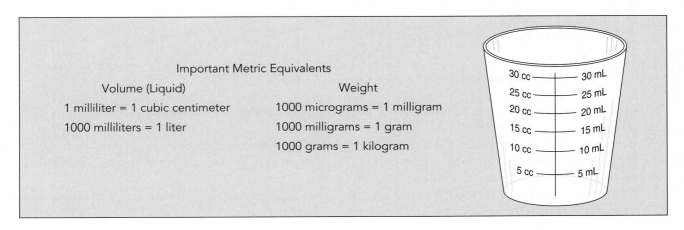

Important Metric Equivalents

Volume (Liquid)	Weight
1 milliliter = 1 cubic centimeter	1000 micrograms = 1 milligram
1000 milliliters = 1 liter	1000 milligrams = 1 gram
	1000 grams = 1 kilogram

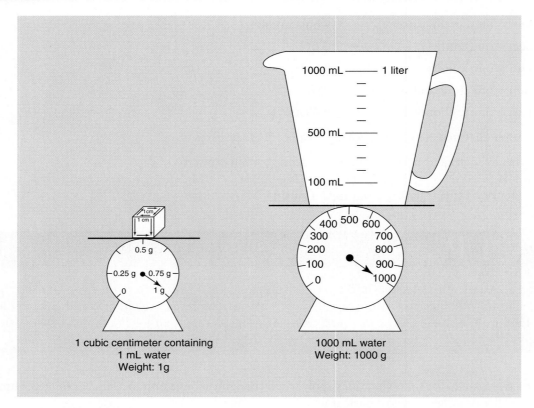

Figure 12-1   The relationship between metric units of weight and volume

Changing grams to milligrams (there are 1000 milligrams in 1 gram):

Example: How many milligrams are there in 0.25 grams?

Solution: Multiply 0.25 grams by 1000 to determine that there are 250 milligrams in 0.25 grams.

The rule for converting between decimals and percents can be expanded to include multiplying and dividing by 10, 100, or 1000 by moving the decimal point to the left or right for the same number of places as there are zeros.

The multiplication by 1000 can be accomplished by simply moving the decimal point three places to the right, so .025 grams equals 250 milligrams.

To change grams to milligrams and liters to milliliters, move the decimal point three places to the right, because the basic unit is multiplied by 1000.

Changing milliliters to liters (there are 1000 milliliters in 1 liter):

Example: How many liters are there in 750 milliliters?

Solution: Divide 750 milliliters by 1000. The division by 1000 can be accomplished by simply moving the decimal point three places to the left, so 0.75 liters equals 750 milliliters.

To change milliliters to liters and milligrams to grams, move the decimal point three places to the left, because the basic unit is divided by 1000.

In writing in the metric system, the amount to be given always precedes the unit of measure, regardless of whether the full unit name or an abbreviation is used. The amount to be given is always written as a whole number or a decimal. Fractions should never be used in the metric system.

The abbreviations L for liter and g for gram are used (gm is an obsolete abbreviation). Those terms that represent more or less than the basic unit are abbreviated by using the first letter of the prefix and the first letter of the basic unit, writing them in small letters without a period. An exception to this rule is the abbreviation for microgram. Because the letters mg stand for milligram, microgram is abbreviated as μg or mcg.)

The abbreviation for kilograms is kg, the abbreviation for milligrams is mg, and the abbreviation for milliliter is ml. The abbreviation mL is increasingly being used for milliliter and is the abbreviation used in this book. Although used infrequently, the abbreviation for cubic centimeter is cc. Thus, 10 mL is 10 milliliters, 5 kg is 5 kilograms, 8 mL is 8 milliliters, four and one-fourth grams is written as 4.25 g, and three-fourths milliliter is written as 0.75 mL.

Problem Set 12.1

Write the following amounts correctly:

1. $7\frac{1}{2}$ mgm   _____

2. mcg 0.25   _____

3. g VIISS   _____

4. Gm 42   _____

5. $\frac{1}{5}$ mL   _____

Convert:

6. 5 g   _____ mg

7. 2 mcg   _____ mg

8. 0.25 g   _____ mg

9. 0.3 mg   _____ mcg

10. 11.25 L   _____ mL

11. 2.75 kg   _____ g

12. 325 mL   _____ L

13. 350 mg   _____ g

14. 5250 g   _____ kg

15. 2500 mg   _____ g

Answers   **1.** 7.5 mg   **2.** 0.25 mcg   **3.** 7.5 g   **4.** 42 g   **5.** 0.2 mL   **6.** 5000 mg   **7.** 0.002 mg   **8.** 250 mg   **9.** 300 mcg   **10.** 11,250 mL   **11.** 2750 g   **12.** 0.325 L   **13.** 0.35 g   **14.** 5.25 kg   **15.** 2.5 g

 VIP

In the metric system:

- When changing from a larger unit to a smaller unit, move the decimal point the appropriate number of places to the right.

- When changing from a smaller unit to a larger unit, move the decimal point the appropriate number of places to the left.

Self-Evaluation Test 12.1
The Metric System

Convert the following to the equivalent unit indicated. (Make certain the answers to all the conversions are in the correct form.)

1. 5 L   _____ mL

2. 7 kg   _____ g

3. 15 L   _____ mL

4. 10 mg   _____ g

5. 0.5 g   _____ mg

6. 375 g   _____ kg

7. 0.4 mg   _____ mcg

8. 750 mL   _____ L

9. 250 mL   _____ L

10. 100 mg   _____ g

11.	0.02 kg	_____ g	14.	0.01 mg	_____ mcg
12.	45 mcg	_____ mg	15.	0.125 mg	_____ mcg
13.	0.33 g	_____ mg			

Answers   1. 5000 mL   2. 7000 g   3. 15,000 mL   4. 0.01 g   5. 500 mg   6. 0.375 kg   7. 400 mcg   8. 0.75 L   9. 0.25 L   10. 0.1 g
11. 20 g   12. 0.045 mg   13. 330 mg   14. 10 mcg   15. 125 mcg

If you had fewer than three errors on Self-Evaluation Test 12.1, proceed to the next chapter. If you had four or more errors, review the material on the metric system and complete Self-Evaluation Test 12.2 before continuing.

Self-Evaluation Test 12.2
The Metric System

Convert the following to the equivalent unit indicated. (Make certain the answers to all the conversions are in the correct form.)

1.	0.5 L	_____ mL	9.	60 mcg	_____ mg
2.	200 g	_____ kg	10.	750 mg	_____ g
3.	0.25 g	_____ mg	11.	0.025 L	_____ mL
4.	90 mg	_____ g	12.	0.325 g	_____ mg
5.	9.5 kg	_____ g	13.	0.02 mg	_____ mcg
6.	100 μg	_____ mg	14.	0.006 kg	_____ g
7.	850 mL	_____ L	15.	0.75 mg	_____ mcg
8.	650 mL	_____ L			

Answers   1. 500 mL   2. 0.2 kg   3. 250 mg   4. 0.09 g   5. 9500 g   6. 0.1 mg   7. 0.85 L   8. 0.65 L   9. 0.06 mg   10. 0.75 g
11. 25 mL   12. 325 mg   13. 20 mcg   14. 6 g   15. 750 mcg

The Self-Evaluation Tests on the metric system should be repeated until fewer than three errors occur.

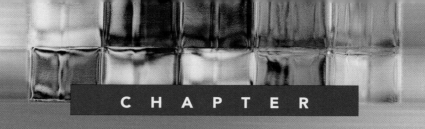

13

Determining Equivalents and Converting Between the Systems of Measurement

Learning Outcomes

After successfully completing this chapter, the learner should be able to:

- *Recognize the equivalents for basic units of measure among the various systems of measurement.*

- *Recognize how to set up and label the terms in a proportion used to convert between systems of measurement.*

- *Use proportions to convert a specific amount in one system of measurement to a specific amount in another system of measurement.*

GENERAL INFORMATION

The nurse may be called on to administer a medication that has been ordered in a unit of measure from the apothecaries' system but is supplied in a unit of measure from the metric system. To administer the drug correctly, the nurse must know how to convert the metric measure into the apothecaries' measure.

Whenever we convert from one system of measurement to another, we are dealing with approximate equivalents rather than with exact equivalents. When we convert a unit of measure in the apothecaries' system into a unit of measure in the metric system, the result is an approximate equivalent. **In computing dosage, the approximate equivalent must never differ by more than 10% from the prescribed dosage.**

The conversion between systems of measurement can best be computed by establishing a numerical relationship between the systems. This can be accomplished by setting up a proportion (using either the ratio or fraction form) or by using some type of conversion factor formula.

V I P

In proportions:

The terms on both sides of the equal sign must be set up in the same order. Either term may be the numerator or denominator as long as they are set up in the same order on both sides of the equal sign. For example:

(ratio form)   apothecaries : metric = apothecaries : metric

(fraction form) $\dfrac{\text{apothecaries}}{\text{metric}} = \dfrac{\text{apothecaries}}{\text{metric}}$

or use

(ratio form)   metric : apothecaries = metric : apothecaries

(fraction form) $\dfrac{\text{metric}}{\text{apothecaries}} = \dfrac{\text{metric}}{\text{apothecaries}}$

ALL TERMS IN A PROPORTION MUST BE LABELED TO AVOID ERRORS.

In setting up the proportion, one side uses a specific unit of measure from one system and its approximate equivalent from the other system. The other side of the proportion is set up by using the known quantity being converted and the unknown quantity (x). To know what the x is equal to when finished, make certain all terms in the proportion are labeled. For example:

$$\frac{\text{Specific unit of measure from one system}}{\substack{\text{Approximate equivalent unit of measure} \\ \text{from the other system}}} = \frac{\substack{\text{Known quantity being converted} \\ \text{from one system}}}{\substack{\text{Unknown quantity to be determined} \\ \text{from the other system (x)}}}$$

Calculation Alert

For consistency, the proportion method using the fraction form is used for moving between the systems of measurement and for computing proper dosage within the same system throughout the remainder of this book.

CONVERTING BETWEEN THE MEASURES OF WEIGHT IN THE METRIC AND APOTHECARIES' SYSTEMS

Fifteen grains of a substance weighs a little less than 1 gram, and 16 grains weighs a little more; therefore, either 15 or 16 grains may be used as the approximate equivalent of 1 gram. The choice of 15 or 16 grains as the equivalent is determined by trying both figures and using the one that divides evenly or with the most easily measurable fraction remaining. For example, to convert 30 grains to grams, use 15 grains equals 1 gram as the equivalent, because 30 can be divided evenly by 15. To convert 64 grains to grams, use 16 grains equals 1 gram as the equivalent, because 64 can be divided evenly by 16. To convert 2.5 grams to grains, use 16 grains equals 1 gram as the equivalent, thus avoiding a fraction in the answer.

In summary, either 15 or 16 grains can be used as the equivalent of 1 gram, because there is no hard-and-fast rule governing the use of either number. Either number will produce an answer within the 10% difference permitted in conversion.

When setting up the proportion to convert between systems, use a specific unit from one system and its approximate equivalent from the other system as one side of the proportion. The other side of the proportion is set up by using the known quantity you are converting and the unknown quantity (x) from the other system.

Example: Convert 45 grains to grams.

Solution: Use as the known side of the proportion the equivalent for grains to grams (15 or 16 grains/1 gram).

$$\frac{15 \text{ grains}}{1 \text{ gram}} = \frac{45 \text{ grains}}{x \text{ grams}}$$
$$15x = 45$$
$$x = 3 \text{ grains} \qquad \text{Therefore, 45 grains = 3 grams}$$

Example: Convert 60 grains to grams.

Use as the known side of the proportion the approximate equivalents for grains and grams. Because 60 can be divided evenly by 15, use 15 grains = 1 gram.

Solution:
$$\frac{15 \text{ grains}}{1 \text{ gram}} = \frac{60 \text{ grains}}{x \text{ grams}}$$
$$15x = 60$$
$$x = 4 \text{ grams} \qquad \text{Therefore, 60 grains = 4 grams}$$

Example: Convert 96 grains to grams.

Solution:
$$\frac{16 \text{ grains}}{1 \text{ gram}} = \frac{96 \text{ grains}}{x \text{ grams}}$$
$$16x = 96$$
$$x = 6 \text{ grams} \qquad \text{Therefore, 96 grains = 6 grams}$$

To convert milligrams to grains or grains to milligrams, change the milligrams to grams and follow the procedure for changing grams to grains. The conversion can also be accomplished by changing the grains to grams and then changing the grams to milligrams.

Example: Convert 500 milligrams to grains.

Solution: First, convert 500 milligrams to grams by moving the decimal point three places to the left. (Remember, to change a milligram to a gram, divide by 1000.)

500 milligrams = 0.5 grams

Then convert the grams to grains using the proportion:
$$\frac{\text{grains}}{\text{grams}} = \frac{\text{grains}}{\text{grams}}$$
$$\frac{15 \text{ grains}}{1 \text{ gram}} = \frac{x \text{ grains}}{0.5 \text{ grams}}$$
$$x = 7\frac{1}{2} \text{ grains} \qquad \text{Therefore, 500 milligrams} = 7\frac{1}{2} \text{ grains}$$

Example: Convert 30 grains to milligrams.

Solution: First, convert the grains to grams using the proportion:

$$\frac{15 \text{ grains}}{1 \text{ gram}} = \frac{30 \text{ grains}}{x \text{ grams}}$$
$$x = 2 \text{ grams}$$

Then convert the grams to milligrams by moving the decimal point three places to the right. (Remember, to change a gram to a milligram, multiply by 1000.)

2 grams = 2000 milligrams Therefore, 30 grains equals 2000 milligrams

Another method for converting milligrams to grams or grains to milligrams, which is sometimes easier, is to convert the milligrams directly to grains or grains directly to milligrams by using the approximate equivalent 60 to 65 milligrams = 1 grain. These numbers will produce an answer within the 10% difference permitted in conversion.

Example: Convert 5 grains to milligrams.

Use the approximate equivalents for grains and milligrams.

Solution: $\dfrac{1 \text{ grain}}{60 \text{ milligrams}} = \dfrac{5 \text{ grains}}{x \text{ milligrams}}$

$x = 300$ milligrams   Therefore, 5 grains equals 300 milligrams

(If the equivalent 1 grain equals 65 milligrams had been used, the answer would have been 5 grains = 325 milligrams. This answer would be less than 10% of the difference permitted in conversion.)

Example: Convert 600 milligrams to grains.

Solution: $\dfrac{60 \text{ mg}}{1 \text{ gr}} = \dfrac{600 \text{ mg}}{x \text{ gr}}$

$60x = 600$

$x = 10$ grains   Therefore, 600 milligrams equals 10 grains

Calculation Alert

In computation, the household-system pound (which is the avoirdupois pound) is used to convert pounds to kilograms:

1 kilogram = 2.2 pounds

Example: Convert 78 pounds to kilograms.

Solution: $\dfrac{2.2 \text{ lb}}{1 \text{ kg}} = \dfrac{78 \text{ lb}}{x \text{ kg}}$

$2.2x = 78$

$x = 35.45$ kg   Therefore, 78 pounds equals 35.45 kilograms

If you need to convert from one system to another and are unsure of equivalent values, always check a standard table of approximate equivalents before proceeding. Always begin by determining the approximate equivalent of one of the units to be converted.

Problem Set 13.1

Convert to the apothecaries' or metric system. Answers may vary depending upon the number used for conversion, but must be within the 10% difference permitted.

1. 70 kg _____ pounds

2. gr $\dfrac{3}{4}$ _____ milligrams

3. 400 μg _____ grains

4. 750 mg _____ grains

5. 0.325 g _____ grains

6. gr $\dfrac{1}{100}$ _____ milligrams

7. 2500 mg _____ grains

8. 20 drams _____ grams

9. 32 pounds _____ kilograms

10. 480 grams _____ ounces

Answers   **1.** 154 pounds   **2.** 45 or 50 mg   **3.** $\frac{1}{150}$ grain   **4.** 12 grains   **5.** 5 grains   **6.** 0.6 mg   **7.** 40 grains   **8.** 80 grams   **9.** 14.5 kilograms   **10.** 16 ounces

VIP

Important equivalents to memorize:

1 grain = 60 milligrams	15 or 16 grains = 1 gram
1 dram = 4 grams	1 ounce = 30 or 32 grams
	2.2 pounds = 1 kilogram

To help remember the fact that 1 grain is equivalent to 60 milligrams, think of the fact that 1 hour is equivalent to 60 minutes. It should then be easy to recall that:

15 minutes = $\frac{1}{4}$ hour : 15 milligrams = $\frac{1}{4}$ grain

30 minutes = $\frac{1}{2}$ hour : 30 milligrams = $\frac{1}{2}$ grain

45 minutes = $\frac{3}{4}$ hour : 45 milligrams = $\frac{3}{4}$ grain

60 minutes = 1 hour : 60 milligrams = 1 grain

Self-Evaluation Test 13.1
Review of Conversions Between the Measures of Weight in the Apothecaries' and Metric Systems

Convert the following to the equivalent. (Make certain the answers to all the conversions are within the 10% difference permitted)

1. gr x _____ grams
2. oz v _____ grams
3. 0.5 g _____ grains
4. 250 g _____ ounces
5. 240 g _____ drams
6. 640 g _____ ounces
7. 0.6 mg _____ grains
8. 100 μg _____ grains
9. 180 mg _____ grains
10. gr $\frac{1}{200}$ _____ micrograms
11. $\frac{1}{6}$ grain _____ milligrams
12. 10 grams _____ grains
13. 8 pounds _____ kilograms
14. 60 grains _____ milligrams
15. $\frac{1}{150}$ grain _____ micrograms

Answers   **1.** 0.6 grams   **2.** 150 or 160 grams   **3.** $7\frac{1}{2}$ grains   **4.** 8 ounces   **5.** 60 drams   **6.** 20 ounces   **7.** $\frac{1}{100}$ grain   **8.** $\frac{1}{600}$ grain   **9.** 3 grains   **10.** 300 micrograms   **11.** 10 milligrams   **12.** 150 or 160 grains   **13.** 3.6 kilograms   **14.** 3600 milligrams   **15.** 400 micrograms

If you had fewer than three errors on Self-Evaluation Test 13.1, move on to the next section. If you had four or more errors, review the material on converting between the measures of weight in the metric and apothecaries' systems and complete Self-Evaluation Test 13.2 before continuing.

Self-Evaluation Test 13.2
Review of Conversions Between the Measures of Weight in the Apothecaries' and Metric Systems

Convert the following to the equivalent unit indicated. (Make certain the answers to all the conversions are within the 10% difference permitted.)

1. oz x _____ grams
2. 25 g _____ grains
3. 16 oz _____ grams
4. 25 oz _____ grams
5. gr $\frac{3}{4}$ _____ milligrams
6. 10 lb _____ kilograms
7. gr $\frac{1}{8}$ _____ milligrams

8. 0.2 mg _____ grains
9. 600 μg _____ grain
10. 0.4 mg _____ grain
11. 4 drams _____ grams
12. 8 grains _____ gram
13. 25 grains _____ milligrams
14. 100 drams _____ grams
15. $\frac{1}{300}$ grain _____ micrograms

Answers   1. 300 or 320 grams   2. 375 or 400 grains   3. 480 grams   4. 750 grams   5. 45 or 50 milligrams   6. 4.5 kilograms
7. 8 milligrams   8. $\frac{1}{300}$ grain   9. $\frac{1}{100}$ grain   10. $\frac{1}{150}$ grain   11. 16 grams   12. 0.5 gram   13. 1500 milligrams   14. 400 grams
15. 200 micrograms

The Self-Evaluation Tests on the review of conversion between the units of weight in the metric and apothecaries' systems should be repeated until fewer than three errors occur. If you continue to make mistakes, try to identify whether your errors are related to problems in the basic mathematical skills or in not knowing the value of the stated units. Review the material on the systems of measurement and repeat the two tests.

CONVERTING BETWEEN THE MEASURES OF VOLUME (LIQUID) IN THE METRIC AND APOTHECARIES' SYSTEMS

In the table of liquid measure in the apothecaries' system, 1 minim of water weighs about 1 grain, so that 1 minim is considered to be equal to 1 grain. In the metric system, 1 cubic centimeter or 1 milliliter of water weighs approximately 1 gram, so that 1 cubic centimeter or 1 milliliter is considered equal to 1 gram. Syringes and other equipment may be calibrated in cc, but dosage is usually ordered in milliliter.

Because 1 milliliter is considered equal to 1 gram and 1 minim is considered equal to 1 grain, and knowing that 1 gram is equal to 15 or 16 grains, by substituting equivalents it can be concluded that 1 milliliter equals 15 or 16 minims.

The same proportions can be used for these conversions by simply substituting the unit names of the liquid measures for the unit names of the weight measures. For example:

$$\frac{\text{Minims}}{\text{Milliliters}} = \frac{\text{Minims}}{\text{Milliliters}}$$

From the apothecaries' table of weights, it is known that 60 grains equals 1 dram, a grain is equal to a minim, 60 minims equals 1 fluid dram, and 15 minims equals 1 milliliter. With this information, it can be determined that 1 dram equals 4 grams and 1 fluid dram equals 4 milliliters.

Problem Set 13.2

Convert to the apothecaries' or metric system. Answers may vary depending upon the number used for conversion, but must be within the 10% difference permitted.

1. 5 mL _____ minims
2. 120 mL _____ fluid ounces
3. 240 mL _____ fluid ounces
4. 400 mL _____ fluid drams
5. 96 fl oz _____ milliliters

6. $\frac{1}{2}$ fl oz _____ milliliters
7. 1000 mL _____ fluid ounces
8. 150 minims _____ milliliters
9. 4 fluid drams _____ milliliters
10. 10 fluid ounces _____ milliliters

Answers   **1.** 75 or 83 minims   **2.** 4 fluid ounces   **3.** 8 fluid ounces   **4.** 100 fluid drams   **5.** 2880 or 3072 milliliters   **6.** 15 milliliters   **7.** 32 fluid ounces   **8.** 9 milliliters   **9.** 16 milliliters   **10.** 300 milliliters

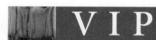

V I P

Important equivalents to memorize:

1 minim = 0.06 milliliters
1 fluid dram = 4 milliliters
16 fluid ounces = 500 mL

15 or 16 minims = 1 milliliter
1 fluid ounce = 30 or 32 milliliters
1 quart = 1000 mL or 1 L

Self-Evaluation Test 13.3
Review of Conversions Between the Measures of Volume in the Apothecaries' and Metric Systems

Convert the following to the equivalent unit indicated. (Make certain the answers to all the conversions are within the 10% difference permitted.)

1. 8 mL _____ minims
2. 15 mL _____ minims
3. 45 mL _____ fluid ounces
4. 2 fl oz _____ milliliters
5. 600 mL _____ fluid ounces
6. 6 quarts _____ milliliters
7. 1000 mL _____ pints
8. 4500 mL _____ quarts

9. 8 minims _____ milliliters
10. 6 minims _____ milliliters
11. 2 fluid drams _____ milliliters
12. 28 fluid drams _____ milliliters
13. 5000 milliliters _____ quarts
14. 48 fluid ounces _____ milliliters
15. 250 fluid ounces _____ liters

Answers   **1.** 120 or 128 minims   **2.** 225 or 240 minims   **3.** $1\frac{1}{2}$ fluid ounces   **4.** 60 or 64 milliliters   **5.** 20 fluid ounces

6. 6000 milliliters   **7.** 2 pints   **8.** $4\frac{1}{2}$ quarts   **9.** 0.5 milliliters   **10.** 0.4 milliliters   **11.** 8 milliliters   **12.** 112 milliliters   **13.** 5 quarts

14. 1440 or 1536 milliliters   **15.** 8 liters

If you had fewer than three errors on Self-Evaluation Test 13.3, move on to the next section. If you had four or more errors, review the material on converting between the measures of volume in the metric and apothecaries' systems and complete Self-Evaluation Test 13.4 before continuing.

Self-Evaluation Test 13.4
Review of Conversions Between the Measures of Volume in the Apothecaries' and Metric Systems

Convert the following to the equivalent unit indicated. (Make certain the answers to all the conversions are within the 10% difference permitted.)

1.	10 mL	_____ minims	9.	2500 mL	_____ quarts
2.	60 mL	_____ fluid drams	10.	45 minims	_____ milliliters
3.	0.2 mL	_____ minims	11.	10 minims	_____ milliliters
4.	fl oz iv	_____ milliliters	12.	12 milliliters	_____ minims
5.	4 pints	_____ milliliters	13.	225 milliliters	_____ fluid ounces
6.	5 liters	_____ fluid ounces	14.	8 fluid drams	_____ milliliters
7.	1 gallon	_____ milliliters	15.	64 fluid ounces	_____ milliliters
8.	fl oz xxx	_____ milliliters			

Answers   1. 150 or 160 minims   2. 15 fluid drams   3. 3 minims   4. 120 or 128 milliliters   5. 2000 milliliters   6. 160 fluid ounces

7. 4000 milliliters   8. 900 or 960 milliliters   9. $2\frac{1}{2}$ quarts   10. 3 milliliters   11. 0.6 or 0.7 milliliters   12. 180 or 192 minims

13. $7\frac{1}{2}$ fluid ounces   14. 32 milliliters   15. 1920 or 2048 milliliters

The Self-Evaluation Tests on the review of conversion between the units of volume in the metric and apothecaries' systems should be repeated until fewer than three errors occur. If you continue to make mistakes, try to identify whether your errors are related to problems in the basic mathematical skills or in not knowing the value of the stated units. Review the material on the systems of measurement and repeat the two tests.

CONVERTING BETWEEN THE METRIC OR APOTHECARIES' SYSTEM OF MEASUREMENT AND THE HOUSEHOLD SYSTEM

The household system should not be used for medications because it is very inaccurate. It is frequently used in the calculation of a patient's fluid intake and output.

1 drop = 1 minim

75 drops = 1 teaspoon

75 minims = 1 teaspoon

15 minims = 1 mL

4 mL = 1 teaspoon

However, the drop is so approximate that a full teaspoon is considered to contain 4 or 5 mL. Inasmuch as 3 or 4 teaspoons equals 1 tablespoon (depending on the size of the spoon), there are 15 or 16 milliliters in 1 tablespoon.

60 or 64 mL = 4 Tbs

2 Tbs = 1 oz

30 or 32 mL = 1 oz

180 mL = 6 oz

240 mL = 8 oz

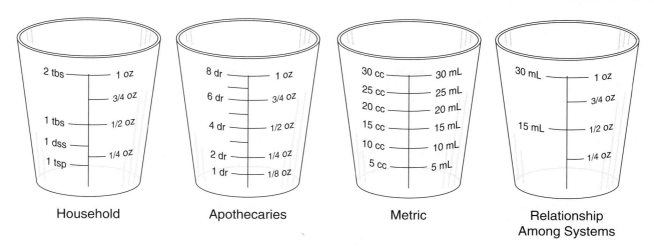

Figure 13-1   Measuring cups reflecting systems of measurement

Self-Evaluation Test 13.5
Review of Metric, Apothecaries', and Household Systems

Convert the following to the equivalent unit indicated. (Make certain the answers to all the conversions are in the correct form.)

1. 5 L   _____ mL
2. 4 tsp   _____ gtt
3. 24 oz   _____ glasses
4. 10 μg   _____ mg
5. gr xxx   _____ dram
6. 0.25 L   _____ mL
7. 1.25 g   _____ mg
8. 1500 g   _____ kg

9. 300 mL   _____ L
10. 750 mg   _____ g
11. 2500 mL   _____ L
12. 48 drams   _____ ounces
13. 0.004 mg   _____ μg
14. 24 ounces   _____ teacups
15. 32 ounces   _____ pints

Answers   **1.** 5000 mL **2.** 300 gtt **3.** 3 glasses **4.** 0.01 mg **5.** $\frac{1}{2}$ dram **6.** 250 mL **7.** 1250 mg **8.** 1.5 kg **9.** 0.3 L **10.** 0.75 g **11.** 2.5 L **12.** 6 ounces **13.** 4 μg **14.** 4 teacups **15.** 2 pints

If you had four or more errors on Self-Evaluation Test 13.5, review the material about the metric, apothecaries', and household systems and complete Self-Evaluation Test 13.6 before continuing.

Self-Evaluation Test 13.6
Review of Metric, Apothecaries', and Household Systems

Convert the following to the equivalent unit indicated. (Make certain the answers to all the conversions are in the correct form.)

1. 4 L   _____ mL
2. 5 μg   _____ mg
3. 7.5 g   _____ mg

4. 6.7 kg   _____ g
5. fl dr s̄s̄   _____ minims
6. 500 mL   _____ L

7. fl dr xvi _____ fl oz

8. 150 mg _____ g

9. 0.325 g _____ mg

10. 0.015 mg _____ μg

11. 3500 mg _____ g

12. $\frac{1}{2}$ glass _____ fl oz

13. 8 ounces _____ drams

14. 96 ounces _____ quarts

15. $1\frac{1}{2}$ teacups _____ ounces

Answers 1. 4000 mL 2. 0.005 mg 3. 7500 mg 4. 6700 g 5. 30 minims 6. 0.5 L 7. 2 fl oz 8. 0.15 g 9. 325 mg 10. 15 μg 11. 3.5 g 12. 4 fl oz 13. 64 drams 14. 3 quarts 15. 9 ounces

The Self-Evaluation Tests on the review of the metric, apothecaries', and household systems should be repeated until fewer than three errors occur. If you continue to make mistakes, try to identify whether your errors are related to problems in the basic mathematical skills or in not knowing the value of the stated units. Review the material on the systems of measurement and repeat the two tests.

VIP

A knowledge of the units of weight and volume in the systems is vital for safety. By remembering the tables of weight and volume and learning the system equivalents, any problem of conversion can be calculated. Moving from one system to the other can be accomplished with relative ease.

Review Test 13.1
System of Measurements

Fill in the approximate equivalents in the following table of weights and volume (liquid) measures.

Apothecaries'		Metric		Household (approximate values)
Liquid	**Weight**	**Liquid**	**Weight**	
1 minim	1 grain	0.06 mL	0.06 g; **(1)** _____ mg	**(2)** _____ drop
(3) _____ m	**(4)** _____ gr	1 mL	1 g	$\frac{1}{4}$ tsp
1 fl dram	1 dram	**(5)** _____ mL	**(6)** _____ g	1 tsp
4 fl drams	4 drams	16 mL	16 g	**(7)** _____ Tbs
1 fl ounce	1 ounce	**(8)** _____ mL	**(9)** _____ g	1 oz
		(10) _____ mL	**(11)** _____ g	16 oz or 1 pound
(12) _____ pt		500 mL	500 g	16 fl oz
1 quart		**(13)** _____ mL	**(14)** _____ g	1 quart

Table of Approximate Equivalents

Apothecaries'		Metric	
Weight			
$\frac{1}{600}$ grain	100 mcg (μg)	0.1 mg	0.0001 g
$\frac{1}{300}$ grain	200 mcg (μg)	0.2 mg	0.0002 g
$\frac{1}{200}$ grain	300 mcg (μg)	0.3 mg	0.0003 g
$\frac{1}{150}$ grain	400 mcg (μg)	0.4 mg	0.0004 g
$\frac{1}{100}$ grain	600 mcg (μg)	0.6 mg	0.0006 g
$\frac{1}{60}$ grain		1 mg	0.001 g
$\frac{1}{30}$ grain		2 mg	0.002 g
$\frac{1}{20}$ grain		3 mg	0.003 g
$\frac{1}{10}$ grain		6 mg	0.006 g
$\frac{1}{8}$ grain		8 mg	0.008 g
$\frac{1}{6}$ grain		10 mg	0.01 g
$\frac{1}{5}$ grain		12 mg	0.012 g
$\frac{1}{4}$ grain		15 mg	0.015 g
$\frac{1}{3}$ grain		20 mg	0.02 g
$\frac{3}{8}$ grain		25 mg	0.025 g
$\frac{1}{2}$ grain		30 mg	0.03 g
$\frac{2}{3}$ grain		40 mg	0.04 g
$\frac{3}{4}$ grain		45 mg	0.045 g

*One grain equals approximately 60–65 mg.

(continues)

Table of Approximate Equivalents (Continued)

Apothecaries'	Metric	
1 grain	60 mg*	0.06 g
$1\frac{1}{4}$ grains	75 mg	0.075 g
$1\frac{1}{2}$ grains	100 mg	0.1 g
2 grains	120 mg	0.12 g
$2\frac{1}{2}$ grains	150 mg	0.15 g
3 grains	200 mg	0.2 g
4 grains	250 mg	0.25 g
5 grains	300 mg	0.3 g
$7\frac{1}{2}$ grains	500 mg	0.5 g
12 grains	750 mg	0.75 g
15 or 16 grains	1000 mg	1.0 g
Liquid		
15 or 16 minims	1 mL	
1 fluid dram	4 mL	
1 fluid ounce	30 mL (32 mL may be used)	
16 fluid ounces (1 pint)	500 mL	
32 fluid ounces (1 quart)	1000 mL or 1 L	

unit 3

Preparing for the Safe Administration of Medications

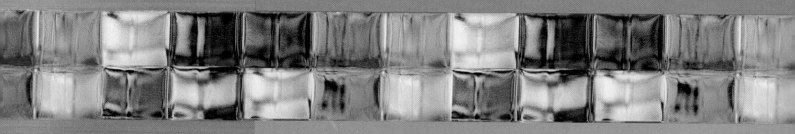

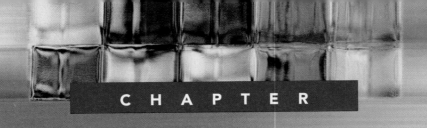

14

Abbreviations Used in Administering Medications

Learning Outcomes

After successfully completing this chapter, the learner should be able to:

- *Identify the commonly used abbreviations concerned with the calculation and administration of medications.*

- *Correctly interpret the physician's written medication orders containing commonly used abbreviations.*

GENERAL INFORMATION

The nurse is responsible for interpreting the physician's written medication order, which frequently contains a number of abbreviations. Therefore, to correctly administer medications, the nurse must be aware of and learn the more commonly used abbreviations. Medication orders must make sense and abbreviations must be viewed within the appropriate context. If there are any questions about the order as written, the order must be checked and clarified with the prescriber.

For quick and easy reference, many common, useful abbreviations are listed on the inside front cover of this textbook.

COMMONLY USED ABBREVIATIONS

The commonly used abbreviations for measurement of medications include:

capsule	cap
cubic centimeter	cc
dram	dr or ʒ
drop	gtt
fluid dram	fl dr or fl ʒ
grain	gr
gram	g
kilogram	kg
liter	L
microgram	mcg or μg
milliequivalent	mEq
milligram	mg
milliliter	ml or mL
millimole $\left(\dfrac{1}{1000} \text{ of a mole} \right)$	mmol
minim	m̨ or M
one-half	s̄s̄
ounce	oz or ʒ
fluid ounce	fl oz or fl ʒ
teaspoon	tsp
tablespoon	Tbs
tablet	tab
unit	U

The commonly used abbreviations for method of administration of medications include:

both ears	AU
left ear	AS
right ear	AD
both eyes	OU
left eye	OS
right eye	OD
by mouth	po or PO
gastrostomy tube	GT
drops per minute	gtt/min
hypodermic	H
inhalation	I or INH
intradermal	ID
intramuscular	IM
intravenous	IV

intravenous piggyback	IVPB
intravenous push	IVP or IV push
keep vein open (a very slow rate of infusion to keep an IV open)	KVO
nasogastric tube	NGT
subcutaneous	SC or SQ or subq
sublingual	SL
topical	T
total parenteral nutrition	TPN

The commonly used abbreviations for times of administration of medications include:

after meals	pc	every 12 hours	q12h
at once, immediately	stat	every other day	qod
before meals	ac	four times a day	qid
every day, once a day	qd or od	hour of sleep	hs
every hour	qh or q1h	once if necessary	sos
every 2 hours	q2h	three times a day	tid
every 3 hours	q3h	twice a day	bid
every 4 hours	q4h	when necessary;	prn
every 6 hours	q6h	as needed	
every 8 hours	q8h		

The commonly used miscellaneous abbreviations associated with medications include:

after	$\overline{p}$	nothing by mouth	NPO
ampule	amp	quantity sufficient	qs
as desired	ad lib	solution	sol
before	$\overline{a}$	suspension	susp
discontinue	dc	tincture	tinct
elixir	elix	with	$\overline{c}$
fluid	fl	without	$\overline{s}$
of each	$\overline{a}\overline{a}$	National Formulary	NF
liquid	liq	United States Pharmacopoeia	USP

Review Test 14.1
Abbreviations and Interpreting the Physician's Orders

Write out the meaning of these orders; include all facts as presented:

1. Morphine sulfate 8 mg sc, q4h, prn _____

2. Atropine sulfate 0.4 mg IM, stat _____

3. Vitamin B_{12} 1000 mcg IM, qod _____

4. Potassium penicillin 500,000 U q4h, IVPB _____

5. Codeine sulfate gr $\frac{1}{4}$ and aspirin gr x po, q6h _____

6. Maalox Tbs 1 po, q2h _____

7. Gentamycin sulfate 45 mg IVPB, q12h _____

8. Persantine 50 mg po, tid _____

9. Timoptic eye gtt 0.25%, 1 gtt, OS, qid _____

10. Digoxin 0.125 mg po, od _____

11. Nitroglycerin gr $\frac{1}{150}$, SL, prn _____

12. Compazine 10 mg, IM, stat _____

13. Inderal 40 mg, PO, TID _____

14. Ampicillin 1 g IVPB, q6h _____

15. Kanamycin sulfate 1000 mg, PO, q1h × 4 _____

Answers   **1.** Morphine sulfate 8 milligrams subcutaneously, every 4 hours, if necessary   **2.** Atropine sulfate 0.4 milligrams intramuscularly, at once   **3.** Vitamin B_{12} 1000 micrograms intramuscularly, every other day   **4.** Potassium penicillin 500,000 units every 4 hours, by intravenous piggyback   **5.** Codeine sulfate grains $\frac{1}{4}$ and aspirin grains 10 by mouth, every 6 hours   **6.** Maalox 1 tablespoon by mouth, every 2 hours   **7.** Gentamycin sulfate 45 milligrams by intravenous piggyback, every 12 hours   **8.** Persantine 50 milligrams by mouth, three times a day   **9.** Timoptic eye drops, 0.25% one drop in left eye, four times a day   **10.** Digoxin 0.125 milligrams, by mouth, daily   **11.** Nitroglycerin grains $\frac{1}{150}$, sublingually, as necessary   **12.** Compazine 10 milligrams, intramuscularly, at once   **13.** Inderal 40 milligrams, by mouth, three times a day   **14.** Ampicillin 1 gram by intravenous piggyback, every 6 hours   **15.** Kanamycin sulfate 1000 milligrams (1 gram), by mouth, every hour for 4 doses

If you had fewer than three errors on Review Test 14.1, proceed to the next chapter. If you had four or more errors, review the material on abbreviations and interpreting physician's orders and complete Review Test 14.2 before continuing.

Review Test 14.2
Abbreviations and Interpreting the Physician's Orders

1. Seconal 100 mg IM, hs, sos _____

2. Regular insulin U 5 sc, ac and hs _____

3. Potassium chloride liquid 5%, 40 mEq, PO, qd _____

4. Ferrous sulfate tab 1 PO, pc _____

5. Magnesium hydroxide fl oz 1 1c̄ cascara elix fl dr 1 po, stat _____

6. Ibuprofen 600 mg po qid _____

7. Sodium phenobarbital gr ii IM q4h _____

8. Xanax 0.5 mg PO tid _____

9. Hydrocortisone sodium succinate 100 mg IVPB stat _____

10. Hydromorphone hydrochloride SC 2 mg q4-6h prn _____

11. Ciprofloxacin 250 mg, PO, q12h _____

12. Prozac oral sol 20 mg, po, bid _____

13. Heparin 5000 U, IVP, stat _____

14. Fentanyl 0.05 mg, IM, $\frac{1}{2}$ hr preop _____

15. Homatropine opth sol 2%, 2 gtt OU, q 5 min × 2 doses _____

Answers   **1.** Seconal 100 milligrams intramuscularly, at bedtime, once if necessary   **2.** Regular insulin 5 units subcutaneously, before meals and at bedtime   **3.** Potassium chloride liquid 5% 40 milliequivalents, by mouth, daily   **4.** Ferrous sulfate tablets one by mouth, after meals   **5.** Magnesium hydroxide 1 fluid ounce with cascara elixir 1 fluid dram by mouth, at once   **6.** Ibuprofen 600 milligrams, by mouth, four times a day   **7.** Sodium phenobarbital, grains two, intramuscularly, every 4 hours   **8.** Xanax 0.5 milligrams by mouth, three times a day   **9.** Hydrocortisone sodium succinate 100 milligrams by intravenous piggyback, at once   **10.** Hydromorphone hydrochloride subcutaneously, two milligrams every 4 to 6 hours if necessary   **11.** Ciprofloxacin 250 milligrams, by mouth, every 12 hours   **12.** Prozac oral solution, 20 milligrams, by mouth, twice a day   **13.** Heparin 5000 units, intravenous push, at once   **14.** Fentanyl 0.05 milligrams, intramuscularly, $\frac{1}{2}$ hr before surgery   **15.** Homatropine ophthalmic solution 2%, 2 drops, both eyes, every 5 minutes for 2 doses

The Review Tests on abbreviations and interpreting physician's orders should be repeated until fewer than three errors occur.

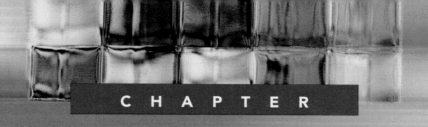

CHAPTER

15

Administering Medications and Interpreting Drug Labels

Learning Outcomes

After successfully completing this chapter, the learner should be able to:

- ■ *List the components necessary for a legal drug order.*
- ■ *List the five rights of medication administration.*
- ■ *Identify the nurse's legal responsibilities in administering any medication.*
- ■ *State the components of proper recording of medication administration.*
- ■ *Identify the information that can be found on a manufacturer's drug label.*
- ■ *Read and interpret the information on a manufacturer's drug label.*

GENERAL INFORMATION

Before a nurse can administer any medication, there must be a written, legal order for the medication. Those capable of writing a legal order include a physician, dentist, physician's assistant, or nurse practitioner (depending on state law). In addition to being written and signed by the prescriber, a legal drug order must indicate:

- ■ Patient's full name
- ■ Date the order was written
- ■ Name of the medication: may be generic or trade name (combination drugs are usually ordered by trade or brand name)
- ■ Dose

- Frequency of administration
- Route of administration
- Duration of order, if applicable (orders for some types of drugs, such as narcotics, have an automatic expiration time)

If any of these facts are missing, the order is incomplete and should be questioned by the nurse. On the physician's order sheet in most hospitals, the time the order was written is also included. This fact (though not legally required) prevents overriding or conflicting orders and reduces the chance of administration errors.

Although the unit dose is commonly used in hospitals throughout the United States, the nurse is still ultimately responsible for safely administering the patient's medication. (A *unit dose* is a prepackaged single dose of a medication that contains a frequently ordered strength and is labeled accordingly by the manufacturer. See aluminum hydroxide gel and Fosamax labels.

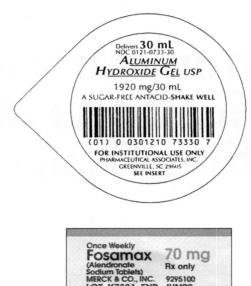

Whenever administering medications, the nurse should carefully check that the five "rights" of medication administration are ensured. These rights are the:

- Right patient
- Right medication
- Right dose
- Right route of administration
- Right time

The nurse is also legally responsible for knowing the usual dose, the expected action, any interactions with drugs or food, the side effects, and the adverse reactions of any drug administered, and should not administer any medication without this knowledge.

Only a single dose of medication should be prepared or poured at any one time and poured medications should never be out of the nurse's view. *A nurse should never administer a medication prepared by anyone else.*

Recording the administration of medications is a legal responsibility and should occur as soon after administration as possible. Recording should include time, medication, dose, patient response, and the nurse's signature. If the medication was a prn medication, the indication for administration should also be included. The recording should be dated and signed by the nurse who administered the medication. (See the sample medication records in Chapter 24.)

VIP

Before administering any medication:

- Check if the patient has any allergies.
- Read and interpret the legal medication order.
- Read and interpret the label and check the label with the prescriber's order.
- Know the expected action and side effects of any medications administered.
- Be certain the amount prescribed is within a safe or therapeutic range.
- Check with the physician any time the total prescribed dose exceeds the manufacturer's recommended daily dose of any medication.
- Make certain it is the right patient; right medication; right dose; right route of administration; and right time.

THE MEDICATION LABEL

The nurse must recognize and identify vital information present on the hospital pharmacy drug dispensing label, the drug dispensing label on prescriptions, and the manufacturer's drug label.

The hospital pharmacy drug dispensing label usually includes:

- The patient's name and room number
- The date the prescription was filled
- The generic and/or brand name of the drug
- The strength of the drug in the supplied form

The drug dispensing label on prescriptions usually includes:

- The patient's name
- The prescriber's name
- The name and address of the pharmacy
- The date the prescription was filled
- The prescription number
- The generic and/or brand name of the drug
- Form of drug
- Route of administration
- The strength of drug in the supplied form, and the total amount dispensed
- The expiration date, if applicable
- Directions for use

The manufacturer's drug label usually contains the following information:

- Manufacturer's name and company's location
- The drug's generic name—the official chemical name of the drug under which it is licensed
- The drug's trade or brand name—the registered name given to a generic drug or combination of drugs by the manufacturer, usually followed by the symbol ®
- The names of any additional substances added to mix, preserve, or enhance the drug

■ The lot or control number

■ The expiration date

■ Form in which drug is supplied

■ Route of administration

■ Strength of drug in supplied form

■ Total amount of drug in container

■ Specific storage and dispensing directions

■ Method for mixing or preparing medication for administration, if applicable

■ Dosage information

■ Precautions or warnings

The following manufacturers' labels demonstrate these facts. See circled areas for manufacturer's name and company's location, the drug's generic name, the drug's trade or brand name, and the names of any additional substances.

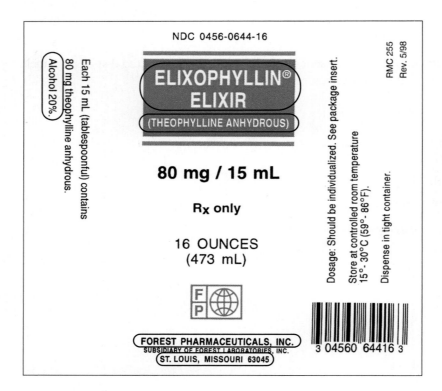

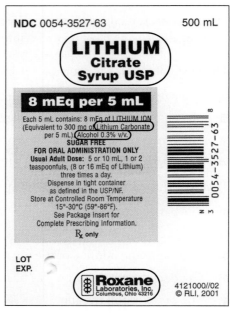

See circled areas for the lot or control number and the expiration date.

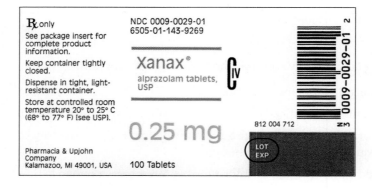

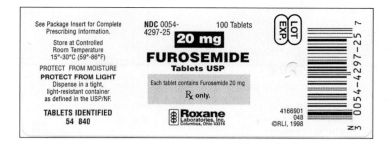

See circled areas for form in which drug is supplied, route of administration (when stated), strength of drug in supplied form, total amount of drug in container.

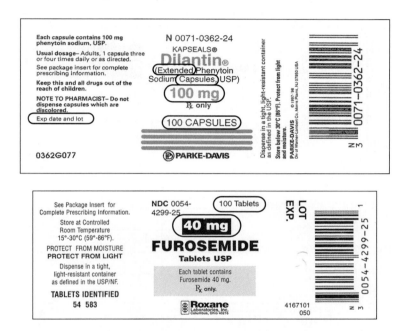

See circled areas for specific storage and dispensing directions, including how drug is to be mixed or prepared for administration, *if applicable;* and dosage information.

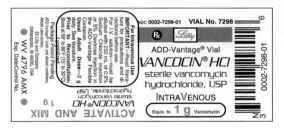

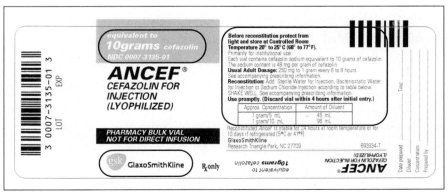

Review Test 15.1
Manufacturers' Drug Labels

Identify the following information from the pictured labels:

A.

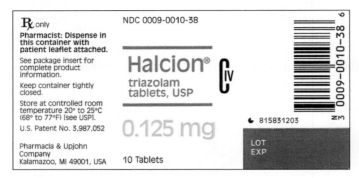

1. The drug's trade or brand name _____

2. The drug's generic name _____

3. Manufacturer's name _____

4. Any additional substances added _____

5. Form of drug and route of administration _____

6. Strength of drug _____

7. Total amount of drug in container _____

8. Storage and dispensing directions _____

B.

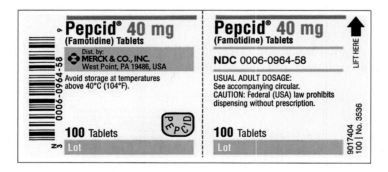

1. The drug's trade or brand name _____

2. The drug's generic name _____

3. Manufacturer's name _____

4. Any additional substances added _____

5. Form of drug and route of administration _____

6. Strength of drug _____

7. Total amount of drug in container _____

8. Storage and dispensing directions _____

C.

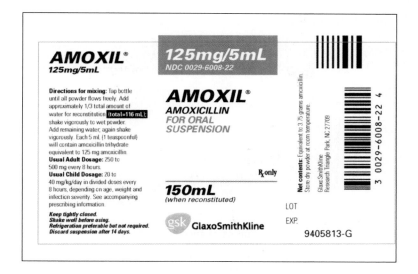

1. The drug's trade or brand name _____

2. The drug's generic name _____

3. Manufacturer's name _____

4. Any additional substances added _____

5. Form of drug and route of administration
   (note directions for mixing) _____

6. Strength of drug _____

7. Total amount of drug in container _____

8. Storage directions _____

D.

N 0071-2214-20

Dilantin-125®
(Phenytoin Oral
Suspension, USP)
125 mg per 5 mL potency

℞ only

**IMPORTANT–SHAKE WELL
BEFORE EACH USE**

8 fl oz (237 mL)

Ⓟ **PARKE-DAVIS**

6505-00-890-1110

**THIS PRODUCT MUST BE SHAKEN WELL
ESPECIALLY PRIOR TO INITIAL USE.**
Each 5 mL contains phenytoin, 125 mg with
a maximum alcohol content not greater than
0.6 percent.
Usual Dosage–Adults, 1 teaspoonful (5 mL)
three times daily; pediatric patients, see
package insert.
**Advice to Pharmacist and
Patient**–Patient must be
advised to use an accurate
measuring device when
using this product.
See package insert for complete prescribing information.
**Store at Controlled Room
Temperature 20°-25°C
(68°-77°F) [see USP]. Protect from freezing and light.
Keep this and all drugs out
of the reach of children.**

PARKE-DAVIS
Div of Warner-Lambert Co
Morris Plains, NJ 07950 USA
©1996-'99

N 3 0071-2214-20 8

Exp date and lot

2214G141

1. The drug's trade or brand name _____

2. The drug's generic name _____

3. Manufacturer's name _____

4. Any additional substances added _____

5. Form of drug and route of administration _____

6. Strength of drug _____

7. Total amount of drug in container _____

8. Storage directions _____

E.

851640   NDC 0026-8564-64

CIPRO® I.V.

(ciprofloxacin)

SINGLE DOSE VIAL
contains: **40 mL** sterile
1% solution

400 mg ciprofloxacin

DILUTE BEFORE USE.
For Intravenous (iv) Infusion

℞ **Only**

FOR ADMINISTRATION,
DILUTE with 200 mLs of suitable diluent.
For complete product information, including Dosage and
Administration, see accompanying package insert.
INACTIVE INGREDIENTS:
Lactic acid as solubilizer. HCl to adjust pH and
Water for Injection,USP.
Store between 41-86°F (5-30°C).
Protect from light.
Avoid freezing.
PL500264   ©2001 Bayer Corporation   10538   Printed in USA

Manufactured for
Bayer Corporation
Pharmaceutical Division
400 Morgan Lane
West Haven, CT 06516

71004780, R.0

Bayer

Batch:
Expires:

1. The drug's trade or brand name _____

2. The drug's generic name _____

3. Manufacturer's name _____

4. Any additional substances added _____

5. Form of drug and route of administration _____

6. Strength of drug _____

7. Total amount of drug in container _____

8. Storage directions _____

F.

NDC 0006-3275
2 mL INJECTION
COGENTIN®
(BENZTROPINE MESYLATE)
2 mg per 2 mL
Dist. by:
MERCK & CO., INC.
West Point, PA 19486, USA

USUAL ADULT DOSAGE:
See accompanying circular.

9113907

Lot

Exp.

1. The drug's trade or brand name _____

2. The drug's generic name _____

3. Manufacturer's name _____

4. Any additional substances added _____

5. Form of drug and route of administration _____

6. Strength of drug _____

7. Total amount of drug in container _____

8. Storage directions _____

G.

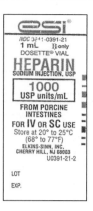

1. The drug's trade or brand name _____

2. The drug's generic name _____

3. Manufacturer's name _____

4. Any additional substances added _____

5. Form of drug and route of administration _____

6. Strength of drug _____

7. Total amount of drug in each vial _____

8. Storage directions _____

H.

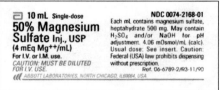

1. The drug's trade or brand name _____

2. The drug's generic name _____

3. Manufacturer's name _____

4. Any additional substances added _____

5. Form of drug and route of administration _____

6. Strength of drug _____

7. Total amount of drug in container _____

8. Storage directions _____

I.

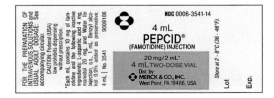

1. The drug's trade or brand name _____

2. The drug's generic name _____

3. Manufacturer's name _____

4. Any additional substances added _____

5. Form of drug and route of administration _____

6. Strength of drug _____

7. Total amount of drug in container _____

8. Storage directions _____

J.

Delivers **15 mL**
NDC 0121-0465-15
Potassium Chloride
Oral Solution USP 10%
20 mEq per 15 mL
Sugar Free   Alcohol 5%
DILUTE BEFORE USING

(01) 0 0301210 46515 4
Rx ONLY
FOR INSTITUTIONAL USE ONLY
PHARMACEUTICAL ASSOCIATES, INC.
GREENVILLE, SC 29605
SEE INSERT

1. The drug's trade or brand name _____

2. The drug's generic name _____

3. Manufacturer's name _____

4. Any additional substances added _____

5. Form of drug and route of administration _____

6. Strength of drug _____

7. Total amount of drug in container _____

8. Storage directions _____

Answers   **A. 1.** Halcion **2.** triazolam **3.** Pharmacia & Upjohn **4.** none listed **5.** tablet, oral **6.** 0.125 mg **7.** 10 tablets
8. Store at controlled room temperature 20° to 25°C (68° to 77°F).
  B. 1. Pepcid **2.** famotidine **3.** Merck & Co., Inc. **4.** none listed **5.** tablet, oral **6.** 40 mg **7.** 100 tablets **8.** Avoid storage at
temperatures above 40°C (104°F).
  C. 1. Amoxil **2.** amoxicillin for oral suspension **3.** GlaxoSmithKline **4.** water when reconstituted **5.** powder for oral suspension
6. Each teaspoon = 125 mg/5 mL **7.** 150 mL (when reconstituted) **8.** Keep tightly closed. Directions for mixing. Shake well before using.
Refrigeration preferable but not required. Discard suspension after 14 days.
  D. 1. Dilantin-125 **2.** phenytoin oral suspension **3.** Parke-Davis **4.** alcohol 0.6% **5.** liquid oral suspension **6.** 125 mg per 5 mL
7. 8 fl oz (237 mL) **8.** Store at Controlled Room Temperature 20°–25°C (68°–77°F). . . . Protect from freezing and light, use accurate measuring
device.
  E. 1. Cipro I.V. **2.** ciprofloxacin **3.** Bayer **4.** lactic acid, hydrochloric acid (HCl), water **5.** liquid, IV **6.** 400 mg per 40 mL vial
7. 400 mg **8.** Store between 41–86°F (5–30°C). Protect from light. Avoid freezing. Dilute with 200 mLs of suitable diluent.
  F. 1. Cogentin **2.** benztropine mesylate **3.** Merck & Co., Inc. **4.** none listed **5.** liquid, injection **6.** 2 mg per 2 mL **7.** 2 mL
8. none listed
  G. 1. Heparin **2.** heparin sodium **3.** Elkins-Sinn, Inc. **4.** none listed **5.** liquid, IV or SC use **6.** 1000 units/mL **7.** 1000 units per mL
single dose vial **8.** Store at 20° to 25°C (68° to 77°F).
  H. 1. NA **2.** 50% magnesium sulfate **3.** Abbott Laboratories **4.** May contain H_2SO_4 and/or NaOH; calcium **5.** liquid, IV or IM use
6. 4 mEq Mg++/mL **7.** 10 mL (40 mEq) single dose vial **8.** Must be diluted for I.V. use.
  I. 1. Pepcid **2.** famotidine **3.** Merck & Co., Inc. **4.** L-aspartic acid, mannitol, water, benzyl alcohol **5.** liquid, IV **6.** 20 mg/2 mL
7. 4 mL (40 mg) **8.** Store at 2–8°C (38°–48°F). (See circular for preparation.)
  J. 1. NA **2.** potassium chloride oral solution **3.** Pharmaceutical Associates, Inc. **4.** alcohol 5%; sugar free **5.** liquid, oral solution
6. 20 mEq per 15 mL **7.** 15 mL **8.** Dilute before using

All errors should be corrected by rereading the labels for the pertinent information.

unit
4

Oral and Parenteral Medications

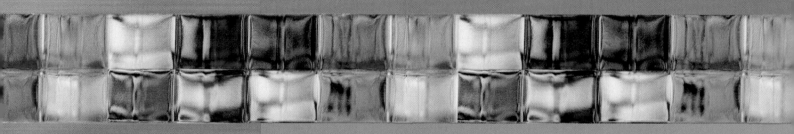

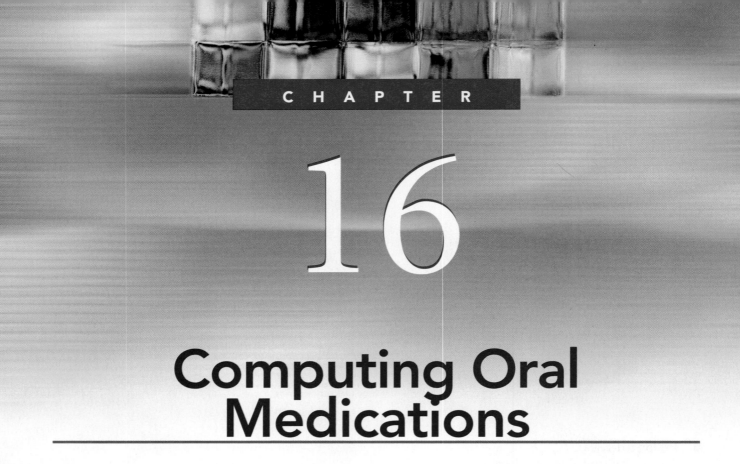

16

Computing Oral Medications

Learning Outcomes

After successfully completing this chapter, the learner should be able to:

- *Identify the various forms of oral medications.*
- *Set up proportions and label terms.*
- *Convert an available on-hand dose of an oral medication to a desired dose.*
- *Calculate the amount of medication to be poured to administer a desired dose.*

GENERAL INFORMATION

The nurse is responsible for giving any medication in the form and route prescribed, although some substitutions in the form may be legally permitted; for example, substituting a liquid form for a tablet form if the nurse finds the patient cannot or will not swallow a tablet. The route of administration prescribed cannot be changed by the nurse and the order must be rewritten.

Oral medications are manufactured in a variety of forms to ensure maximum drug action to best suit the needs of the patient. The oral route of administration is the most commonly prescribed because it can easily be self-administered or administered by the nurse without the need for any invasive techniques.

Certain drugs are manufactured in units rather than in measurements from the apothecaries' or metric system. These drugs are listed as having a stated number of USP units. This designation means that the composition of the unit conforms to the specifications laid down by the United States Pharmacopoeia.

Some drugs are manufactured in milliequivalents (mEq) rather than in measurements from the apothecaries' or metric system. A milliequivalent is one-thousandth of a chemical equivalent.

ORAL MEDICATIONS

Oral medications are supplied in the form of tablets, capsules, and liquids.

Tablets

A compressed or solid form of a drug that is molded by the manufacturer into a variety of shapes and sizes. Example: amlodipine (Norvasc)

- Scored tablets—a tablet with a marked or indicated line in the center intended to facilitate breaking the tablet in half if necessary. Unscored tablets should not be broken. Example: furosemide (Lasix)
- Enteric-coated tablets (controlled-release tablets)—a tablet with an outer covering or coating that is designed to withstand gastric acid and to dissolve in the small intestine. This controlled release is used for drugs, such as aspirin, that are irritating to the gastric mucosa. Enteric-coated tablets should never be crushed or chewed. Example: enteric-coated aspirin (Ecotrin)
- Sublingual (buccal) tablets—a tablet designed to be placed beneath the tongue or in the buccal patch for rapid absorption of the drug into the bloodstream. Example: nitroglycerin (Nitrostat)

Capsules

A round or oval gelatinous container that is filled with a powdered or liquid form of the medication. Example: docusate sodium (Colace)

- Prolonged-release capsules—capsules that contain pellets or compressed bits of the medication that have been coated and allow the drug to be released over time. Crushing or removing this medication from the capsule negates the purpose of the capsule. These capsules are usually identified with letters following the trade name. Example: Procan SR (Procan Sustained Release); Cardizem CD (Cardizem Continuous Dose); Sinemet CR (Sinemet Continuous Release).

Liquids

A fluid containing medication that is used primarily for oral administration.

- Elixir—a liquid containing water, alcohol, and sweetener that is used as a vehicle for delivering oral medications. Example: digoxin (Lanoxin Elixir)
- Syrup—a liquid containing water with concentrated sugar that is used as a vehicle for delivering oral medications, especially those with an unpleasant taste. Example: guaifenesin (Robitussin syrup)
- Suspension—a liquid medium in which small, fine particles of a drug have been dispersed but cannot be dissolved. Because the drug cannot be dissolved in the liquid, suspensions must be stirred or shaken before being administered. Example: sulfamethoxazole and trimethoprim (Septra suspension)
- Solution—a liquid, usually water or normal saline, in which one or more medications have been dissolved. Example: potassium iodide (Lugol's Solution)

Frequently, the nurse administering medications does not find the exact dosage of drug that has been ordered. In such instances, the nurse is often called on to move freely within a system of measurement and to convert from one system to another—remembering that in computing dosage, the approximate equivalent must never differ by more than 10% from the prescribed dosage. The first step in computing medication dosage is to make certain the strength of the drug ordered and the strength of the drug available are in the same unit of measure. Once this is done, the problem can be set up as a proportion.

RATIO AND PROPORTION REVIEW

A ratio expresses the numerical relationship between two quantities and a proportion is an equation that contains two ratios of equal value.

Proportions can be set up in a variety of ways as long as the ratios on both sides of the equal sign are written in the same order or sequence.

In a true proportion, the product of the means equals the product of the extremes (or the product of the extremes equals the product of the means). This is an important principle that is used to determine the value of an unknown term.

This unknown term is most commonly signified by the letter x. When solving for an unknown, always divide both sides of the equation by the number preceding the x.

SETTING UP THE PROPORTION

One side of the proportion represents the dosage of the drug, and the other side is the number of tablets, capsules, milliliters, or minims that contain the stated dosage. To avoid confusion, it is vital to label all terms of the proportion.

The *desired dosage* is the dosage of the drug to be administered. The *have dosage* is the dosage of the drug available. The *desired amount* is the number of tablets, capsules, milliliters, or minims that contains the desired dosage. The *have amount* is the number of tablets, capsules, milliliters, or minims in which the available dosage is supplied.

$$\frac{\text{Desired Dosage}}{\text{Have Dosage}} = \frac{\text{Desired Amount}}{\text{Have Amount}}$$

or

Desired Dosage : Have Dosage = Desired Amount : Have Amount

Example: A patient is to receive albuterol syrup (Proventil) 4 mg tid by mouth. Available is a bottle labeled 2 mg = 5 mL (see label). How much medication should the patient receive?

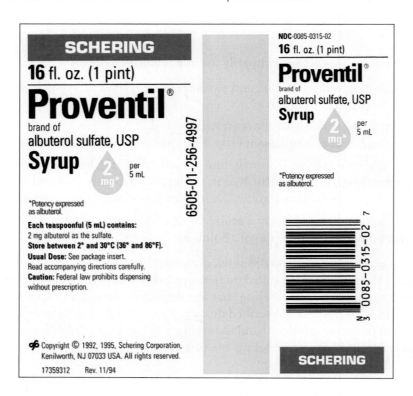

Solution: Because the desired dosage and the available dosage are in the same unit of measure, no conversion is necessary in this problem. Being certain to label all terms, set up the problem using the proportion:

$$\frac{\text{Desired Dosage}}{\text{Have Dosage}} = \frac{\text{Desired Amount}}{\text{Have Amount}}$$

$$\frac{4\text{ mg}}{2\text{ mg}} = \frac{x\text{ mL}}{5\text{ mL}}$$

$$2x = 20$$

$$x = 10\text{ mL}$$

To administer albuterol syrup (Proventil) 4 mg, the patient should receive 10 mL of Proventil labeled 2 mg = 5 mL.

Example: A patient is to receive allopurinol (Zyloprim) 0.2 g daily by mouth. Zyloprim is available in 100 mg tablets (see label). How many 100 mg tablets should the patient receive?

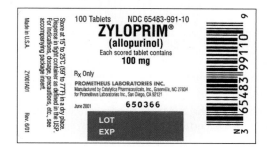

Solution: Proceed by first converting the dosage desired, 0.2 g, and the dosage available, 100 mg, to one unit of measure. This can be accomplished by moving the decimal place three places to the right, changing 0.2 g to 200 mg. Being certain to label all terms, set up the problem using the proportion:

$$\frac{\text{Desired Dosage}}{\text{Have Dosage}} = \frac{\text{Desired Amount}}{\text{Have Amount}}$$

$$\frac{200\text{ mg}}{100\text{ mg}} = \frac{x\text{ tablets}}{1\text{ tablet}}$$

$$100x = 200$$

$$x = 2\text{ tablets}$$

To administer 0.2 g of Zyloprim, the patient should receive 2 tablets of 100 mg strength.

Example: A patient is to receive penicillin V potassium (V-Cillin K) 800,000 units. V-Cillin K is available in 250 mg tablets (see label). How many 250 mg tablets should the patient receive?

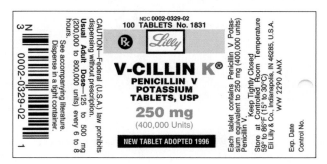

Solution: Proceed by first converting the dosage desired, 800,000 units, and the dosage available, 250 mg, to one unit of measure. This conversion can be completed by reading the drug label, which states 250 mg = 400,000 units. Being certain to label all terms, set up the problem using the proportion:

$$\frac{\text{Desired Dosage}}{\text{Have Dosage}} = \frac{\text{Desired Amount}}{\text{Have Amount}}$$

$$\frac{800,000\text{ units}}{400,000\text{ units}} = \frac{x\text{ tablets}}{1\text{ tablet}}$$

$$400,000x = 800,000$$

$$x = 2\text{ tablets}$$

To administer 800,000 units of V-Cillin K, the patient should receive 2 tablets of 250 mg (400,000 unit) strength.

Example: A patient is to receive potassium chloride 30 mEq 10% oral solution. The label on the container reads: potassium chloride 20 mEq equals 15 mL 10% oral solution (see label). How many mL should the nurse administer?

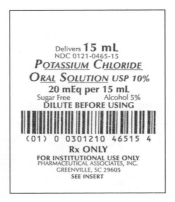

Solution: Because the desired dosage and the available dosage are in the same unit of measure, no conversion is necessary in this problem. Being certain to label all terms, set up the problem using the proportion:

$$\frac{\text{Desired Dosage}}{\text{Have Dosage}} = \frac{\text{Desired Amount}}{\text{Have Amount}}$$

$$\frac{30 \text{ mEq}}{20 \text{ mEq}} = \frac{x \text{ mL}}{15 \text{ mL}}$$

$$20x = 450$$

$$x = 22.5 \text{ mL}$$

To administer potassium chloride oral solution 10% 30 mEq, the patient should receive 22.5 mL of potassium chloride oral solution 10% 20 mEq equals 15 mL.

Example: A patient is to receive codeine sulfate 1 grain po q4h for pain. Codeine sulfate is available in 30 mg tablets (see label). How many 30 mg tablets should the patient receive?

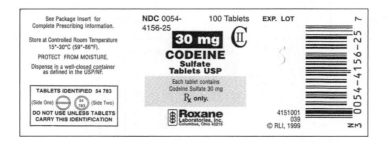

Solution: Proceed by first converting the dosage desired, 1 grain, and the dosage available, 30 mg, to one unit of measure. This can be accomplished by converting the 1 grain to mg by using the approximate equivalent 1 grain = 60 milligrams. Being certain to label all terms, set up the problem using the proportion:

$$\frac{\text{Desired Dosage}}{\text{Have Dosage}} = \frac{\text{Desired Amount}}{\text{Have Amount}}$$

$$\frac{60 \text{ mg}}{30 \text{ mg}} = \frac{x \text{ tablets}}{1 \text{ tablet}}$$

$$30x = 60$$

$$x = 2 \text{ tablets}$$

To administer 1 grain of codeine sulfate, the patient should receive two tablets of 30 mg strength.

Problem Set 16.1

1. A patient is to receive erythromycin (EryPed) 250 mg q6h PO. The drug on hand is labeled:

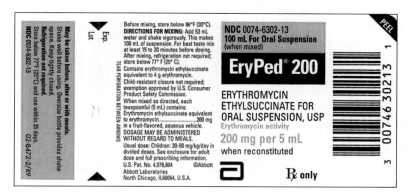

The nurse should administer _____ mL.

2. A patient is to receive phenytoin oral suspension (Dilantin-125) 250 mg PO. The drug on hand is labeled:

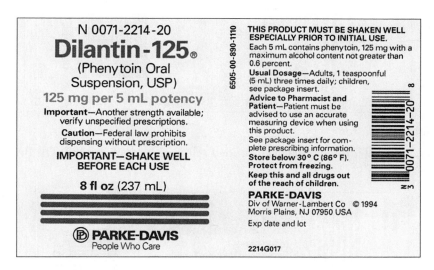

The nurse should administer _____ mL.

3. A patient is to receive lactulose solution 30 g PO. The drug on hand is labeled:

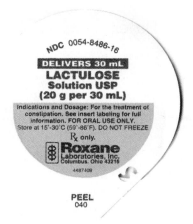

The nurse should administer _____ mL.

4. A patient is to receive digoxin (Lanoxin) 0.125 mg PO. The drug on hand is labeled:

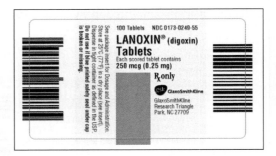

The nurse should administer _____ tablet(s).

5. A patient is to receive ciprofloxacin tablets (Cipro) 0.5 g PO. The drug on hand is labeled:

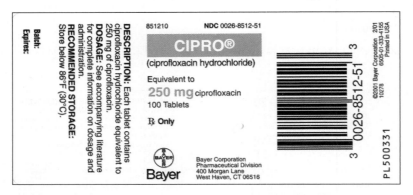

The nurse should administer _____ tablet(s).

6. A patient is to receive nifedipine (Adalat) extended release tablets 60 mg PO. The drug on hand is labeled:

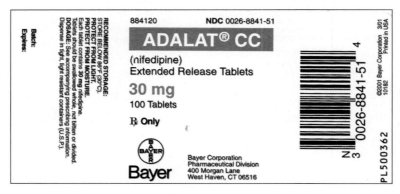

The nurse should administer _____ tablet(s).

7. A patient is to receive prednisone (PredniSONE) 7.5 mg PO. The drug on hand is labeled:

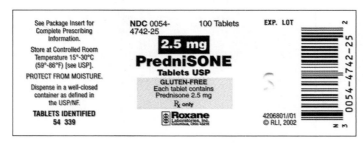

The nurse should administer _____ tablet(s).

8. A patient is to receive cefdinir oral suspension (Omnicef oral suspension) 100 mg PO. The drug on hand is labeled:

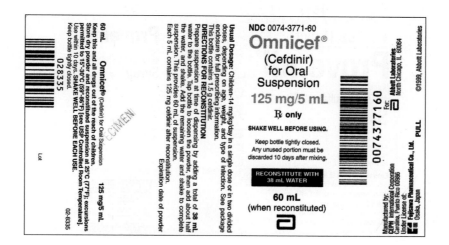

The nurse should provide the patient with _____ mL.

9. A patient is to receive penicillin V potassium tablets (V-CILLIN K) 600,000 units PO. The drug on hand is labeled:

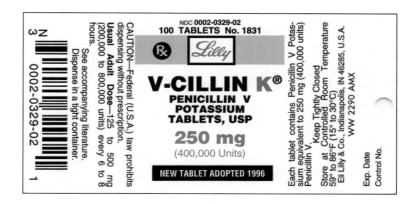

The nurse should administer _____ tablets.

10. A patient is to receive potassium chloride 10% oral solution 40 mEq PO. The drug on hand is labeled:

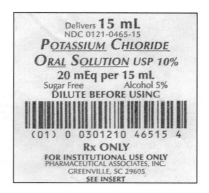

The nurse should administer _____ mL.

11. A patient is to receive albuterol sulfate syrup (Proventil Syrup) 0.004 g PO. The drug on hand is labeled:

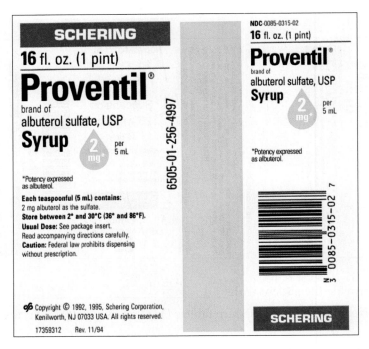

The nurse should administer _____ mL.

12. A patient is to receive amoxicillin for oral suspension (Amoxil) 500 mg PO. The drug on hand is labeled:

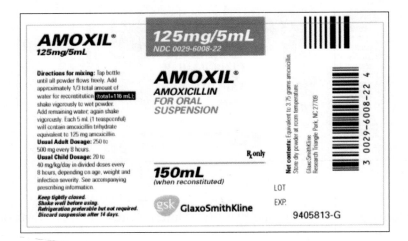

The nurse should administer _____ mL.

13. A patient is to receive potassium chloride extended-release tablets (Slow-K) 1200 mg PO. The drug on hand is labeled:

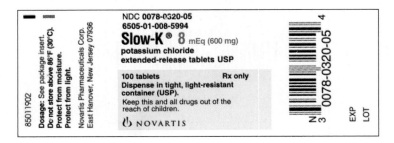

The nurse should administer _____ tablet(s).

14. A patient is to receive levothyroxine sodium (Synthroid) 0.2 mg PO. The drug on hand is labeled:

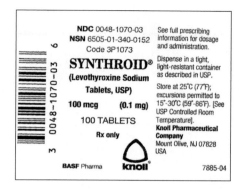

The nurse should administer _____ tablet(s).

15. A patient is to receive phenobarbital gr $\frac{3}{4}$ PO. The drug on hand is labeled:

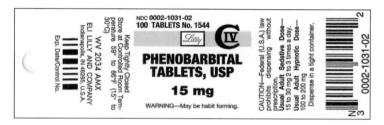

The nurse should administer _____ tablet(s).

Answers   **1.** The patient should receive 6.2 mL from the bottle labeled EryPed (erythromycin oral suspension) 200 mg per 5 mL.   **2.** The patient should receive 10 mL from the bottle labeled Dilantin-125 (phenytoin) oral suspension 125 mg per 5 mL.   **3.** The patient should receive 45 mL of the lactulose solution labeled 20 g per 30 mL.   **4.** The patient should receive $\frac{1}{2}$ tablet from the container labeled Lanoxin (digoxin), each scored tablet contains 250 mcg.   **5.** The patient should receive 2 tablets from the container labeled Cipro (ciprofloxacin hydrochloride), equivalent to 250 mg.   **6.** The patient should receive 2 tablets from the container labeled Adalat (nifedipine), extended release tablets 30 mg. **7.** The patient should receive 3 tablets from the container labeled PredniSONE (prednisone), each tablet contains prednisone 2.5 mg.   **8.** The patient should receive 4 mL from the bottle labeled Omnicef Oral Suspension 125 mg per 5 mL.   **9.** The patient should receive $1\frac{1}{2}$ tablets from the container labeled V-CILLIN K, each tablet contains 400,000 units.   **10.** The patient should receive 30 mL from the bottle labeled potassium chloride oral solution 10% 20 mEq per 15 mL.   **11.** The patient should receive 10 mL from the bottle labeled Proventil 2 mg per 5 mL.   **12.** The patient should receive 20 mL from the bottle labeled Amoxil (amoxicillin for oral suspension) 125 mg per 5 mL.   **13.** The patient should receive 2 tablets from the container labeled Slow-K (potassium chloride extended release tablets) 8 mEq (600 mg).   **14.** The patient should receive 2 tablets from the container labeled Synthroid (levothyroxine sodium) tablets 100 mcg (0.1 mg).   **15.** The patient should receive 3 tablets from the container labeled phenobarbital tablets 15 mg.

VIP

- Oral medications are supplied as tablets, capsules, and liquids.

- Before computing any dosage of medication, the strength of the drug ordered and the strength of the drug available must be in the same unit of measure. Remember, in computing dosage, the approximate equivalent must never differ by more than 10% from the prescribed dosage.

  Set the problem as a proportion.

  $$\frac{\text{Desired dosage}}{\text{Have dosage}} = \frac{\text{Desired amount}}{\text{Have amount}}$$

- One side of the proportion represents the dosage of the drug, and the other side is the number of tablets, capsules, milliliters, or minims that contain the stated dosage.

- It is vital to label all terms of the proportion.

Review Test 16.1
Oral Medications

1. The patient is to receive nitroglycerin (Nitrostat) gr $\frac{1}{100}$ SL. On hand are sublingual tablets of Nitrostat labeled:

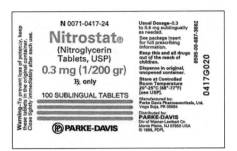

The nurse should administer _____ tablet(s).

2. The patient is to receive alprazolam (Xanax) 0.75 mg PO. On hand are tablets of Xanax labeled:

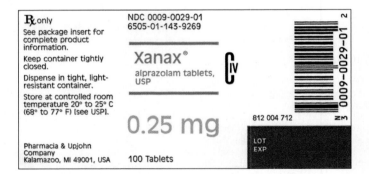

The nurse should administer _____ tablet(s).

3. The patient is to receive digoxin (Lanoxin) 0.5 mg PO. On hand are tablets of Lanoxin labeled:

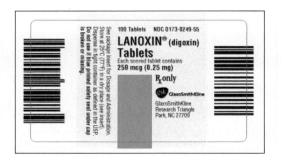

The nurse should administer _____ tablet(s).

4. The patient is to receive Augmentin (amoxicillin/clavulanate potassium) oral suspension 0.5 g PO. On hand is a bottle of Augmentin labeled:

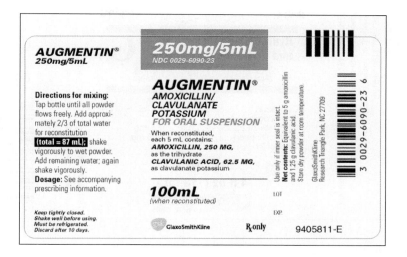

The nurse should administer _____ mL.

5. The patient is to receive mercaptopurine (Purinethol) 0.1 g PO. On hand is a bottle of Purinethol tablets labeled:

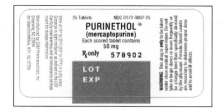

The nurse should administer _____ tablet(s).

6. The patient is to receive secobarbital (Seconal sodium) gr iss PO. On hand is a bottle of Seconal capsules labeled:

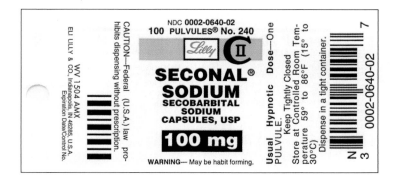

The nurse should administer _____ capsule(s).

7. The patient is to receive hydrocodone 10 mg with acetaminophen 667 mg PO. On hand is a bottle of hydrocodone bitartrate and acetaminophen elixir labeled:

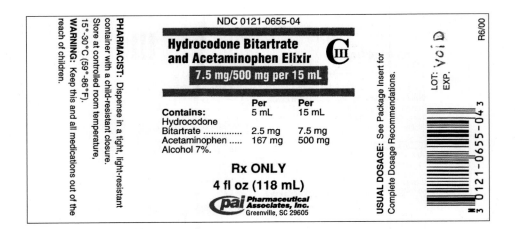

The nurse should administer _____ mL.

8. The patient is to receive extended phenytoin sodium capsules (Dilantin) gr v orally. On hand is a bottle of Dilantin capsules labeled:

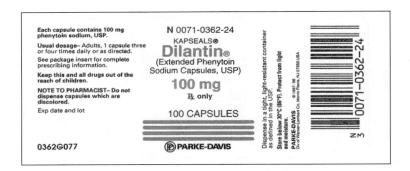

The nurse should administer _____ capsule(s).

9. The patient is to receive famotidine (Pepcid) 1 grain PO. On hand is a bottle of Pepcid tablets labeled:

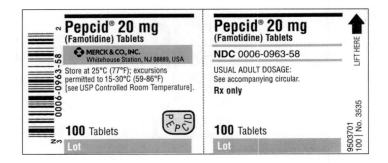

The nurse should administer _____ tablet(s).

10. The patient is to receive triazolam (Halcion) 0.25 mg PO. The bottle of Halcion tablets is labeled:

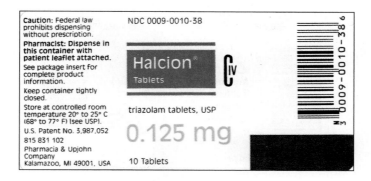

The nurse should administer _____ tablet(s).

11. The patient is to receive lithium citrate syrup 12 mEq PO. The bottle of lithium syrup is labeled:

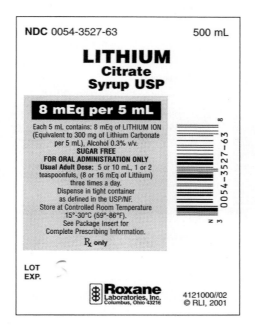

The nurse should administer _____ mL.

12. The patient is to receive glyburide (Micronase) tablets 0.01 g PO. The bottle of Micronase tablets is labeled:

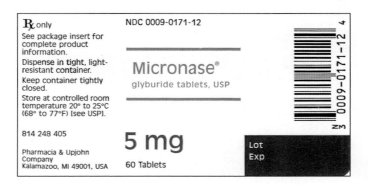

The nurse should administer _____ tablet(s).

13. The patient is to receive ondansetron (Zofran) 6 mg PO. The bottle of Zofran tablets is labeled:

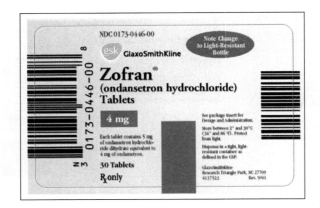

The nurse should administer _____ tablet(s).

14. The patient is to receive ranitidine hydrochloride (Zantac) tablets 0.3 g PO. The bottle of Zantac tablets is labeled:

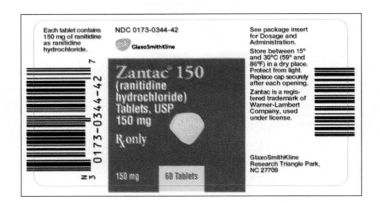

The nurse should administer _____ tablet(s).

15. The patient is to receive losartan (Cozaar) 37.5 mg PO. On hand is a bottle of Cozaar labeled:

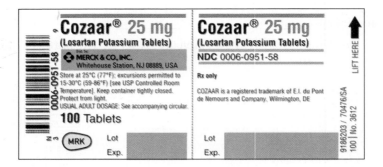

The nurse should administer _____ tablet(s).

Answers   **1.** 2 tablets   **2.** 3 tablets   **3.** 2 tablets   **4.** 10 mL   **5.** 2 tablets   **6.** 1 capsule   **7.** 20 mL   **8.** 3 capsules   **9.** 3 tablets

10. 2 tablets   **11.** 7.5 mL   **12.** 2 tablets   **13.** $1\frac{1}{2}$ tablets   **14.** 2 tablets   **15.** $1\frac{1}{2}$ tablets

If you had fewer than three errors on Review Test 16.1, move on to the next chapter. If you had four or more errors, review the material on oral medications and complete Review Test 16.2 before continuing.

Review Test 16.2
Oral Medications

1. The patient is to receive sertraline hydrochloride (Zoloft) 75 mg PO. On hand are tablets of Zoloft labeled 50 mg.

   The nurse should administer _____ tablet(s).

2. The patient is to receive ciprofloxacin hydrochloride (Cipro) 0.5 g PO. On hand are tablets of Cipro labeled 250 mg.

   The nurse should administer _____ tablet(s).

3. The patient is to receive rantidine hydrochloride syrup (Zantac syrup) 300 mg PO. On hand is a bottle of Zantac syrup labeled 1 mL contains 15 mg.

   The nurse should administer _____ mL.

4. The patient is to receive codeine phosphate oral solution grains 1 PO. The bottle of codeine phosphate oral solution is labeled 15 mg equals 5 mL.

   The nurse should administer _____ mL.

5. The patient is to receive warfarin sodium (Coumadin) 10 mg PO. On hand are tablets of Coumadin labeled 2.5 mg.

   The nurse should administer _____ tablet(s).

6. The patient is to receive glimepiride (Amaryl) 2 mg PO. On hand are tablets of Amaryl labeled 4 mg.

   The nurse should administer _____ tablet(s).

7. The patient is to receive conjugated estrogenic substances (Premarin) 3.75 mg PO. On hand are tablets of Premarin labeled 1.25 mg.

   The nurse should administer _____ tablet(s).

8. The patient is to receive naproxen (Naprosyn) 0.375 g PO. On hand are tablets of Naprosyn 250 mg.

   The nurse should administer _____ tablet(s).

9. The patient is to receive nystatin (Mycostatin) oral tablets 1,000,000 units tid PO. On hand are Mycostatin tablets labeled 500,000 units.

   The nurse should administer _____ tablet(s).

10. The patient is to receive diazepam (Valium) oral solution 10 mg PO. The container is labeled 5 mL contains 5 mg of Valium.

    The nurse should administer _____ mL.

11. The patient is to receive morphine sulfate oral solution gr $\frac{1}{4}$ PO. The container is labeled 20 mg equals 10 mL.

    The nurse should administer _____ mL.

12. The patient is to receive triamterene (Dyrenium) 0.2 g PO. On hand are tablets of Dyrenium labeled 100 mg.

    The nurse should administer _____ tablet(s).

13. The patient is to receive lithium carbonate syrup (Lithium Citrate Syrup) 600 mg PO. The bottle is labeled 5 mL contains 8 mEq (300 mg of lithium carbonate).

    The nurse should administer _____ mL.

14. The patient is to receive syrup docusate sodium (Colace) 30 mg PO. The container is labeled 20 mg equals 5 mL.

    The nurse should administer _____ mL.

15. The patient is to receive prednisone 12.5 mg PO. On hand are tablets of prednisone labeled 5 mg.

    The nurse should administer _____ tablet(s).

Answers   1. $1\frac{1}{2}$ tablets   2. 2 tablets   3. 20 mL   4. 20 mL   5. 4 tablets   6. $\frac{1}{2}$ tablet   7. 3 tablets   8. $1\frac{1}{2}$ tablets   9. 2 tablets

10. 10 mL   11. 7.5 mL   12. 2 tablets   13. 10 mL   14. 7.5 mL   15. $2\frac{1}{2}$ tablets

The Review Tests on oral medications should be repeated until fewer than three errors occur.

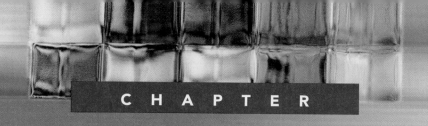

17

Computing Parenteral Medications

Learning Outcomes

After successfully completing this chapter, the learner should be able to:

■ *Identify the markings on standard syringes.*

■ *Calculate the amount of medication to be drawn up in a syringe to administer a desired dose.*

■ *Interpret the meaning of parenteral medication orders written in other than the metric or apothecaries' systems of measurement.*

■ *Calculate dosage for drugs to be administered parenterally.*

■ *State how much sterile fluid should be added to a vial of medication to produce a specific dose.*

■ *Explain the role of the displacement factor when mixing drugs supplied in powdered form.*

■ *Calculate the amount of unit dosage to be administered with or without the use of specially marked syringes.*

GENERAL INFORMATION

Recall that certain drugs are manufactured and supplied in units or milliequivalents (mEq) rather than in measurements from the apothecaries' or metric systems. Although some of these drugs are administered orally, many are administered parenterally. The parenteral drugs ordered in units include insulin, heparin, some hormones, and some forms of penicillin. Those ordered in milliequivalents include potassium chloride, ammonium chloride, and magnesium sulfate. The dosage for these drugs is usually prescribed in units or milliequivalents.

Many medications are manufactured for parenteral use. The most common parenteral routes are intravenous (IV) (included in Unit 4), intramuscular (IM), and subcutaneous (SC, SQ, Subq). Parenteral medications are usually supplied as vials, ampules, single-dose syringes, or IV piggybacks (see Figure 17-1). The drug forms most commonly available are solutions prepared by the manufacturer or powders that must be reconstituted (made into a liquid) by the pharmacist or the nurse.

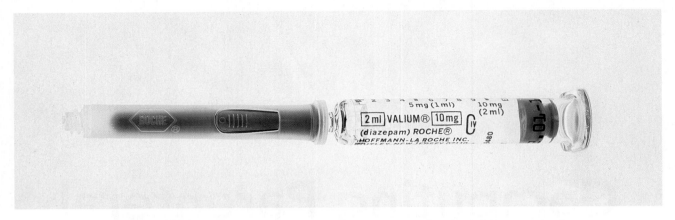

Figure 17-1   Prefilled single-dose syringe (Courtesy of Roche Laboratories, Inc.)

Intravenous drugs are usually administered with a large syringe (5 mL or more) for IV push or mixed in an IV fluid or IV piggyback, whereas intramuscular and subcutaneous medications are usually administered with a small syringe (3 mL or less). For adults: intramuscular injections should not exceed 3 mL, and subcutaneous injections should not exceed 1 mL. Administration of more fluid than this is painful and can cause tissue damage. These facts are important to remember when reconstituting powdered medication, as the prescribed dose often influences the amount of diluent (fluid used to dissolve the powder) to be added.

Small syringes—for example, the 1 and 3 mL—are marked in both milliliters and minims, as shown in Fig. 17-2.

Observe the 3 mL syringe (Figure 17-2 A):

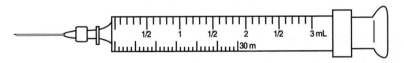

Figure 17-2 A   3 mL syringe

The milliliter side is divided into 0.1 mL intervals and is numerically marked at 0.5, or $\frac{1}{2}$ mL, intervals. The minim side is divided into 1 minim intervals, with wider markings at each 5 minim interval, but is usually not numerically marked until 30 minims. In this syringe 16 minims = 1 mL.

Observe the 1 mL, or tuberculin, syringe (Figure 17-2 B):

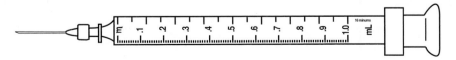

Figure 17-2 B   1 mL tuberculin syringe

The milliliter side is divided into 0.01 mL intervals and numerically marked at 0.1 intervals. The minim side is divided into 1 minim intervals, with wider markings at each 2 minim interval, and numerically marked at 16 minims. In this syringe, 16 minims = 1 mL. This syringe is most frequently used for more accurate measurement of small amounts of drugs.

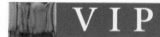

V I P

- Small syringes are marked both in minims and milliliters.
- Always determine the amount of liquid the desired dose is contained in, because syringes do not contain any markings for weights such as milligrams or grams.

SETTING UP THE PROPORTION

Once again ratio and proportion are used. One side of the proportion represents the dosage of the drug, and the other side is the number of milliliters or minims that contains the stated dosage. To avoid confusion, it is vital to label all terms of the proportion.

The desired dosage is the dosage of the drug to be administered. The "have" dosage is the dosage of the drug available. The desired amount is the number of milliliters or minims that contains the desired dosage. The "have" amount is the number of milliliters or minims in which the available dosage is supplied.

$$\frac{\text{Desired Dosage}}{\text{Have Dosage}} = \frac{\text{Desired Amount}}{\text{Have Amount}}$$

or

Desired Dosage : Have Dosage = Desired Amount : Have Amount

PART 1 Premied Parenteral Medications

Example: A patient is to receive prochlorperazine (Compazine) 7 mg by injection IM. Available is a multidose vial of Compazine labeled 5 mg = 1 mL (see Compazine label). How much of the Compazine 5 mg = 1 mL should the nurse administer?

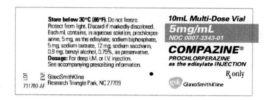

Solution: With the desired dosage and the available dosage in the same unit of measure, the problem can be set up by using the proportion:

$$\frac{\text{Desired Dosage}}{\text{Have Dosage}} = \frac{\text{Desired Amount}}{\text{Have Amount}}$$

$$\frac{7 \text{ mg}}{5 \text{ mg}} = \frac{x \text{ mL}}{1 \text{ mL}}$$

$$5x = 7$$

$$x = 1.4 \text{ mL}$$

In looking at the problem, it should be recognized that more than 1 mL but less than 2 mL of solution will be needed to administer the required dosage. In situations of this type, the 1.4 mL can be used, or the 1 mL in the original proportion can first be converted to minims.

1 mL = 15 or 16 minims

$$\frac{7 \text{ mg}}{5 \text{ mg}} = \frac{x \text{ minims}}{16 \text{ minims}}$$

$$5x = 112$$

$$x = 22.4 \text{ or } 22 \text{ minims}$$

To administer Compazine 7 mg by IM injection, the nurse would inject 1.4 milliliters or 22 minims. The syringe should look like Figure 17-3.

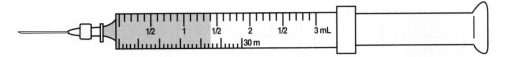

Figure 17-3

NOTE

The difference using either of the two approaches (mL or minims) is extremely small and well within the 10% conversion factor; therefore, either approach can be used for setting up this type of problem.

Example: A patient is to receive morphine sulfate 7 mg by injection SC. Available is a vial labeled morphine sulfate 10 mg/mL (see morphine sulfate label). How much of the morphine 10 mg/mL should the nurse administer?

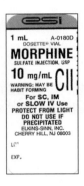

Solution: With the desired dosage and the available dosage in the same unit of measure, the problem can be set up by using the proportion (use either milliliters or minims):

$$\frac{\text{Desired Dosage}}{\text{Have Dosage}} = \frac{\text{Desired Amount}}{\text{Have Amount}}$$

$$\frac{7 \text{ mg}}{10 \text{ mg}} = \frac{x \text{ mL}}{1 \text{ mL}} \qquad or \qquad \frac{7 \text{ mg}}{10 \text{ mg}} = \frac{x \text{ minims}}{16 \text{ minims}}$$

$$10x = 7 \qquad\qquad 10x = 112$$

$$x = 0.7 \text{ mL} \qquad\qquad x = 11.2 \text{ or } 11 \text{ minims}$$

To administer morphine sulfate 7 mg SC, the nurse would inject 0.7 mL or 11 minims. The model syringe should look like Figure 17-4.

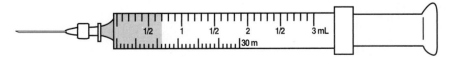

Figure 17-4

Example: A patient is to receive lorazepam injection (Ativan) 1.5 mg IM. Available is a vial of Ativan labeled 2 mg in 1 mL (see Ativan label). How much of the Ativan 2 mg = 1 mL should the nurse administer?

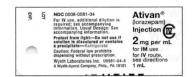

Solution: With the desired dose and the available dose in the same unit of measure, the problem can be set up by using the proportion:

$$\frac{\text{Desired Dosage}}{\text{Have Dosage}} = \frac{\text{Desired Amount}}{\text{Have Amount}}$$

$$\frac{1.5 \text{ mg}}{2 \text{ mg}} = \frac{x \text{ mL}}{1 \text{ mL}} \quad \text{or} \quad \frac{1.5 \text{ mg}}{2 \text{ mg}} = \frac{x \text{ mL}}{1 \text{ mL}}$$

$$2x = 1.5 \qquad\qquad 2x = 1.5$$

$$x = 0.75 \text{ or } 0.8 \text{ mL} \qquad x = 0.75 \text{ or } 0.8 \text{ mL}$$

To administer Ativan 1.5 mg IM, the nurse would inject 0.8 mL. Mark the syringe in Figure 17-5 to show the required dose.

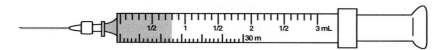

Figure 17-5
Note: This illustration of a 3 mL syringe will be repeated throughout the chapter so students can mark the correct drug dosages.

The syringe should look like Figure 17-6.

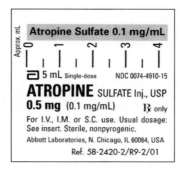

Figure 17-6

Example: A patient is to receive atropine sulfate 80 mcg IM. Available is a vial labeled atropine 0.1 mg/mL (see atropine label). How much of the atropine 0.1 mg/mL should the nurse administer?

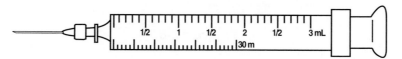

Atropine Sulfate 0.1 mg/mL

5 mL Single-dose   NDC 0074-4910-15
ATROPINE SULFATE Inj., USP
0.5 mg (0.1 mg/mL)   ℞ only
For I.V., I.M. or S.C. use. Usual dosage:
See insert. Sterile, nonpyrogenic.
Abbott Laboratories, N. Chicago, IL 60064, USA
Ref. 58-2420-2/R9-2/01

Solution: First convert the desired dosage and the available dosage to the same unit of measure.

80 mcg = 0.08 mg *or* 0.1 mg = 100 mcg

With the desired dosage and the available dosage in the same unit of measure, the problem can be set up by using the proportion:

$$\frac{\text{Desired Dosage}}{\text{Have Dosage}} = \frac{\text{Desired Amount}}{\text{Have Amount}}$$

$$\frac{80 \text{ mcg}}{100 \text{ mcg}} = \frac{x \text{ mL}}{1 \text{ mL}} \quad \text{or} \quad \frac{0.08 \text{ mg}}{0.1 \text{ mg}} = \frac{x \text{ mL}}{1 \text{ mL}}$$

$$100x = 80 \qquad\qquad 0.1x = 0.08$$

$$x = 0.8 \text{ mL} \qquad\qquad x = 0.8 \text{ mL}$$

To administer atropine 80 mcg IM, the nurse would inject 0.8 mL. Mark the syringe in Figure 17-7 to show the required dose.

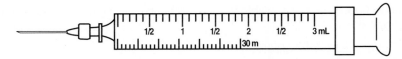

Figure 17-7

The syringe should look like Figure 17-8.

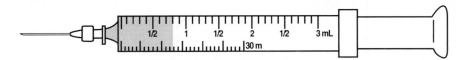

Figure 17-8

Example: A patient is to receive meperidine hydrochloride 75 mg by injection IM. Available is a vial labeled meperidine 100 mg/mL (see meperidine label). How much of the meperidine 100 mg/mL should the nurse administer?

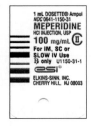

Solution: With the desired dosage and the available dosage in the same unit of measure, the problem can be set up by using the proportion:

$$\frac{\text{Desired Dosage}}{\text{Have Dosage}} = \frac{\text{Desired Amount}}{\text{Have Amount}}$$

$$\frac{75 \text{ mg}}{100 \text{ mg}} = \frac{x \text{ mL}}{1 \text{ mL}}$$

$$100x = 75$$

$$x = 0.75 \text{ mL}$$

To administer meperidine 75 mg IM, the nurse would inject 0.75 mL. Mark the model syringe in Figure 17-9 to show the required dose.

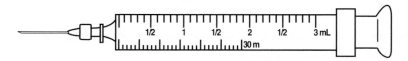

Figure 17-9

The syringe should look like Figure 17-10.

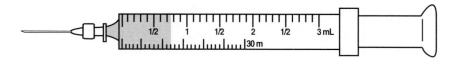

Figure 17-10

Problem Set 17.1

1. A patient is to receive hydroxyzine hydrochloride Vistaril 70 mg IM. The multidose vial on hand is labeled:

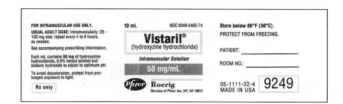

The nurse should inject _____ mL.

Set the model syringe or mark the syringe in Figure 17-11 to show the required dose.

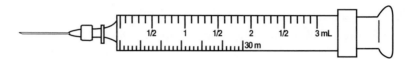

Figure 17-11

2. A patient is to receive furosemide 20 mg IM. The multidose vial on hand is labeled:

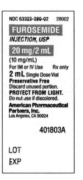

The nurse should inject _____ mL.

Mark the syringe in Figure 17-12 to show the required dose.

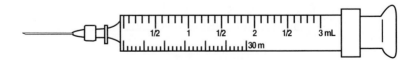

Figure 17-12

3. A patient is to receive dexamethasone (Decadron) 4.8 mg by injection IM. The vial on hand is labeled:

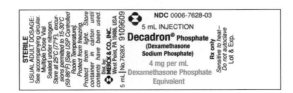

The nurse should inject _____ mL.

Set the model syringe or mark the syringe in Figure 17-13 to show the required dose.

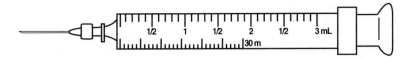

Figure 17-13

4. A patient is to receive clindamycin phosphate (Cleocin Phosphate) 250 mg by injection IM. The multidose vial on hand is labeled:

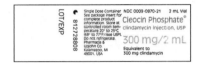

The nurse should inject _____ mL.

Mark the syringe in Figure 17-14 to show the required dose.

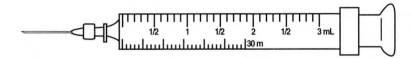

Figure 17-14

5. A patient is to receive prochlorperazine (Compazine) 8 mg IM. The vial on hand is labeled:

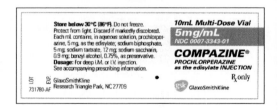

The nurse should inject _____ mL.

Mark the syringe in Figure 17-15 to show the required dose.

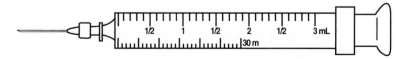

Figure 17-15

6. A patient is to receive morphine sulfate 15 mg by injection IM. The vial on hand is labeled:

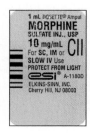

The nurse should inject _____ mL.

Mark the syringe in Figure 17-16 to show the required dose.

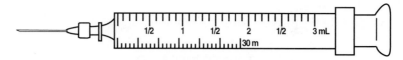

Figure 17-16

7. A patient is to receive cimetidine hydrochloride (Tagamet) 0.2 g by injection IM. The multidose vial on hand is labeled:

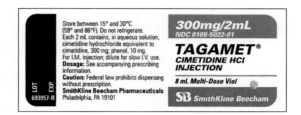

The nurse should inject _____ mL.

Mark the syringe in Figure 17-17 to show the required dose.

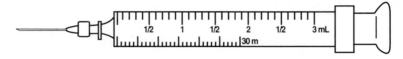

Figure 17-17

8. A patient is to receive lorazepam (Ativan) 1 mg IM. The multidose vial on hand is labeled:

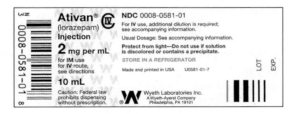

The nurse should inject _____ mL.

Mark the syringe in Figure 17-18 to show the required dose.

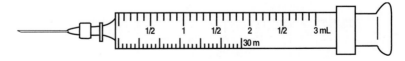

Figure 17-18

9. A patient is to receive 50% magnesium sulfate 1000 mg IM. The multidose vial is labeled 50% magnesium sulfate Inj. 4 mEq per mL:

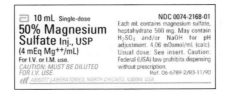

How many mg of magnesium sulfate are contained in each mL? _____

The nurse should inject _____ mL.

Mark the syringe in Figure 17-19 to show the required dose.

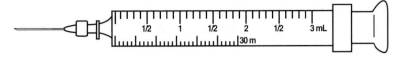

Figure 17-19

10. A patient is to receive meperidine 75 mg IM. The vial on hand is labeled:

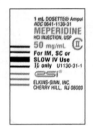

The nurse should inject _____ mL.

Mark the syringe in Figure 17-20 to show the required dose.

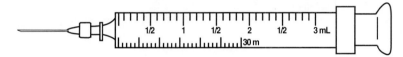

Figure 17-20

Answers: **1.** To administer Vistaril 70 mg by IM injection, the nurse should withdraw 1.4 mL from the multidose vial labeled Vistaril 50 mg/mL. The syringe should look like Figure 17-21.

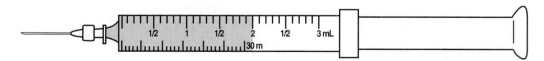

Figure 17-21

2. To administer furosemide 20 mg/2 mL by IM injection, the nurse should withdraw 2 mL from the multidose vial. The syringe should look like Figure 17-22.

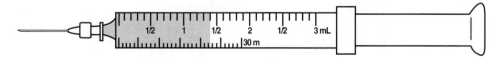

Figure 17-22

3. To administer Decadron 4.8 mg by IM injection, the nurse should withdraw 1.2 mL from the vial labeled Decadron 4 mg per mL. The syringe should look like Figure 17-23.

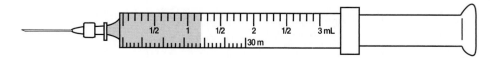

Figure 17-23

4. To administer Cleocin Phosphate 250 mg by IM injection, the nurse should withdraw 1.7 mL from the multidose vial labeled Cleocin Phosphate 300 mg/2 mL. The syringe should look like Figure 17-24.

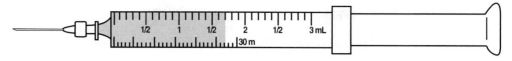

Figure 17-24

5. To administer Compazine 8 mg by IM injection, the nurse should withdraw 1.6 mL from the vial labeled Compazine 5 mL/mL. The syringe should look like Figure 17-25.

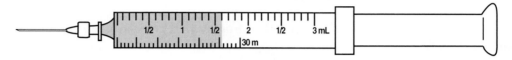

Figure 17-25

6. To administer morphine 15 mg by IM injection, the nurse should withdraw 1.5 mL from vials labeled morphine 10 mg per mL (2 vials). The syringe should look like Figure 17-26.

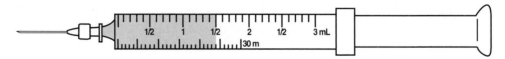

Figure 17-26

7. To administer Tagamet 0.2 g by IM injection, the nurse should withdraw 1.3 mL from the multidose vial labeled Tagamet 300 mg/2 mL (remember, 0.2 g = 200 mg). The syringe should look like Figure 17-27.

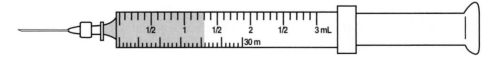

Figure 17-27

8. To administer Ativan 1 mg by IM injection, the nurse should withdraw 0.5 mL from the multidose vial labeled Ativan 2 mg per mL. The syringe should look like Figure 17-28.

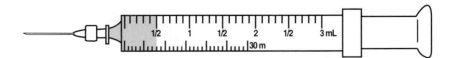

Figure 17-28

9. Each mL of 50% magnesium sulfate contains 500 mg. To administer 1000 mg by IM injection, the nurse should withdraw 2 mL from the vial labeled 50% magnesium sulfate 4 mEq Mg++/mL. The syringe should look like Figure 17-29.

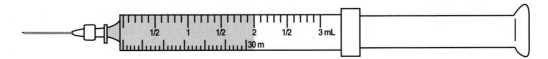

Figure 17-29

10. To administer meperidine 75 mg by IM injection, the nurse should withdraw 1.5 mL from the vials labeled meperidine 50 mg/mL (2 vials). The syringe should look like Figure 17-30.

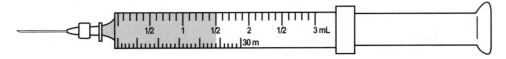

Figure 17-30

PART 2 Reconstitution of Powdered Parenteral Medication

Some drugs are extremely unstable in liquid form. Other drugs require constant refrigeration once they are dissolved to maintain stability. To store and ship these drugs with relative ease, they are generally supplied in a powdered form and must be dissolved in a diluent before they can be used. It is always important to read the literature packaged with the drug for instructions regarding the type and amount of diluent to be added.

Some drugs dissolve completely in the diluent and do not add any volume to the amount of diluent added. Other powdered drugs take up actual fluid space and increase the amount of total fluid (volume) in the mixed form of the drug beyond the amount of diluent added. This is called the displacement factor and must be accounted for in order to administer the correct amount of medication. Whether a drug has a displacement factor can always be determined from the manufacturer's label or from the product information insert.

Whenever a nurse reconstitutes a medication where all the medication will not be administered in a single dose or discarded, a label must be attached to the bottle containing the following information:

- The amount and type of diluent added
- The strength of the resulting mixture
- The date and time reconstitution occurred
- The initials of the nurse performing the reconstitution
- The patient's name and room number, if applicable

Example: The directions on the label of a vial containing 1 g of a powdered drug read:

Add 3.5 mL of sterile water (diluent) to produce a solution where 1 mL = 0.25 g of the drug.

Solution: If 1 mL = 0.25 g of the drug, 4 mL = 1 g of the drug. Because only 3.5 mL of diluent was added, it is obvious that the drug itself must have a displacement factor of 0.5 mL. The presence of the displacement factor emphasizes the importance of reading the manufacturer's label. This bottle should be labeled:

3.5 mL of sterile water added

1 mL = 0.25 g

Mixed 5/30 at 10:30 AM

DFS

V I P

- Always read the manufacturer's label or the drug insert before mixing the drug.
- Follow directions for the type and amount of diluent to be added, if provided by the manufacturer.
- When reconstituting powdered medication for intramuscular use, and the amount of diluent to be added is not stated by the manufacturer, try to limit the amount of diluent to be added so that the desired dose of medication is contained in between 1 mL and 2 mL of the resulting solution. This limits the amount of fluid that must be injected.

■ If the drug has a displacement factor, use the manufacturer's figures of drug strength in setting up the proportion.

■ Label the vial of mixed medication with the type and amount of diluent added, strength of the reconstituted solution, the date and time mixed, and the nurse's initials.

Example: A patient is to receive hydrocortisone sodium succinate (Solu-Cortef) 85 mg by injection IM. Available is a multidose vial that contains 100 mg of hydrocortisone sodium succinate powder for injection (see Solu-Cortef label). How would the nurse reconstitute the powdered medication and how much of the resulting solution should the patient receive?

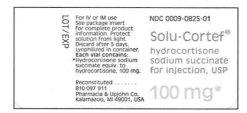

Solution: Before proceeding, always read and follow any directions supplied by the manufacturer either on the vial itself or on the product information sheet supplied with the vial. These directions may specify the sterile diluent to be used and/or the amount of the sterile diluent to be added.

It is not necessary to convert in this problem, because the desired dosage and the available dosage are in the same unit of measure. The next step is to set up the proportion; however, in this instance the medication for injection must be changed from a powder into a liquid. The reconstitution of the medication is accomplished by dissolving the powder in a sterile diluent, usually sterile water. When dissolving any powdered medication, to avoid a too heavily concentrated solution (and in the absence of specific manufacturer's direction as to the amount of fluid to be added), a minimum of 1 mL of diluent should be used. The maximum amount of medication for intramuscular injection is usually 3 mL, and it is rarely necessary or desirable to use more than this amount. In this situation, the patient is to receive 85 mg and the vial contains 100 mg of powder, so only part of the contents of the vial will be used. If 2 mL of sterile water is added to the vial, a solution of hydrocortisone sodium succinate where 100 mg = 2 mL will result. The problem can be set up using the proportion:

$$\frac{\text{Desired Dosage}}{\text{Have Dosage}} = \frac{\text{Desired Amount}}{\text{Have Amount}}$$

$$\frac{85 \text{ mg}}{100 \text{ mg}} = \frac{x \text{ mL}}{2 \text{ mL}}$$

$$100x = 170$$

$$x = 1.7 \text{ mL}$$

To administer 85 mg of hydrocortisone sodium succinate by IM injection, the nurse should add 2 mL of sterile water to the vial and inject 1.7 mL. The remaining solution should be discarded.

Mark the syringe in Figure 17-31 to show the required dose.

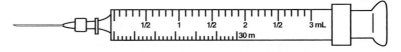

Figure 17-31

The syringe should look like Figure 17-32.

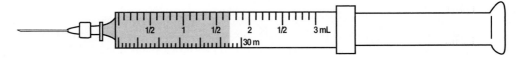

Figure 17-32

Example: A patient is to receive cefazolin sodium (Ancef) 250 mg by injection IM. Available is a multidose vial of powdered drug labeled Ancef 1 g powder for injection (see Ancef label). How would the nurse reconstitute the powdered medication and how much of the resulting solution should the patient receive?

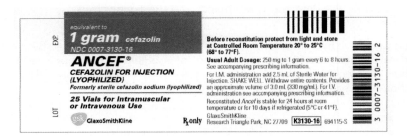

equivalent to
1 gram *cefazolin*
NDC 0007-3130-16
ANCEF®
CEFAZOLIN FOR INJECTION (LYOPHILIZED)
Formerly sterile cefazolin sodium (lyophilized)

25 Vials for Intramuscular or Intravenous Use

gsk **GlaxoSmithKline**

R̲ only

Before reconstitution protect from light and store at Controlled Room Temperature 20° to 25°C (68° to 77°F).

Usual Adult Dosage: 250 mg to 1 gram every 6 to 8 hours. See accompanying prescribing information.

For I.M. administration add 2.5 mL of Sterile Water for Injection. SHAKE WELL. Withdraw entire contents. Provides an approximate volume of 3.0 mL (330 mg/mL). For I.V. administration see accompanying prescribing information.

Reconstituted *Ancef* is stable for 24 hours at room temperature or for 10 days if refrigerated (5°C or 41°F).

GlaxoSmithKline
Research Triangle Park, NC 27709 [K3130-16] 694115-S

Solution: To see if the available vial of drug contains the desired dose, convert the 1 g to mg:

1 g = 1000 mg

Next determine how much diluent should be added. In this instance, simply follow the directions of the manufacturer and add 2.5 mL of sterile water to produce a solution where 3 mL of solution contains 1 g of Ancef (330 mg = 1 mL). Recognize that the dissolved powdered Ancef has added 0.5 mL to the volume of the solution produced (displacement factor). After adding the diluent, use the manufacturer's figures in setting up the proportion, not the amount of diluent actually added. The proportion can be set up as follows:

$$\frac{\text{Desired Dosage}}{\text{Have Dosage}} = \frac{\text{Desired Amount}}{\text{Have Amount}}$$

$$\frac{250 \text{ mg}}{330 \text{ mg}} = \frac{x \text{ mL}}{1 \text{ mL}}$$

$$330x = 250$$

$$x = 0.75 \text{ or } 0.8 \text{ mL}$$

To administer Ancef 250 mg using a multidose vial labeled 1 g, the nurse should add 2.5 mL of sterile water to the vial and withdraw 0.8 mL of solution for administration to the patient. When a diluent is added to a multidose vial, it is important that the vial be carefully labeled with the strength of the solution it contains and the date and time of mixing. The label attached to this vial should read: 250 mg or 0.25 g = 0.8 mL.

Mark the syringe in Figure 17-33 to show the required dose.

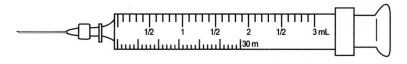

Figure 17-33

The syringe should look like Figure 17-34.

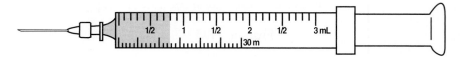

Figure 17-34

Example: A patient is to receive penicillin G potassium (Pfizerpen) 250,000 units for injection IM. Available is a multidose vial of powdered drug labeled penicillin G potassium for injection 5 million (see Pfizerpen label). How would the nurse reconstitute the powdered medication and how much of the resulting solution should the patient receive?

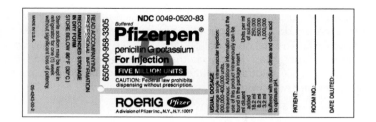

Solution: First determine how much diluent should be added. In this instance, simply follow the directions on the manufacturer's label on the vial of Pfizerpen 5 million units that reads: add 18.2 mL of diluent to provide 250,000 units per milliliter. It is important that the vial be labeled, once the diluent has been added, with the units per milliliter and the date and time the solution was mixed. To administer potassium penicillin G 250,000 units using a multidose vial of powder labeled 5,000,000 units, the nurse should follow the manufacturer's direction and add 18.2 mL of sterile water and withdraw 1 mL of solution for administration to the patient. The vial should be labeled 250,000 units = 1 mL. Recognize that the dissolved powdered penicillin has added 1.8 mL for a total volume of 20 mL. After adding the diluent, use the manufacturer's figures in setting up the proportion. The proportion can be set up as follows:

$$\frac{\text{Desired Dosage}}{\text{Have Dosage}} = \frac{\text{Desired Amount}}{\text{Have Amount}}$$

$$\frac{250,000 \text{ units}}{5,000,000 \text{ units}} = \frac{x \text{ mL}}{20 \text{ mL}}$$

$$5,000,000x = 5,000,000$$

$$x = 1 \text{ mL}$$

Mark the syringe in Figure 17-35 to show the required dose.

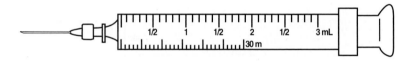

Figure 17-35

The syringe should look like Figure 17.36.

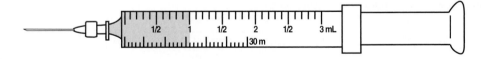

Figure 17-36

Example: A patient is to receive chlordiazepoxide HCl (Librium) 75 mg by injection IM. Available is a duplex package that contains a vial of powdered drug labeled Librium 100 mg and a 2 mL ampule of special intramuscular diluent (see Librium label). How would the nurse reconstitute the powdered medication and how much of the resulting solution should the patient receive?

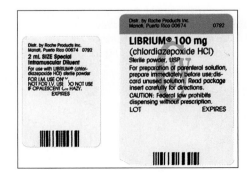

Solution: First determine how much diluent should be added. In this instance, simply follow the directions on the package insert that reads: add 2 mL of special intramuscular diluent to the 100 mg of powdered Librium to provide 100 mg per 2 mL. The vial need not be labeled once the diluent has been added because any unused solution must be discarded. Recognize that the dissolved powdered Librium has not added anything to the volume of the solution produced. After adding the diluent, use the manufacturer's figures in setting up the proportion. The proportion can be set up as follows:

$$\frac{\text{Desired Dosage}}{\text{Have Dosage}} = \frac{\text{Desired Amount}}{\text{Have Amount}}$$

$$\frac{75 \text{ mg}}{100 \text{ mg}} = \frac{x \text{ mL}}{2 \text{ mL}}$$

$$100x = 150$$

$$x = 1.5 \text{ mL}$$

To administer Librium 75 mg using a vial of powder labeled 100 mg, the nurse should follow the manufacturer's direction and add 2 mL of sterile water and withdraw 1.5 mL of solution for administration to the patient.

Mark the syringe in Figure 17-37 to show the required dose.

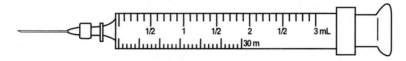

Figure 17-37

The syringe should look like Figure 17-38.

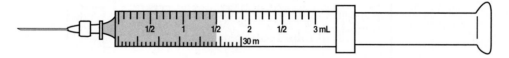

Figure 17-38

Example: A patient is to receive cefamandole (Mandol) 250 mg by injection IM. Available is a vial of powdered drug labeled Mandol 1 g. How would the nurse reconstitute the powdered medication and how much of the resulting solution should the patient receive?

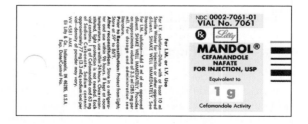

Solution: Convert the 1 g of Mandol to mg : 1 g = 1000 mg

First determine how much diluent should be added. In this instance, simply follow the directions: using the 1 g vial, add 3 mL of an approved diluent to produce a solution where 3.5 mL = 1 g or 1000 mg. Recognize that the dissolved powdered medication has added 0.5 mL to the total volume of the solution produced. After adding the diluent, use the manufacturer's figures in setting up the proportion. The proportion can be set up as follows:

$$\frac{\text{Desired Dosage}}{\text{Have Dosage}} = \frac{\text{Desired Amount}}{\text{Have Amount}}$$

$$\frac{250 \text{ mg}}{1000 \text{ mg}} = \frac{x \text{ mL}}{3.5 \text{ mL}}$$

$$1000x = 875$$

$$x = 0.875 \text{ or } 0.9 \text{ mL}$$

To administer Mandol 250 mg using a vial of powder labeled 1 g, the nurse should follow the manufacturer's direction and add 3 mL of diluent and withdraw 0.9 mL of solution for administration to the patient.

Mark the syringe in Figure 17-39 to show the required dose.

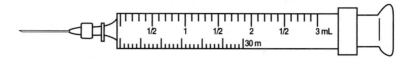

Figure 17-39

The syringe should look like Figure 17-40.

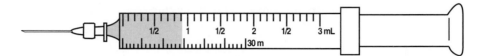

Figure 17-40

Problem Set 17.2

1. A patient is to receive cefazolin (Ancef) 750 mg IM by injection. The vial of powdered medication on hand is labeled Ancef 1 gram. The directions state: For IM administration add 2.5 mL of sterile water and shake to provide an approximate volume of 3 mL.

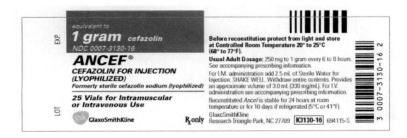

The nurse should inject _____ mL.

Mark the syringe in Figure 17-41 to show the required dose.

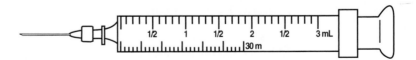

Figure 17-41

2. A patient is to receive cefamandole nafate (Mandol) 500 mg IM by injection. The vial of powdered medication on hand is labeled Mandol 1 gram. The directions state: For IM solution add 3 mL of sterile diluent to provide an approximate volume of 3.5 mL = 1 gram.

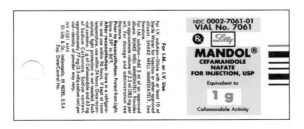

The nurse should inject _____ mL.

Mark the syringe in Figure 17-42 to show the required dose.

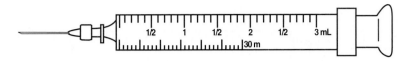

Figure 17-42

3. A patient is to receive cefotaxime sodium (Claforan) 630 mg IM by injection. The vial of powdered medication on hand is labeled Claforan 2 grams. The package insert states, for IM injection, to add 5 mL of sterile water to provide an approximate volume of 6 mL with a concentration of 330 mg per mL.

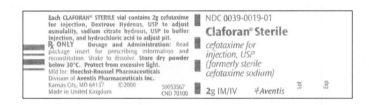

The nurse should inject _____ mL.

Mark the syringe in Figure 17-43 to show the required dose.

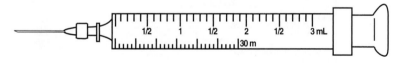

Figure 17-43

4. A patient is to receive cefotaxamine sodium (Claforan) 810 mg IM by injection. The vial of powdered medication is labeled Claforan 1 gram. The package insert states: For IM injection, add 3 mL of sterile water to produce an approximate volume of 3.4 mL containing 300 mg per mL.

The nurse should inject _____ mL.

Mark the syringe in Figure 17-44 to show the required dose.

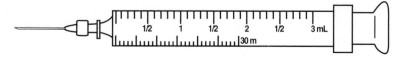

Figure 17-44

5. A patient is to receive methylprednisolone sodium (Solu-Medrol) 250 mg IM by injection. The Act-O-Vial of powdered medication on hand is labeled Solu-Medrol 500 mg. The directions state: For IM solution add 4 mL of provided diluent.

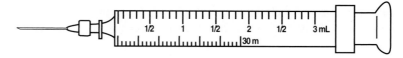

The nurse should inject _____ mL.

Mark the syringe in Figure 17-45 to show the required dose.

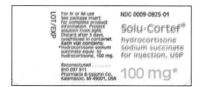

Figure 17-45

6. A patient is to receive hydrocortisone sodium succinate (Solu-Cortef) 0.1 g IM by injection. The vial of powdered medication on hand is labeled Solu-Cortef 100 mg. The directions state: Reconstitute with 2 mL of diluent to provide a volume of 2 mL.

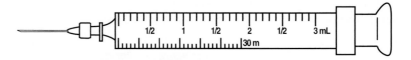

The nurse should inject _____ mL.

Mark the syringe in Figure 17-46 to show the required dose.

Figure 17-46

7. A patient is to receive penicillin G potassium (Pfizerpen) 1,000,000 units IM by injection. The multidose vial of powdered medication on hand is labeled penicillin G potassium 5 million units. The directions state: Reconstitute with 8.2 mL of diluent to provide 500,000 units of medication per mL.

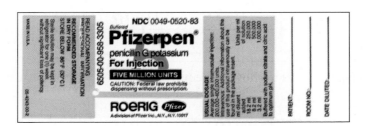

The nurse should inject _____ mL.

Mark the syringe in Figure 17-47 to show the required dose.

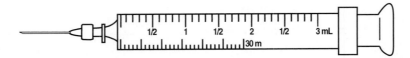

Figure 17-47

8. A patient is to receive penicillin G potassium (Pfizerpen) 450,000 units IM by injection. The vial of powdered medication on hand is labeled penicillin G potassium one million units. The directions state: Reconstitute with 4 mL of diluent to provide 250,000 units per mL.

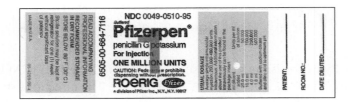

The nurse should inject _____ mL.

Mark the syringe in Figure 17-48 to show the required dose.

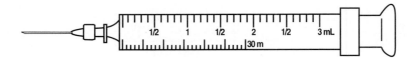

Figure 17-48

9. A patient is to receive chlordiazepoxide HCl (Librium) 25 mg IM by injection. The vial of powdered medication on hand is labeled Librium 100 mg. The directions state: Reconstitute with the 2 mL of special diluent included to provide an approximate volume of 2 mL.

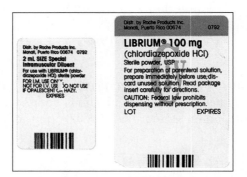

The nurse should inject _____ mL.

Mark the syringe in Figure 17-49 to show the required dose.

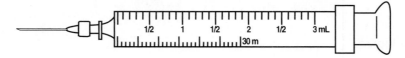

Figure 17-49

10. A patient is to receive cefazolin (Ancef) 500 mg IM by injection. The vial of powdered medication on hand is labeled Ancef 1 gram. The directions state: Reconstitute with 2.5 mL of sterile water for injection to provide an approximate volume of 3 mL.

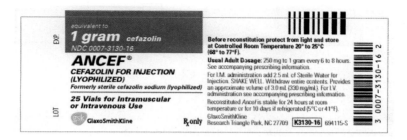

The nurse should inject _____ mL.

Mark the syringe in Figure 17-50 to show the required dose.

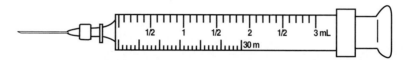

Figure 17-50

Answers: **1.** To administer Ancef 750 mg IM, the nurse should add 2.5 mL of sterile water to the 1 gram vial of powdered medication (because the directions state that this will produce an approximate volume of 3 mL of fluid, the Ancef powder has a displacement factor of 0.5 mL), shake, and withdraw 2.25 mL for injection. The syringe should look like Figure 17-51.

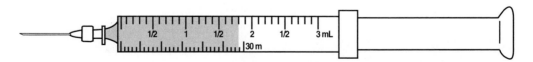

Figure 17-51

2. To administer cefamandole nafate (Mandol) 500 mg by injection from a vial of powdered medication labeled 1 gram, the nurse should add 3 mL of sterile diluent to provide an approximate volume of 3.5 mL, mix, and withdraw 1.75 or 1.8 mL from the vial for injection. The syringe should look like Figure 17-52.

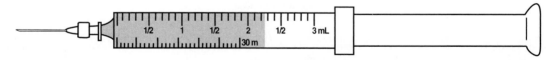

Figure 17-52

3. To administer cefotaxime sodium (Claforan) 630 mg by IM injection, the nurse should add 5 mL of sterile water to a vial of powdered Claforan 2 grams, which provides an approximate volume of 6 mL with a concentration of 330 mg per mL. The nurse should administer 1.9 mL for IM injection. The syringe should look like Figure 17-53.

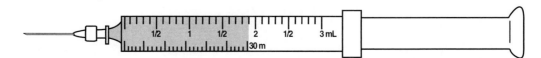

Figure 17-53

4. To administer cefotaxamine sodium (Claforan) 810 mg IM by injection from a vial of powdered medication labeled Claforan 1 gram, the nurse should add 3 mL of sterile water to yield a reconstituted solution of 3.4 mL, shake well, and withdraw 2.7 mL for injection. The syringe should look like Figure 17-54.

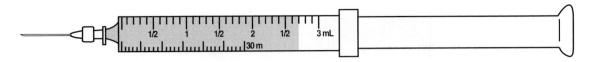

Figure 17-54

5. To administer methylprednisolone sodium (Solu-Medrol) 250 mg IM by injection from an Act-O-Vial of powdered medication labeled Solu-Medrol 500 mg, the nurse should add 4 mL of diluent, mix, and withdraw 2 mL for injection. The syringe should look like Figure 17-55.

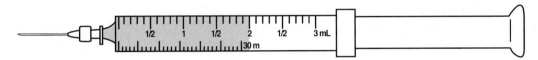

Figure 17-55

6. To administer Solu-Cortef 0.1 g IM by injection from a vial of powdered medication labeled Solu-Cortef 100 mg, the nurse should add 2 mL of diluent, shake well, and withdraw 2 mL for injection. The syringe should look like Figure 17-56.

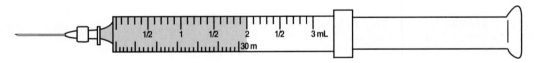

Figure 17-56

7. To administer penicillin G potassium (Pfizerpen) 1,000,000 units of IM by injection from a multidose vial of powdered medication labeled penicillin G potassium 5 million units, the nurse should add 8.2 mL producing a solution of 500,000 units per mL and withdraw 2 mL for injection. The syringe should look like Figure 17-57.

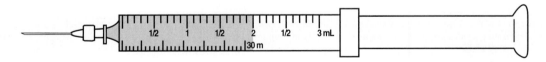

Figure 17-57

8. To administer penicillin G (Pfizerpen) 450,000 units IM by injection from a vial of powdered medication labeled Pfizerpen one million units, the nurse should add 4 mL of sterile water producing a solution of 250,000 units per mL, and withdraw 1.8 mL for injection. The syringe should look like Figure 17-58.

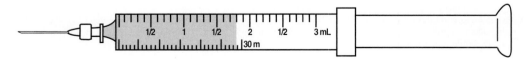

Figure 17-58

9. To administer chlordiazepoxide HCl (Librium) 25 mg IM by injection from a vial of powdered medication labeled Librium 100 mg, the nurse should add the 2 mL of special diluent included, shake to dissolve the powder, and withdraw 0.5 mL for injection. The syringe should look like Figure 17-59.

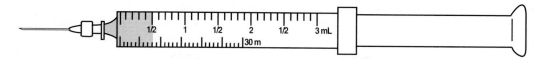

Figure 17-59

10. To administer cefazolin sodium (Ancef) 500 mg IM by injection from a vial of powdered medication labeled Ancef 1 g, the nurse should add 2.5 mL of sterile water for injection (because the directions state that this will produce an approximate volume of 3 mL of fluid, the Ancef powder has a displacement factor of 0.5 mL), shake well to dissolve the powder, and withdraw 1.5 mL for injection. The syringe should look like Figure 17-60.

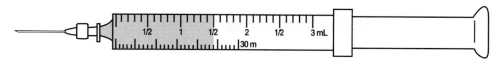

Figure 17-60

PART 3 Special Parenteral Medications

HEPARIN

Heparin sodium is an anticoagulant that inhibits the body's blood-clotting mechanism. The major routes of administration of this drug are intravenous (either intermittent injection or infusion), or deep subcutaneous. It is ineffective when given orally and is never given by intramuscular injection because of the danger of hematomas.

Heparin is supplied as a premixed liquid, measured in USP units. It is available in both single and multidose vials in a wide variety of strengths to reduce cumbersome calculations and dosage errors. The strengths available include: 1000 units per mL, 2500 units per mL, 5000 units per mL, 7500 units per mL, 10,000 units per mL, and 20,000 units per mL.

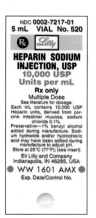
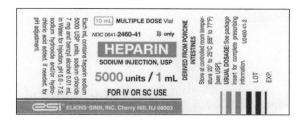
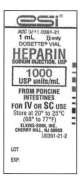

There is also a heparin lock-flush solution that is available in strengths of 10 units/mL and 100 units/mL. This solution is used to maintain patency of indwelling intravenous catheters. Heparin lock-flush solution is not intended to be used for anticoagulation therapy, as it is too dilute to be effective.

The physician will usually order Heparin in units, and an order in any other type of dose should be questioned before administration.

Because of the wide variety of strengths available and the bleeding potential associated with anticoagulant drugs, dosage is usually ordered on a daily basis and requires close monitoring of the patient's blood work. Orders must be carefully checked against the available dosage before calculating the amount to be administered.

These inherent dangers make it extremely important that the nurse exercise every precaution to administer the exact dosage prescribed. For this reason, a tuberculin syringe (a 1 mL syringe marked with tenths and hundredths mL) should be used when administering heparin. Hospital policies differ on the administration of heparin and the nurse is responsible for following these policies.

Example: A patient is to receive 4000 units of heparin sodium by subcutaneous injection. Available is a 4 mL multidose vial labeled 10,000 units = 1 mL (see heparin sodium label). How much of the heparin sodium 10,000 units = 1 mL should the nurse administer?

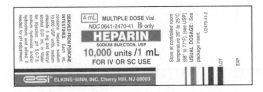

Solution: With the desired dosage and the available dosage in the same unit of measure (units), the problem can be set up by using the proportion:

$$\frac{\text{Desired Dosage}}{\text{Have Dosage}} = \frac{\text{Desired Amount}}{\text{Have Amount}}$$

$$\frac{4000 \text{ units}}{10,000 \text{ units}} = \frac{x \text{ mL}}{1 \text{ mL}}$$

$$10,000x = 4000$$

$$x = 0.4 \text{ mL}$$

To administer heparin sodium 4000 units subcutaneously from a 4 mL multidose vial labeled 10,000 units = 1 mL, the nurse would inject 0.4 mL.

Mark the syringe in Figure 17-61 to show the required dose.

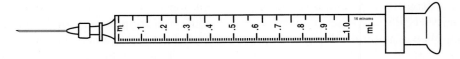

Figure 17-61

The syringe should look like Figure 17-62.

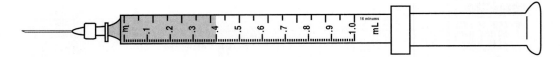

Figure 17-62

Example: A patient is to receive 2000 units of heparin sodium by subcutaneous injection. Available is a 1 mL dosette vial labeled heparin sodium 10,000 units per mL (see heparin sodium label). How much of the heparin sodium 10,000 units/mL should the nurse administer?

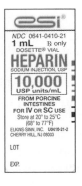

Solution: With the desired dosage and the available dosage in the same unit of measure (units), the problem can be set up by using the proportion:

$$\frac{\text{Desired Dosage}}{\text{Have Dosage}} = \frac{\text{Desired Amount}}{\text{Have Amount}}$$

$$\frac{2000 \text{ units}}{10,000 \text{ units}} = \frac{x \text{ mL}}{1 \text{ mL}}$$

$$10,000x = 2000$$

$$x = 0.2 \text{ mL}$$

To administer heparin sodium 2000 units subcutaneously from a 1 mL dosette vial labeled 10,000 units/mL, the nurse would inject 0.2 mL and discard the rest.

Mark the syringe in Figure 17-63 to show the required dose.

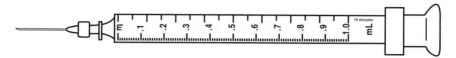

Figure 17-63

The syringe should look like Figure 17-64.

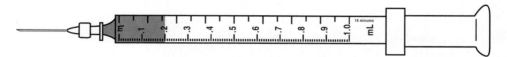

Figure 17-64

Example: A patient is to receive 500 units of heparin sodium by subcutaneous injection. Available is a vial labeled heparin sodium 1000 units per mL (see heparin sodium label). How much of the heparin sodium 1000 units/mL should the nurse administer?

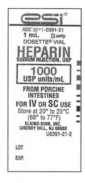

Solution: With the desired dosage and the available dosage in the same unit of measure (units), the problem can be set up by using the proportion:

$$\frac{\text{Desired Dosage}}{\text{Have Dosage}} = \frac{\text{Desired Amount}}{\text{Have Amount}}$$

$$\frac{500 \text{ units}}{1000 \text{ units}} = \frac{x \text{ mL}}{1 \text{ mL}}$$

$$1000x = 500$$

$$x = 0.5 \text{ mL}$$

To administer heparin sodium 500 units subcutaneously from a vial labeled 1000 units/mL, the nurse would inject 0.5 mL and discard the rest.

Mark the syringe in Figure 17-65 to show the required dose.

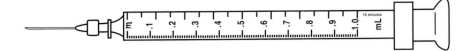

Figure 17-65

The syringe should look like Figure 17-66.

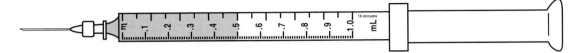

Figure 17-66

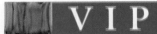

VIP

- Heparin is supplied as a premixed liquid, measured in USP units.
- Heparin orders must be carefully checked against the available dosage before calculating the amount to be administered.
- A tuberculin syringe (a 1 mL syringe marked with tenths and hundredths mL measurements) with a $\frac{1}{2}$ inch needle should be used when administering heparin.
- Heparin sodium for injection and heparin lock-flush solution are different and should never be used interchangeably.

INSULIN

Insulin is a pharmacologic preparation that is used as a substitute for the naturally occurring hormone. Insulin is used in the treatment of some forms of insulin-dependent diabetes mellitus. The major route of administration of this drug is by subcutaneous injection, although regular insulin can be given intravenously. Insulin is destroyed by gastric secretions and therefore cannot be given orally. Insulin is never given intramuscularly because of delayed, irregular absorption and potential damage to muscle tissue.

Insulin is supplied as a premixed liquid, measured in USP units. It is available in multidose vials and insulin delivery pens or cartridges that vary in source, type of action, and strength per mL.

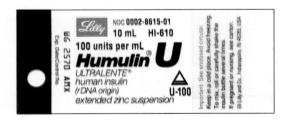

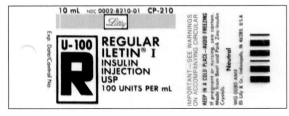

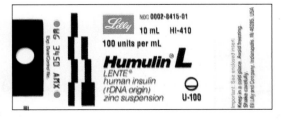

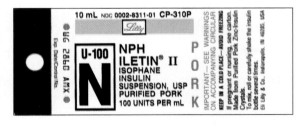

The physician will usually order insulin by source, type, and units. An order without this information must be questioned before administration.

Source of Insulin

The source of insulin refers to the origin of the insulin utilized by the drug manufacturer and is always clearly listed on the label (see Humulin U, Purified Pork R, Iletin, and Humulin L labels). The sources include human, pork, beef, or a combination of pork and beef. Today, the most commonly used source is human insulin, which has fewer side effects. Many manufacturers have incorporated the source of their insulin into their trade names. For example, Eli Lilly calls its human insulin, Humulin. The source of Eli Lilly's Iletin I is a combination of beef and pork, while the source of Iletin II is purified pork.

The nurse must recognize and must teach the patient never to substitute one source or even one brand of insulin for another without medical supervision.

Insulin should be administered at room temperature (avoid extremes of temperature), and should never be used when the expiration date has passed.

Type of Insulin

The type of insulin relates to both the onset and the duration of action, not the source.

Extremely Fast-Acting.   Onset within 10 to 15 minutes, peaks in 30 to 90 minutes, and has a duration of less than 6 hours (Humalog [Insulin lispro rDNA origin]).

Fast-Acting.   Onset within 30 minutes, peaks in $2\frac{1}{2}$ to 5 hours, and ends in 8 hours; signified by the letter "R" for Regular or Semilente (see Regular Iletin and Humulin R labels).

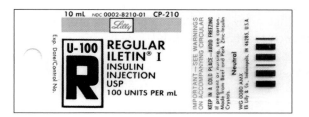
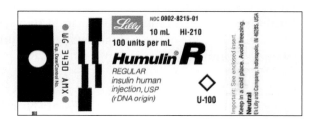

Intermediate-Acting.   Onset $1\frac{1}{2}$ to $2\frac{1}{2}$ hours, peaks in 4 to 15 hours, and ends in 16 to 24 hours; signified by the letter "L" for Lente (an insulin zinc suspension) or "N" for NPH (an isophane insulin suspension).

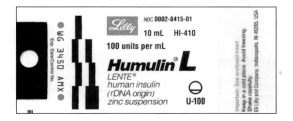
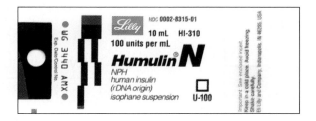

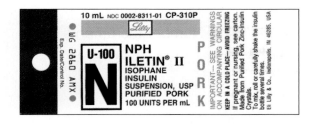

Long-Acting. Onset 4 hours, peaks in 10 to 30 hours, and ends in 36 hours; signified by a letter "U" for Ultralente (an extended insulin zinc suspension) (see Humulin U label).

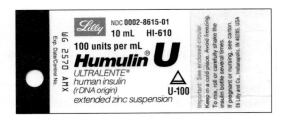

Longer-Acting. Onset 1 hour, no true peak, and a duration of 24 hours; acts as a basal insulin, for example Lantus (insulin glargine [rDNA origin] injection).

Mixtures of Human Insulin. 70/30 is a mixture of 70% NPH insulin and 30% regular; 50/50 is a mixture of 50% NPH insulin and 50% regular insulin (see label).

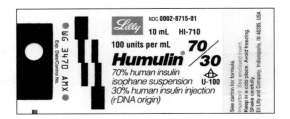

Strength of Insulin

The most commonly prepared strength of insulin is 100 units per milliliter, which is the most frequently used strength. A 500 unit strength insulin is also available for patients who are markedly insulin resistant.

Insulin should be administered with an insulin syringe that is specially calibrated for 100 units in unit increments, with one side of the syringe having odd-number increments and the other side having even-number increments (Figure 17-67).

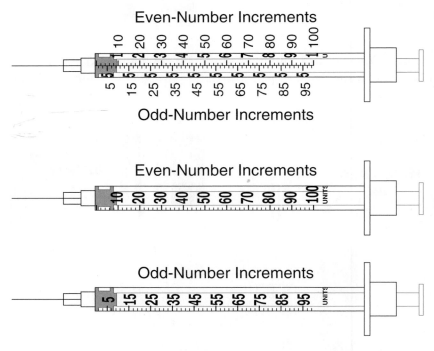

Figure 17-67 Insulin syringes

Low-dose insulin syringes measuring 50 units (0.5 mL) and 30 units (0.3 mL) are also calibrated in increments of 1 unit and should be used for measuring small doses. In an emergency, if an insulin syringe is not available, a 1 mL tuberculin syringe, which is also calibrated for measuring smaller doses accurately, must be used (Figure 17-68). No specific syringe is available for administering 500 units per mL strength insulin, so a tuberculin syringe must be used.

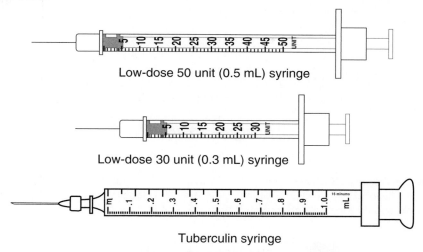

Low-dose 50 unit (0.5 mL) syringe

Low-dose 30 unit (0.3 mL) syringe

Tuberculin syringe

Figure 17-68   Low-dose and tuberculin syringes

Example: A patient is to receive 60 units of regular insulin (Humulin R) by SC injection. Available is a multidose vial of Humulin R insulin labeled 100 units per mL (see Humulin R label). How much of the Humulin R insulin 100 units per mL should the nurse administer?

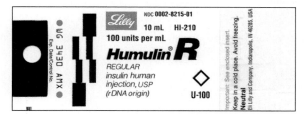

Solution: Because the dosage desired and the dosage available are in units, the problem can be set up using the proportion:

$$\frac{\text{Desired Dosage}}{\text{Have Dosage}} = \frac{\text{Desired Amount}}{\text{Have Amount}}$$

$$\frac{60 \text{ units}}{100 \text{ units}} = \frac{x \text{ mL}}{1 \text{ mL}}$$

$$100x = 60$$

$$x = 0.6 \text{ mL}$$

To administer regular insulin 60 units SC using a multidose vial labeled Humulin R insulin 100 units per mL, the nurse should withdraw 60 units using the insulin syringe, or 0.6 mL using the tuberculin syringe, for administration to the patient.

Mark the syringes in Figure 17-69 to show the required dose in both the insulin and tuberculin syringes.

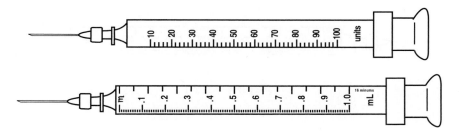

Figure 17-69

The syringes should look like Figure 17-70.

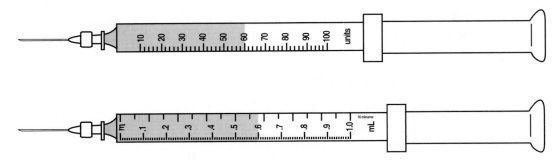

Figure 17-70

Example: A patient is to receive 26 units of Humulin U (Ultralente human insulin). Available is a multidose vial of Humulin U insulin labeled 100 units per mL (see Humulin U label). How much of the Humulin U insulin 100 units per mL should the nurse administer?

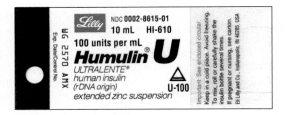

Solution: Because the dosage desired and the dosage available are in units, the problem can be set up using the proportion:

$$\frac{\text{Desired Dosage}}{\text{Have Dosage}} = \frac{\text{Desired Amount}}{\text{Have Amount}}$$

$$\frac{26 \text{ units}}{100 \text{ units}} = \frac{x \text{ mL}}{1 \text{ mL}}$$

$$100x = 26$$

$$x = 0.26 \text{ mL}$$

To administer Humulin U insulin 26 units SC using a multidose vial labeled Humulin U (Ultralente human insulin) 100 units per mL, the nurse should withdraw 26 units using the 100 unit insulin syringe, or 0.26 mL using the tuberculin syringe, for administration to the patient.

Mark the insulin and tuberculin syringes in Figure 17-71 to show the required dose.

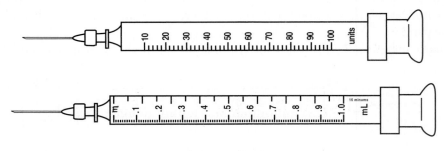

Figure 17-71

The insulin and tuberculin syringes should look like Figure 17-72.

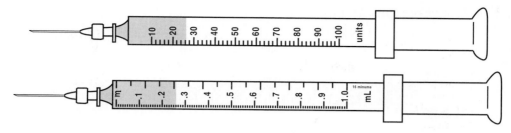

Figure 17-72

Example: A patient is to receive NPH human insulin (Humulin N) 7 units SC by injection. Available is a vial of Humulin N insulin labeled 100 units = 1 mL (see Humulin N label). How much of the Humulin N insulin 100 units per mL should the nurse administer?

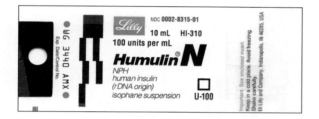

Solution: Because the dosage desired and the dosage available are in units, the problem can be set up using the proportion:

$$\frac{\text{Desired Dosage}}{\text{Have Dosage}} = \frac{\text{Desired Amount}}{\text{Have Amount}}$$

$$\frac{7 \text{ units}}{100 \text{ units}} = \frac{x \text{ mL}}{1 \text{ mL}}$$

$$100x = 7$$

$$x = 0.07 \text{ mL}$$

To administer NPH human insulin (Humulin N) 7 units SC using a multidose vial labeled Humulin N insulin 100 units per mL, the nurse should withdraw 7 units using a 50 unit Lo-Dose 100 unit insulin syringe, or 0.07 mL using the tuberculin syringe, for administration to the patient.

Mark the syringes in Figure 17-73 to show the required dose in both the 50 unit Lo-Dose 100 unit insulin and tuberculin syringes.

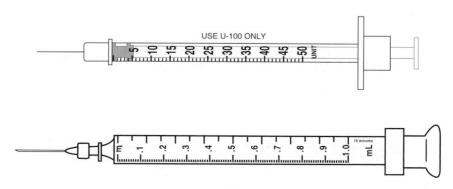

Figure 17-73

The syringes should look like Figure 17-74.

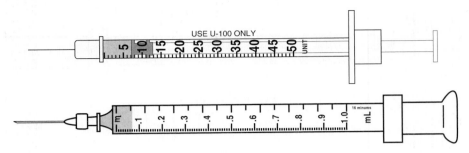

Figure 17-74

Example: A patient is to receive Humulin 70/30 insulin 80 units by SC injection. (Humulin 70/30 insulin 100 units per mL contains 70% or 70 units of NPH human insulin and 30% or 30 units of Regular human insulin). Available is a vial of Humulin 70/30 insulin labeled 100 units per 1 mL (see Humulin 70/30 label). How much of the Humulin 70/30 insulin 100 units per mL should the nurse administer?

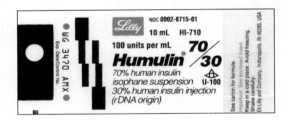

Solution: Because the dosage desired and the dosage available are in units, the problem can be set up using the proportion:

$$\frac{\text{Desired Dosage}}{\text{Have Dosage}} = \frac{\text{Desired Amount}}{\text{Have Amount}}$$

$$\frac{80 \text{ units}}{100 \text{ units}} = \frac{x \text{ mL}}{1 \text{ mL}}$$

$$100x = 80$$

$$x = 0.8 \text{ mL}$$

To administer Humulin 70/30 insulin 80 units SC using a multidose vial labeled Humulin 70/30 insulin 100 units per mL, the nurse should withdraw 80 units using the insulin syringe, or 0.8 mL using the tuberculin syringe, for administration to the patient.

Mark the syringes in Figure 17-75 to show the required dose in both the insulin and tuberculin syringes.

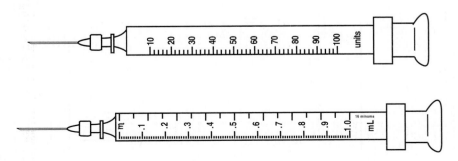

Figure 17-75

The syringes should look like Figure 17-76.

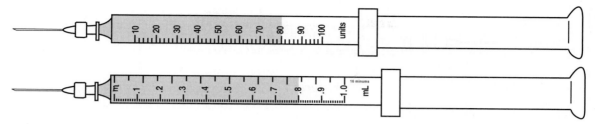

Figure 17-76

Problem Set 17.3

1. A patient is to receive heparin sodium 4000 units SC by injection. The multidose vial is labeled:

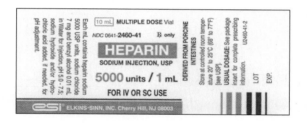

The nurse, using a tuberculin syringe, should administer _____ mL SC.
Mark the syringe in Figure 17-77 to show the required dose.

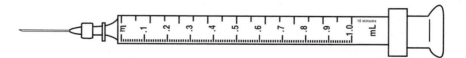

Figure 17-77

2. A patient is to receive heparin sodium 600 units SC by injection. The single-dose vial is labeled:

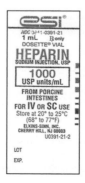

The nurse, using a tuberculin syringe, should administer _____ mL SC.

Mark the syringe in Figure 17-78 to show the required dose.

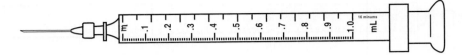

Figure 17-78

3. A patient is to receive heparin sodium 7500 units SC by injection. The single-dosette vial is labeled:

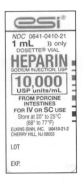

The nurse, using a tuberculin syringe, should administer _____ mL SC.

Mark the syringe in Figure 17-79 to show the required dose.

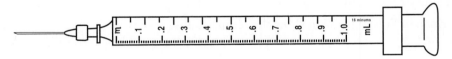

Figure 17-79

4. A patient is to receive heparin sodium 5000 units SC by injection. The multidose vial is labeled:

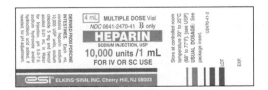

The nurse, using a tuberculin syringe, should administer _____ mL SC.

Mark the syringe in Figure 17-80 to show the required dose.

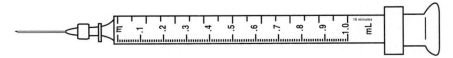

Figure 17-80

5. A patient is to receive heparin sodium 3000 units SC by injection. The multidose vial is labeled:

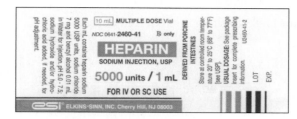

The nurse, using a tuberculin syringe, should administer _____ mL SC.

Mark the syringe in Figure 17-81 to show the required dose.

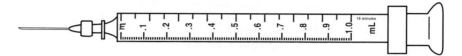

Figure 17-81

6. A patient is to receive Humulin L insulin 36 units SC by injection. The multidose vial of Humulin L insulin is labeled:

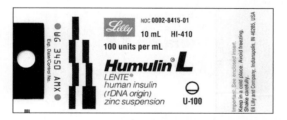

The nurse, using an insulin syringe, should administer _____ units;
or, using a tuberculin syringe, should administer _____ mL SC.

Mark the syringes in Figure 17-82 to show the required dose.

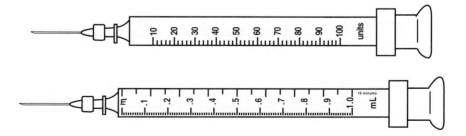

Figure 17-82

7. A patient is to receive Regular Iletin I insulin 13 units SC by injection. The multidose vial of Regular Iletin I insulin is labeled:

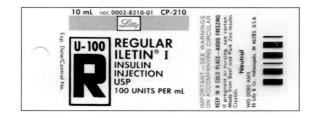

The nurse, using a Lo-Dose insulin syringe, should administer _____ units; or, using a tuberculin syringe, should administer _____ mL SC.

Mark the syringes in Figure 17-83 to show the required dose.

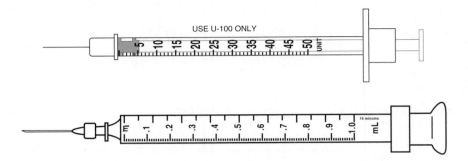

Figure 17-83

8. A patient is to receive Humulin U insulin 42 units SC by injection. The multidose vial of Humulin U insulin is labeled:

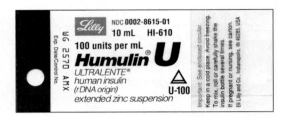

The nurse, using an insulin syringe, should administer _____ units; or, using a tuberculin syringe, should administer _____ mL SC.

Mark the syringes in Figure 17-84 to show the required dose.

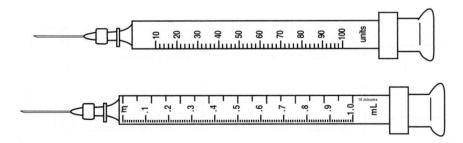

Figure 17-84

9. A patient is to receive Humulin 70/30 insulin 76 units SC by injection. The multidose vial of Humulin 70/30 insulin is labeled:

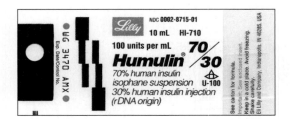

The nurse, using an insulin syringe, should administer _____ units; or, using a tuberculin syringe, should administer _____ mL SC.

Mark the syringes in Figure 17-85 to show the required dose.

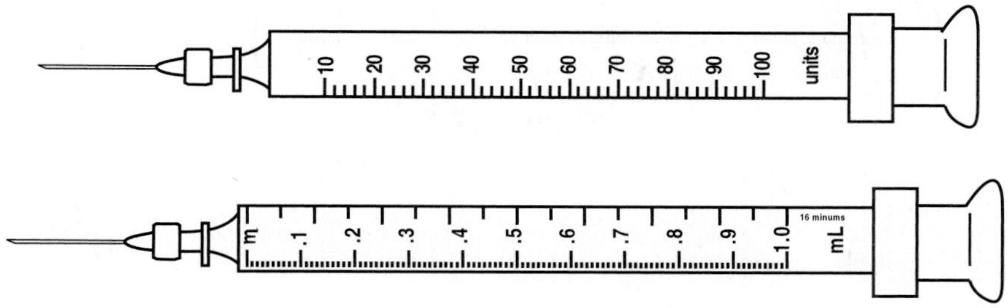

Figure 17-85

10. A patient is to receive Regular human insulin (Humulin R) 32 units SC by injection. The multidose vial of Humulin R insulin is labeled:

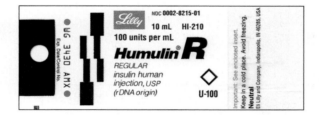

The nurse, using an insulin syringe, should administer _____ units; or, using a tuberculin syringe, should administer _____ mL SC.

Mark the syringes in Figure 17-86 to show the required dose.

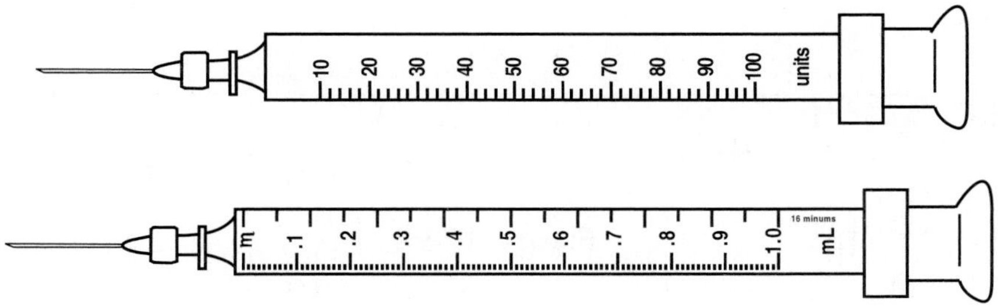

Figure 17-86

Answers: **1.** To administer heparin sodium 4000 units SC by injection from a 5000 unit/mL multidose vial, the nurse should withdraw 0.8 mL for injection. The tuberculin syringe should look like Figure 17-87.

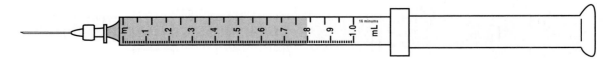

Figure 17-87

2. To administer heparin sodium 600 units SC by injection from a 1000 unit/mL single-dose vial, the nurse should withdraw 0.6 mL for injection. The tuberculin syringe should look like Figure 17-88.

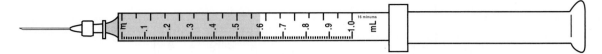

Figure 17-88

3. To administer heparin sodium 7500 units SC by injection from a 10,000 unit/mL single-dosette vial, the nurse should withdraw 0.75 mL for injection. The tuberculin syringe should look like Figure 17-89.

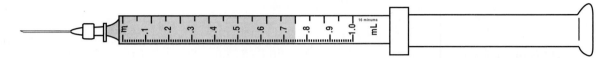

Figure 17-89

4. To administer heparin sodium 5000 units SC by injection from a 10,000 unit/mL multidose vial, the nurse should withdraw 0.5 mL for injection. The tuberculin syringe should look like Figure 17-90.

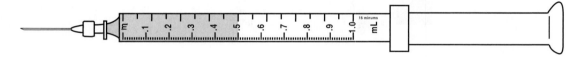

Figure 17-90

5. To administer heparin sodium 3000 units SC by injection from a 5000 unit/mL multidose vial, the nurse should withdraw 0.6 mL for injection. The tuberculin syringe should look like Figure 17-91.

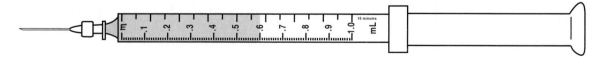

Figure 17-91

6. To administer Humulin L 36 units SC by injection from a 100 unit/mL multidose vial, the nurse should withdraw 36 units using the 100 unit insulin syringe and 0.36 mL using the tuberculin syringe. The syringes should look like Figure 17-92.

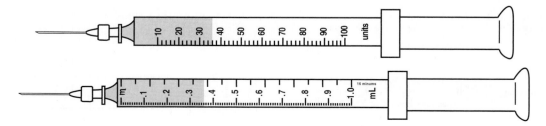

Figure 17-92

7. To administer Regular Iletin I 13 units SC by injection from a 100 unit/mL multidose vial, the nurse should withdraw 13 units using a 100 unit Lo-Dose insulin syringe and 0.13 mL using the tuberculin syringe. The syringes should look like Figure 17-93.

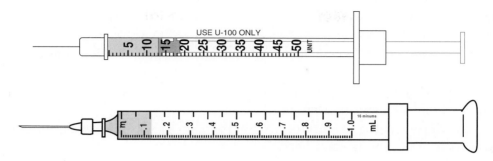

Figure 17-93

8. To administer Humulin U 42 units SC by injection from a 100 unit/mL multidose vial, the nurse should withdraw 42 units using the 100 unit insulin syringe and 0.42 mL using the tuberculin syringe. The syringes should look like Figure 17-94.

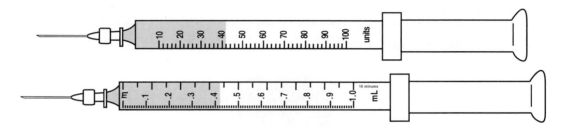

Figure 17-94

9. To administer Humulin 70/30 insulin 76 units SC by injection from a 100 unit/mL multidose vial, the nurse should withdraw 76 units using the 100 unit insulin syringe and 0.76 mL using the tuberculin syringe. The syringes should look like Figure 17-95.

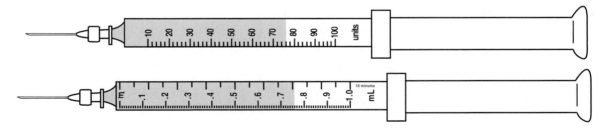

Figure 17-95

10. To administer Humulin R insulin 32 units SC by injection from a 100 unit/mL multidose vial, the nurse should withdraw 32 units using the insulin syringe or 0.32 mL using the tuberculin syringe. The syringes should look like Figure 17-96.

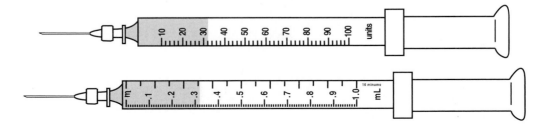

Figure 17-96

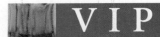

V I P

■ Insulin must be ordered by source, type, and units. An order without this information must be questioned before administration.

■ Never substitute one source or even one brand of insulin for another without medical supervision.

■ Insulin should be administered with a 100 unit insulin syringe that is specially calibrated in increments of units for measuring insulin.

■ Lo-Dose syringes measuring 50 units (0.5 mL) and 30 units (0.3 mL) of 100 unit strength insulin should be used for measuring small doses.

■ If an insulin syringe is not available, a 1 mL tuberculin syringe that is calibrated for measuring smaller doses accurately must be used.

Review Test 17.1
Parenteral Medications

1. A patient is to receive morphine sulfate 12 mg IM by injection. Available is a vial labeled:

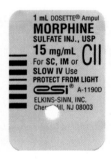

The nurse should administer _____ mL IM.

Mark the syringe in Figure 17-97 to show the required dose.

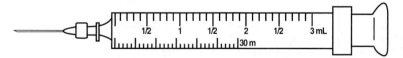

Figure 17-97

2. A patient is to receive tobramycin (Nebcin) 60 mg IM by injection. Available is a vial labeled:

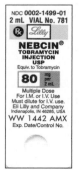

The nurse should administer _____ mL IM.

Mark the syringe in Figure 17-98 to show the required dose.

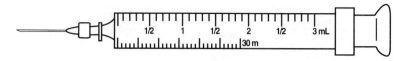

Figure 17-98

3. A patient is to receive meperidine hydrochloride 50 mg IM by injection. Available is a vial labeled:

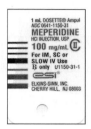

The nurse should administer _____ mL.

Mark the syringe in Figure 17-99 to show the required dose.

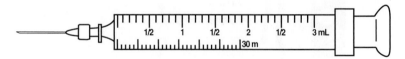

Figure 17-99

4. A patient is to receive cefazolin (Ancef) 500 mg IM every 6 hours. Available is a multidose vial of powdered medication that states: Add 2.5 mL of sterile water to provide a total solution of 3 mL.

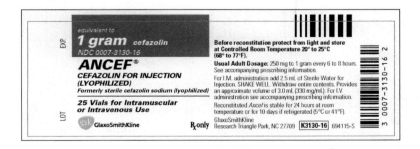

The nurse should administer _____ mL.

Mark the syringe in Figure 17-100 to show the required dose.

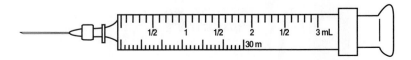

Figure 17-100

5. A patient is to receive hydroxyzine hydrochloride (Vistaril) 75 mg IM. Available is a multidose vial labeled:

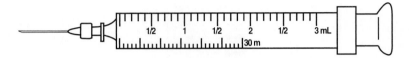

The nurse should administer _____ mL.

Mark the syringe in Figure 17-101 to show the required dose.

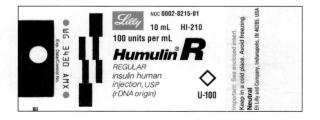

Figure 17-101

6. The patient is to receive 40 units of Humulin N insulin SC by injection. Available is a multidose vial labeled:

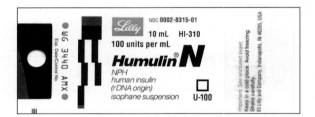

Using a 100 unit syringe, the nurse should administer _____ units.

Using a tuberculin syringe, the nurse should administer _____ mL.

Mark the syringes in Figure 17-102 to show the required dose.

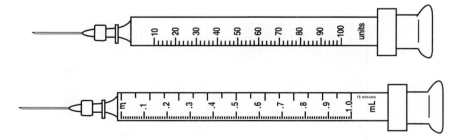

Figure 17-102

7. The patient is to receive Humulin R insulin 5 units SC by injection. Available is a multidose vial labeled:

Using a Lo-Dose insulin syringe measuring 50 units of 100 unit insulin, the nurse should administer _____ units.

Using a tuberculin syringe, the nurse should administer _____ mL.

Mark the syringes in Figure 17-103 to show the required dose.

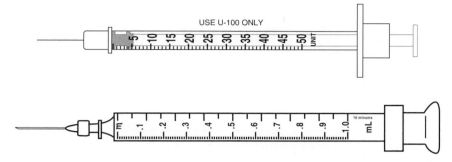

Figure 17-103

8. The patient is to receive penicillin G potassium 750,000 units IM. Available is a multidose vial of powdered medication that states: To reconstitute a 5,000,000 unit vial, add 8.2 mL of diluent to yield a solution that contains 500,000 units per mL.

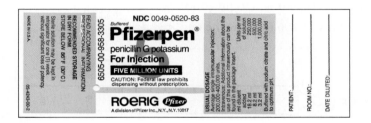

The nurse should administer _____ mL.

Mark the syringe in Figure 17-104 to show the required dose.

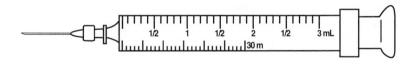

Figure 17-104

9. The patient is to receive atropine sulfate 0.17 mg IM. Available is a vial labeled 0.1 mg/mL.

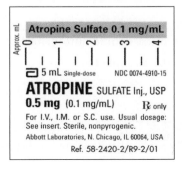

The nurse should administer _____ mL.

Mark the syringe in Figure 17-105 to show the required dose.

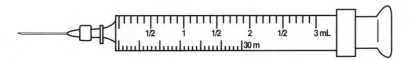

Figure 17-105

10. The patient is to receive heparin sodium 4000 units SC by injection. Available is a multidose vial labeled:

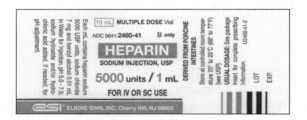

Using a tuberculin syringe, the nurse should administer _____ mL.

Mark the syringe in Figure 17-106 to show the required dose.

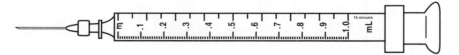

Figure 17-106

11. The patient is to receive heparin sodium 7,500 units SC by injection. Available is a multidose vial of heparin sodium labeled:

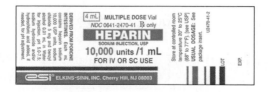

Using a tuberculin syringe, the nurse should administer _____ mL.

Mark the syringe in Figure 17-107 to show the required dose.

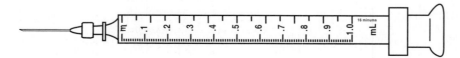

Figure 17-107

12. The patient is to receive Humulin L insulin 85 units SC by injection daily. Available is a multidose vial labeled:

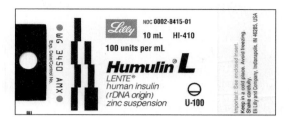

Using a 100 unit insulin syringe, the nurse should administer _____ units.

Using a tuberculin syringe, the nurse should administer _____ mL.

Mark the syringes in Figure 17-108 to show the required dose.

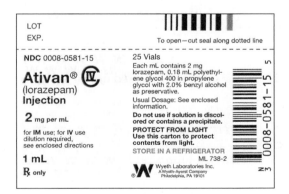

Figure 17-108

13. The patient is to receive lorazepam (Ativan) 0.5 mg IM by injection. Available is a box of single-dose vials labeled:

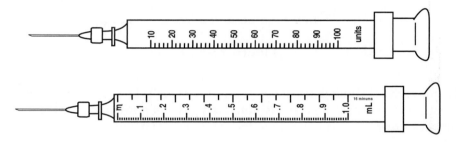

Using a tuberculin syringe, the nurse should administer _____ mL.

Mark the syringe in Figure 17-109 to show the required dose.

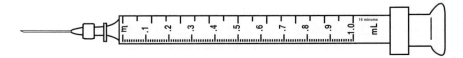

Figure 17-109

14. The patient is to receive methylprednisolone sodium succinate (Solu-Medrol) 240 mg IM. Available is a 4 mL Act-O-Vial of powdered medication with a 4 mL vial of diluent that states: To reconstitute the 500 mg vial of powdered medication, add the 4 mL vial of diluent to yield a solution that contains 125 mg per mL.

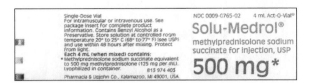

The nurse should administer _____ mL.

Mark the syringe in Figure 17-110 to show the required dose.

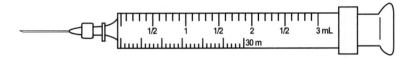

Figure 17-110

15. The patient is to receive cefamandole nafate (Mandol) 750 mg IM by injection. Available is a vial of powdered medication that states: To reconstitute the 1 g vial of powdered medication, add 3 mL of an approved diluent to yield a volume of 3.5 mL that contains 285 mg per mL.

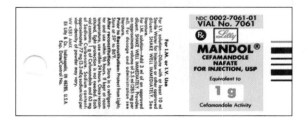

The nurse should administer _____ mL.

Mark the syringe in Figure 17-111 to show the required dose.

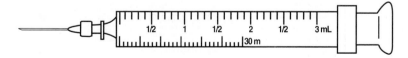

Figure 17-111

Answers: **1.** To administer morphine sulfate 12 mg IM by injection from a single-dose vial labeled 15 mg/mL, the nurse should withdraw 0.8 mL for injection. The syringe should look like Figure 17-112.

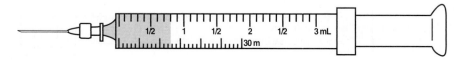

Figure 17-112

2. To administer tobramycin (Nebcin) 60 mg IM by injection from a vial labeled 80 mg = 2 mL, the nurse should withdraw 1.5 mL for injection. The syringe should look like Figure 17-113.

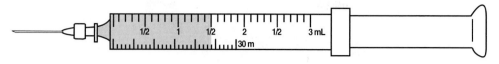

Figure 17-113

3. To administer meperidine hydrochloride 50 mg IM by injection from a vial labeled 100 mg = 1 mL, the nurse should withdraw $\frac{1}{2}$ mL (0.5 mL) for injection. The syringe should look like Figure 17-114.

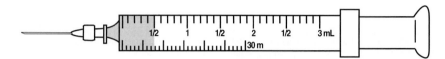

Figure 17-114

4. To administer Ancef 500 mg IM from a 1 g multidose vial of powdered medication that states: Add 2.5 mL of sterile water to provide a total solution of 3 mL, the nurse should add the diluent, mix, and withdraw 1.5 mL for injection. The syringe should look like Figure 17-115.

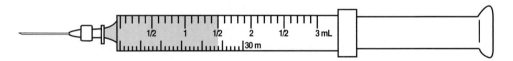

Figure 17-115

5. To administer hydroxyzine hydrochloride (Vistaril) 75 mg IM from a multidose vial of Vistaril labeled 50 mg/mL, the nurse should withdraw 1.5 mL for injection. The syringe should look like Figure 17-116.

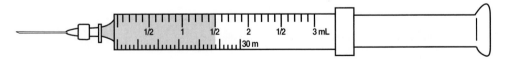

Figure 17-116

6. To administer 40 units of Humulin N insulin SC by injection from a multidose vial of Humulin N labeled 100 units per mL, the nurse should withdraw 40 units using a 100 unit insulin syringe and 0.4 mL using a 1 mL tuberculin syringe for injection. The syringes should look like Figure 17-117.

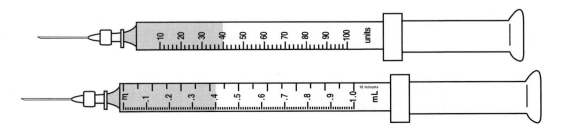

Figure 17-117

7. To administer Humulin R insulin 5 units SC by injection from a multidose vial labeled 100 units per mL, the nurse should withdraw 5 units using a Lo-Dose insulin syringe for 100 unit insulin and 0.05 mL using a 1 mL tuberculin syringe for injection. The syringes should look like Figure 17-118.

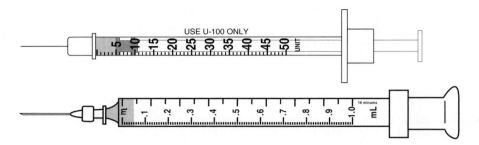

Figure 17-118

8. To administer pencillin G potassium 750,000 units IM from a 5,000,000 unit multidose vial of powdered medication that states: Add 8.2 mL of diluent to provide a solution that contains 500,000 units per mL, the nurse should add the diluent, mix, and withdraw 1.5 mL for injection. The syringe should look like Figure 17-119.

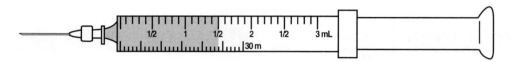

Figure 17-119

9. To administer Atropine sulfate 0.17 mg IM from a vial labeled 0.1 mg/mL, the nurse should withdraw 1.7 mL for injection. The syringe should look like Figure 17-120.

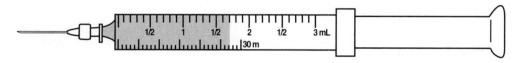

Figure 17-120

10. To administer heparin sodium 4000 units SC from a multidose vial labeled heparin sodium 5000 units/1 mL, the nurse should withdraw 0.8 mL for injection. The syringe should look like Figure 17-121.

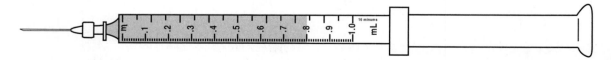

Figure 17-121

11. To administer heparin sodium 7500 units SC from a multidose vial labeled heparin sodium 10,000 units/1 mL, the nurse should withdraw 0.75 mL for injection. The syringe should look like Figure 17-122.

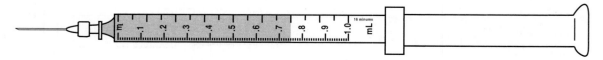

Figure 17-122

12. To administer Humulin L insulin 85 units SC by injection from a multidose vial of Humulin L insulin 100 units per 1 mL, the nurse should withdraw 85 units using a 100 unit insulin syringe and 0.85 mL using a 1 mL tuberculin syringe for injection. The syringes should look like Figure 17-123.

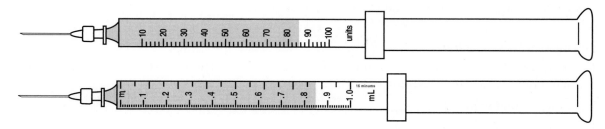

Figure 17-123

13. To administer lorazepam (Ativan) 0.5 mg by injection from a single-dose vial labeled 2 mg per mL, the nurse should withdraw 0.25 mL using a 1 mL tuberculin syringe for injection. The syringe should look like Figure 17-124.

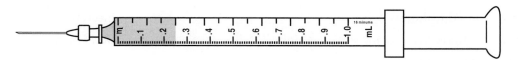

Figure 17-124

14. To administer methylprednisolone sodium succinate (Solu-Medrol) 240 mg IM from a multidose vial of powdered medication that states: Add the 4 mL vial of provided diluent to yield a solution where 125 mg = 1 mL, the nurse should add the diluent, mix, and withdraw 1.9 mL for injection. The syringe should look like Figure 17-125.

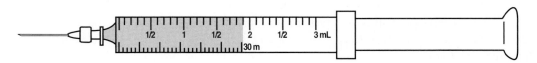

Figure 17-125

15. To administer Mandol 750 mg IM by injection from a multidose vial of powdered medication that states: To reconstitute the 1 g vial of powdered medication, add 3 mL of approved diluent to yield a volume of 3.5 mL that contains 285 mg per mL, the nurse should add the diluent, mix, and withdraw 2.6 mL for injection. The syringe should look like Figure 17-126.

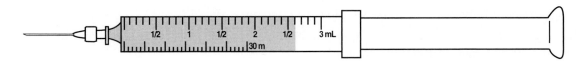

Figure 17-126

If you had fewer than three errors on Review Test 17.1, move on to the next chapter. If you had four or more errors, review the material on parenteral medications and complete Review Test 17.2 before continuing.

Review Test 17.2
Parenteral Medications

1. The patient is to receive secobarbital sodium (Seconal) 65 mg IM. The vial available is labeled 100 mg = 2 mL.

   The nurse should withdraw _____ mL for IM injection.

2. The patient is to receive cefoxitin sodium (Mefoxin) 800 mg IM. The 1 g vial available states: Add 2 mL of diluent to provide a total solution of 2.5 mL.

   The nurse should withdraw _____ mL for IM injection.

3. The patient is to receive furosemide (Lasix) 25 mg IM. The vial is labeled 40 mg = 4 mL.

   The nurse should withdraw _____ mL for IM injection.

4. The patient is to receive carbenicillin disodium (Geopen) 0.5 g IM. The 5 g vial available states: Add 7.0 mL of diluent to yield a solution that contains 1 g per 2 mL.

   The nurse should withdraw _____ mL for IM injection.

5. The patient is to receive fentanyl citrate (Sublimaze) 0.1 mg IM. The 2 mL ampule available is labeled 50 μg per 1 mL.

   The nurse should withdraw _____ mL for IM injection.

6. The patient is to receive codeine sulfate $\frac{3}{4}$ grains IM. The available vial is labeled 60 mg = 1 mL.

   The nurse should withdraw _____ mL for IM injection.

7. The patient is to receive penicillin G sodium 750,000 units IM. Available is a 5,000,000 unit vial of powdered medication that states: Reconstitute with 8 mL of diluent to provide a concentration of 500,000 units per mL.

   The nurse should withdraw _____ mL for IM injection.

8. The patient is to receive heparin sodium 5000 units subcutaneously. The vial available is labeled 7500 units per 1 mL.

   The nurse should withdraw _____ mL for SC injection.

9. The patient is to receive penicillin G potassium 150,000 units IM. Available is a 1,000,000 unit vial of powdered medication that states: Reconstitute with 9.6 mL of diluent to provide a concentration of 100,000 units per 1 mL.

   The nurse should withdraw _____ mL for IM injection.

10. The patient is to receive heparin sodium 8000 units SC by injection. The available multidose vial is labeled heparin sodium 10,000 units per mL.

    The nurse should withdraw _____ mL for SC injection.

11. The patient is to receive Humulin N insulin 20 units SC by injection. The available multidose vial of Humulin N is labeled 100 units per 1 mL.

    Using a 100 unit insulin syringe, the nurse should withdraw _____ units for SC injection.

    Using a tuberculin syringe, the nurse should withdraw _____ mL for SC injection.

12. The patient is to receive Humulin 50/50 insulin 70 U SC by injection. The available multidose vial of Humulin 50/50 is labeled 100 units per 1 mL.

    Using a 100 unit insulin syringe, the nurse should withdraw _____ units for SC injection.

    Using a tuberculin syringe, the nurse should withdraw _____ mL for SC injection.

13. The patient is to receive ceftizoxime sodium (Cefizox) 750 mg IM. Available is a 1 gram vial of powdered medication that states: Reconstitute with 3 mL of sterile water to provide a solution of 3.7 mL that contains 270 mg per 1 mL.

The nurse should withdraw _____ mL for IM injection.

14. The patient is to receive pentamidine isethionate (Pentam 300) 250 mg IM. Available is a 300 mg vial of powdered medication that states: Reconstitute with 3 mL of sterile water to provide a concentration of 100 mg per 1 mL.

    The nurse should withdraw _____ mL for IM injection.

15. The patient is to receive phytonadione (AquaMEPHYTON) 2.5 mg IM by injection. The 5 mL multidose vial available is labeled 1 mg equals 0.5 mL.

    The nurse should withdraw _____ mL for IM injection.

Answers: **1.** 1.3 mL **2.** 2 mL **3.** 2.5 mL **4.** 1 mL **5.** 2 mL **6.** 0.75 or 0.8 mL **7.** 1.5 mL **8.** 0.7 mL **9.** 1.5 mL **10.** 0.8 mL **11.** 20 units; 0.2 mL **12.** 70 units; 0.7 mL **13.** 2.77 or 2.8 mL **14.** 2.5 mL **15.** 1.25 mL

The Review Tests on parenteral medications should be repeated until fewer than three errors occur.

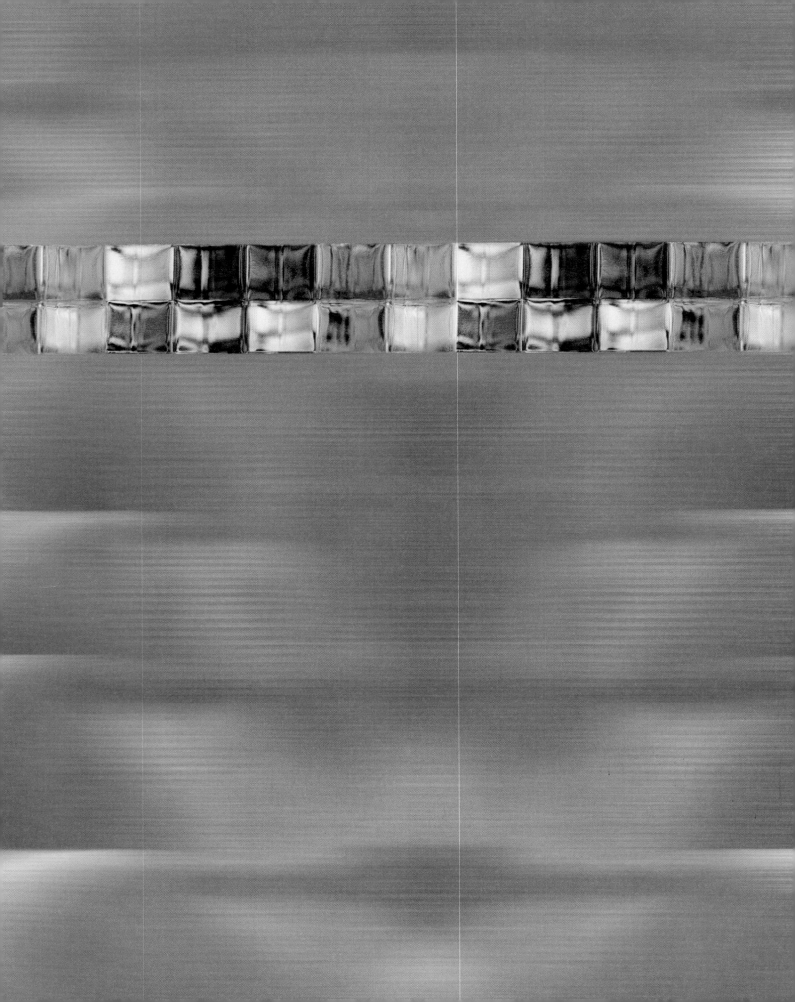

unit
5

Intravenous Fluids and Medications

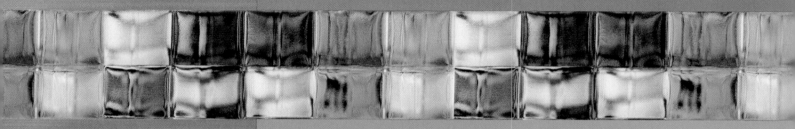

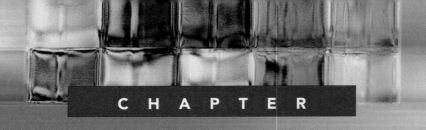

18

Intravenous Fluid Therapy and Computing Flow Rates

Learning Outcomes

After successfully completing this chapter, the learner should be able to:

- *Understand the common abbreviations used in intravenous fluid orders.*
- *Explain the components and percentage strengths of intravenous solutions.*
- *Explain how the different parts of infusion sets function.*
- *Explain the meaning of the drop factor provided on intravenous infusion sets.*
- *Calculate the desired drop rate per minute to provide the intravenous fluid ordered.*
- *Determine the total infusion time for a given amount of fluid to absorb when the rate of absorption per minute or hour is known.*
- *Explain how the manual and electronic delivery systems operate.*

COMMON ABBREVIATIONS FOR INTRAVENOUS SOLUTIONS

Ca	calcium
Cl	chloride
D	dextrose or glucose

D10/NS	10% dextrose in normal saline
D10/W	10% dextrose in water
D5/1/4NS	5% dextrose in one-fourth strength normal saline (0.225% NaCl)
D5/1/3NS	5% dextrose in one-third strength normal saline (0.3% NaCl)
D5/1/2NS	5% dextrose in one-half strength normal saline (0.45% NaCl)
D5/LR	5% dextrose in lactated Ringer's solution
D5/NS	5% dextrose in normal saline (0.9% NaCl)
D5/R	5% dextrose in Ringer's solution
D5/W	5% dextrose in water
1/4NS	one-fourth strength normal saline (0.225% sodium chloride)
1/3NS	one-third strength normal saline (0.3% sodium chloride)
1/2NS	one-half strength normal saline (0.45% sodium chloride)
K	potassium
KCl	potassium chloride
LR	lactated Ringer's solution
M	molar solution (1 mole of solute per liter of solution)
Mg	magnesium
Na	sodium
NaCl	sodium chloride
NS	normal saline (0.9% sodium chloride)
R	Ringer's solution
SW	sterile water for injection

GENERAL INFORMATION

Intravenous solutions are sterile. All the components of the solution must be compatible and soluble in blood, because they are delivered to the body via a vein.

The tonicity of intravenous solutions is directly related to their osmotic pressure equivalent.

Isotonic solutions have an osmotic pressure that is equal to the osmotic pressure of the intracellular (ICF) and extracellular (ECF) body fluids. These solutions simply expand the amount of ECF without exerting any pull (osmotic pressure) on cells in the ICF compartment. Isotonic fluids do not cause any shifts in fluid between the ICF and ECF compartments, because the osmotic pressure in the compartments is not altered. Fluids such as 0.9% normal saline, 5% dextrose in water, 5% dextrose in 0.225% saline, lactated Ringer's solution, and Ringer's solution are isotonic (see Figure 18-1).

Hypertonic solutions have an osmotic pressure that is higher than the osmotic pressure of the intracellular and extracellular body fluids. These hypertonic solutions raise the osmotic pressure in the extracellular fluid and cause fluid to shift from the cells into the extracellular compartments in an attempt to decrease the higher osmotic pressure. Fluids such as 5% dextrose in 0.45% saline, 5% dextrose in 0.9% saline, 3.0% saline, and 10% dextrose in water are hypertonic (see Figure 18-2).

Hypotonic solutions have an osmotic pressure that is lower than the osmotic pressure of the intracellular and extracellular body fluids. These hypotonic solutions provide more water than electrolytes, dilute the extracellular fluid (reduce its osmotic pressure), and cause fluid to shift from the extracellular to the intracellular fluid. Fluids such as saline of less than 0.9% strength (such as 0.45% or 0.225%) are hypotonic.

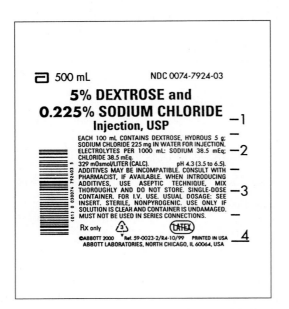

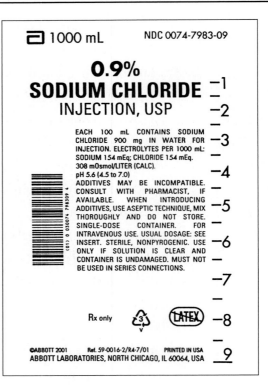

Figure 18-1 Isotonic intravenous fluids

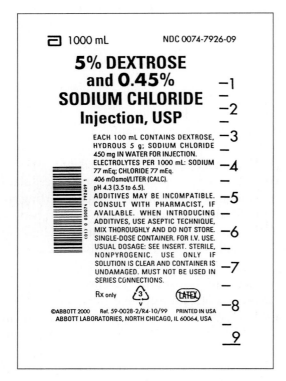

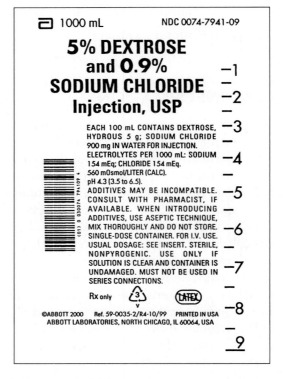

Figure 18-2 Hypertonic intravenous fluids

PERCENTAGE STRENGTH OF SOLUTIONS

The percentage strength of any solution signifies the amount of solute in grams per 100 mL of solution (solute plus solvent). A 5% dextrose in water solution would contain 5 grams of dextrose for every 100 mL of water. A 0.9% saline solution would contain 0.9 grams (900 mg) of sodium chloride and 100 mL of water.

   If the percentage strength of a solution is known, the amount of solute in grams in a specific amount of fluid can be determined by using the familiar ratio-and-proportion method.

Example: Determine the amount of dextrose in 1000 mL of 10% dextrose in water (D10/W).

Solution: One side of the proportion would be the known percentage strength of the solution written in grams over 100 mL and the other side would be the unknown amount of grams over the specific amount of fluid.

$$\frac{10 \text{ g}}{100 \text{ mL}} = \frac{x \text{ g}}{1000 \text{ mL}}$$
$$100x = 10000$$
$$x = 100 \text{ g of dextrose}$$

A 1000 mL container of D10/W would contain 100 grams of dextrose dissolved in 1000 mL of water.

Example: Determine the amount of sodium chloride in 500 mL of 0.9% saline.

Solution:
$$\frac{0.9 \text{ g}}{100 \text{ mL}} = \frac{x \text{ g}}{500 \text{ mL}}$$
$$100x = 450$$
$$x = 4.5 \text{ g of sodium chloride}$$

A 500 mL container of 0.9% saline would contain 4.5 grams of sodium chloride in 500 mL of solution (solute plus solvent).

Example: Determine the amounts of dextrose and sodium chloride in 1000 mL of 5% dextrose in 0.45% saline.

Solution:

$$\frac{5 \text{ g}}{100 \text{ mL}} = \frac{x \text{ g}}{1000 \text{ mL}} \qquad \frac{0.45 \text{ g}}{100 \text{ mL}} = \frac{x \text{ g}}{1000 \text{ mL}}$$
$$100x = 5000 \qquad\qquad 100x = 450$$
$$x = 50 \text{ g of dextrose} \qquad x = 4.5 \text{ g sodium chloride}$$

A 1000 mL container of 5% dextrose in 0.45% saline would contain 50 grams of dextrose and 4.5 grams of sodium chloride dissolved in 1000 mL of solution.

Problem Set 18.1

1. Determine how many grams of sodium chloride would be in 250 mL of a 0.9% sodium chloride solution. _____ grams

2. Determine how many grams of dextrose would be in 500 mL of a 10% dextrose in water solution. _____ grams

3. Determine how many grams of dextrose and how many grams of sodium chloride would be in 1000 mL of a D5/1/2NS solution. _____ grams

4. Determine how many grams of dextrose would be in 2500 mL of a D5/W solution. _____ grams

5. Determine how many grams of sodium chloride would be in 1000 mL of a 0.225% sodium chloride solution. _____ grams

Answers: **1.** 2.25 g sodium chloride   **2.** 50 g dextrose   **3.** 50 g dextrose; 4.5 g sodium chloride   **4.** 125 g dextrose
5. 2.25 g sodium chloride

VIP

- Intravenous fluids may be isotonic, hypertonic, or hypotonic depending on their tonicity (osmotic pressure).
- The percentage strength of any solution signifies the amount of solute in grams per 100 mL of solution (solute plus solvent).

INFUSION SETS

Intravenous or total parenteral nutrition fluids are delivered via an IV infusion set. Infusion sets include tubing with a drip chamber, some type of slide or roller clamp for manually controlling the rate of flow, and an injection port for medication or secondary IVs (see Figure 18-3).

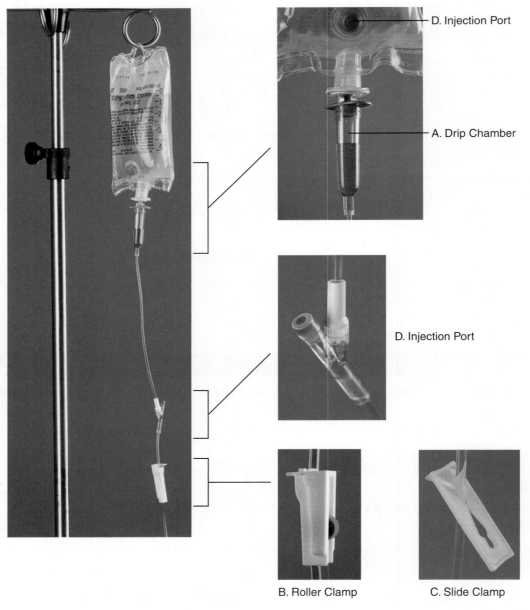

D. Injection Port

A. Drip Chamber

D. Injection Port

B. Roller Clamp

C. Slide Clamp

Figure 18-3 IV infusion set

The drop factor, which is the number of drops that equals 1 mL, differs among infusion sets and depends on the size of the tubing, the type of tubing, and the manufacturer's specifications. The drop factor always appears on the tubing package, and the nurse must be aware of what the drop factor is to accurately administer IV or total parenteral nutrition (TPN) fluids.

Problem Set 18.2

Identify the drop factor for the IV infusion, transfusion sets in Figure 18-4.

1. _____ gtt/mL

2. _____ gtt/mL

3. _____ gtt/mL

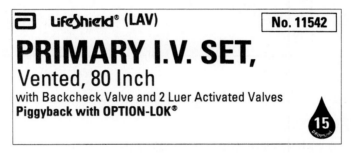

Tubing package 1

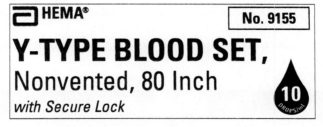

Tubing package 2

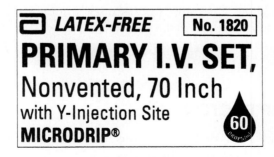

Tubing package 3

Figure 18-4   Tubing packages

Answers: **1.** 15 gtt/mL   **2.** 10 gtt/mL   **3.** 60 gtt/mL

Intravenous drip chambers, which are part of the IV infusion set, enable the nurse to count the number of drops per minute being delivered to the patient. The tubing can be either a macrodrop (standard) intravenous drip chamber or a microdrop (minidrop) intravenous drip chamber (see Figure 18-5).

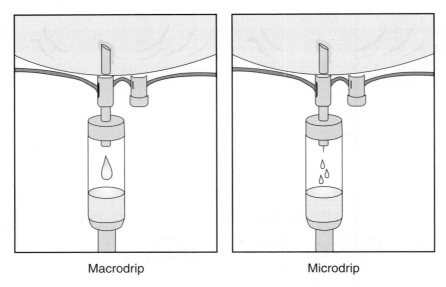

Macrodrip   Microdrip

Figure 18-5 Intravenous drip chambers: Comparison of macro- and microdrips

Intravenous infusion sets with a macrodrop (standard) drip chamber are most commonly used for routine adult IV fluid administration. These macrodrop sets can have a drop factor of 10 gtt/mL, 15 gtt/mL, or 20 gtt/mL. Intravenous infusion sets with a microdrop (minidrop) drip chamber have a drop factor of 60 gtt/mL and allow a slower, more accurate fluid administration rate. These infusion sets are used for children, the elderly, and critically ill patients where exact fluid control is required.

The injection port on the infusion set provides an entry point for administering IV medications or for secondary IVs (piggybacks).

V I P

■ Regardless of the set being used or where the IV was started, it is the nurse's responsibility to know the drop factor. Without this knowledge the nurse cannot regulate the amount of fluid the patient is receiving and needlessly places the patient at risk.

■ If a pump is not being used, the higher an IV bag is hung, the greater the pressure will be, and therefore the faster the IV fluid can flow.

FLOW RATE AND DROP FACTOR

The physician usually orders intravenous or TPN solutions by amount and time. It is the nurse's responsibility to compute the rate the IV will have to infuse to follow this order.

To compute this rate, the nurse must first determine three factors:

■ Number of milliliters the patient is to receive per hour

■ Number of milliliters the patient is to receive per minute

■ Number of drops per minute that will equal the required number of milliliters

The drop factor—the number of drops that equals 1 milliliter—will depend on the size of the drops that a particular IV tubing delivers. This amount will vary with different types of tubing, different sizes of tubing, and different manufacturers. The drop factor is stated on the tubing package, and the nurse is responsible for knowing the drop factor for the infusion set being used.

Determining Number of Milliliters per Hour

When the amount of fluid to be administered in a specific number of hours is known, the number of milliliters the patient is to receive in a specific number of hours (usually one hour) can be determined by using the familiar ratio-and-proportion method.

Example: A patient is to receive 3000 mL of IV fluid over 24 hours. How much fluid should be infused per hour?

Solution: One side of the proportion would be the desired time for the infusion (usually 1 hour) over the total prescribed time in hours and the other side would be the hourly amount in mL over the total volume of fluid to be infused in mL.

Set up the proportion:

$$\frac{\text{Desired time (1 hour)}}{\text{Total prescribed time in hours}} = \frac{\text{Desired hourly amount in mL}}{\text{Total prescribed volume in mL}}$$

$$\frac{1 \text{ hour}}{24 \text{ hours}} = \frac{x \text{ mL}}{3000 \text{ mL}}$$

$$24x = 3000$$

$$x = 125 \text{ mL per hour}$$

The number of mL per hour that the patient is to receive can also be determined by dividing the total number of milliliters the patient is to receive in a specific number of hours by the number of hours during which the solution is to infuse.

Example: A patient is to receive 3000 mL of IV fluid over 24 hours. How much fluid should be infused per hour?

Solution: Divide the 3000 mL of fluid over 24 hours by 24.

3000 mL ÷ 24 = 125 mL

The patient should receive 125 mL per hour.

Example: A patient is to receive 1800 mL of IV fluid over 24 hours. How much fluid should be administered per hour?

Solution: Divide the 1800 mL of fluid over 24 hours by 24.

1800 mL ÷ 24 = 75 mL

The patient should receive 75 mL per hour.

Problem Set 18.3

Determine the mL per hour fluid rate:

1. The patient is to receive 1250 mL of D10/W over 24 hours. The nurse should administer

   _____ mL per hour.

2. The patient is to receive 750 mL of D5/W over 16 hours. The nurse should administer

   _____ mL per hour.

3. The patient is to receive 2000 mL of D5/W over 24 hours. The nurse should administer

   _____ mL per hour.

4. The patient is to receive 1500 mL of Ringer's solution over 12 hours. The nurse should administer

   _____ mL per hour.

5. The patient is to receive 500 mL of D5/1/3NS over 18 hours. The nurse should administer

   _____ mL per hour.

Answers   1. 52 mL/hr   2. 46.9 or 47 mL/hr   3. 83 mL/hr   4. 125 mL/hr   5. 27.8 or 28 mL/hr

Determining Number of Milliliters per Minute

When the number of mL of IV fluid to be infused in an hour (60 minutes) is known, the number of milliliters the patient is to receive in one minute can be determined by using the familiar ratio-and-proportion method.

Example: A patient is to receive 125 mL of IV fluid per hour. How much fluid should be administered per minute?

Solution: One side of the proportion would be the desired time for the infusion (1 minute) over the known infusion time of 60 minutes and the other side would be the amount per minute in mL over the total hourly volume to be infused in mL.

Set up the proportion:

$$\frac{\text{Desired time (1 minute)}}{\text{Total prescribed time in minutes (60)}} = \frac{\text{Desired amount per minute in mL}}{\text{Total prescribed volume in mL}}$$

$$\frac{1 \text{ minute}}{60 \text{ minutes}} = \frac{x \text{ mL}}{125 \text{ mL}}$$

$$60x = 125$$

$$x = 2.08 \text{ or } 2 \text{ mL per minute}$$

The number of mL per minute that the patient is to receive can also be determined by dividing the total number of mL the patient is to receive per hour by the number of minutes (usually 60 minutes).

Example: A patient is to receive 3000 mL of IV fluid over 24 hours or 125 mL per hour.
How much fluid should be administered per minute?

Solution: Divide the 125 mL of fluid per hour by 60.

125 mL ÷ 60 = 2.08 mL

The patient should receive 2.08 or 2 mL per minute.

Example: A patient is to receive 1800 mL of IV fluid over 24 hours or 75 mL per hour.
How much fluid should be administered per minute?

Solution: Divide the 75 mL by 60.

75 mL ÷ 60 = 1.25 mL

The patient should receive 1.25 mL per minute.

Problem Set 18.4

Determine the mL per minute fluid rate:

1. The patient is to receive 120 mL of D5/W per hour. The nurse should administer

    _____ mL per minute.

2. The patient is to receive 75 mL of D5/1/3NS per hour. The nurse should administer

    _____ mL per minute.

3. The patient is to receive 60 mL of D5/1/4NS per hour. The nurse should administer

    _____ mL per minute.

4. The patient is to receive 100 mL of LR solution per hour. The nurse should administer

    _____ mL per minute.

5. The patient is to receive 30 mL of D5/W per hour. The nurse should administer

    _____ mL per minute.

Answers   **1.** 2 mL/min   **2.** 1.25 mL/min   **3.** 1 mL/min   **4.** 1.67 or 1.7 mL/min   **5.** 0.5 mL/min

Determining Number of Drops per Minute

When the number of mL of IV fluid to be administered in one minute and the drop factor of the infusion set being used are known, the number of drops the patient is to receive in one minute can be determined by using the familiar ratio-and-proportion method.

Example: A patient is to receive 2 mL of IV fluid per minute. The infusion set being used has a drop factor of 15 gtt = 1 mL. How many drops a minute should the IV be set to deliver?

Solution: One side of the proportion would be the total amount to be infused in 1 minute over the 1 minute time and the other side would be the desired drop rate over the known drop factor.

Set up the proportion:

$$\frac{\text{Total amount to be infused in 1 minute}}{1 \text{ minute}} = \frac{\text{Desired drop rate}}{\text{Known drop factor}}$$

$$\frac{2 \text{ mL per minute}}{1 \text{ minute}} = \frac{x \text{ drops}}{15 \text{ drops / mL}}$$

$$x = 30 \text{ drops per minute}$$

The number of drops per minute that the patient is to receive can also be determined by multiplying the total number of mL the patient is to receive per minute by the drop factor for the IV set being used.

Example: The patient is to receive 2 mL per minute.
The drop factor of the IV set is 15 gtt = 1 mL.

Solution: Multiply the 2 mL rate per minute by the IV set drop factor of 15 and mark off two decimal places.

```
    2.00
×   15
  1000
   200
 30.00
```

To administer 2 mL per minute using an IV infusion set with a drop factor of 15 gtt/mL, the IV should run at the rate of 30 drops per minute.

Example: The patient is to receive 1.25 mL per minute.
The drop factor of the IV set is 60 gtt = 1 mL.

Solution: Mutliply the 1.25 mL rate per minute by the IV set drop factor of 60 and mark off two decimal places.

```
   1.25
×    60
 75.00
```

To administer 1.25 mL per minute using a microdrop IV infusion set with a drop factor of 60 gtt/mL, the IV should run at the rate of 75 drops per minute.

Once the milliliters of IV fluids per hour the patient is to receive has been determined, the following method may also be used to compute the number of drops per minute the solution should run.

To use this method, the number of milliliters of IV fluid per hour the patient is to receive, the drop factor of the IV set being used, and the following formulas must be known. This method is a fast and accurate way to determine the drop per minute rate and is an excellent way to rapidly check figures from either of the other methods.

- If the drop factor is 10 drops = 1 mL, divide the hourly amount of fluid by 6 = gtt/min
- If the drop factor is 15 drops = 1 mL, divide the hourly amount of fluid by 4 = gtt/min
- If the drop factor is 20 drops = 1 mL, divide the hourly amount of fluid by 3 = gtt/min
- If the drop factor is 60 drops = 1 mL, divide the hourly amount of fluid by 1 = gtt/min

Example: A patient is to receive 80 mL of IV fluid per hour.
The drop factor of the IV set being used is 15 = 1 mL.

Solution: Divide the 80 mL of fluid per hour by 4.
The IV should be set to run at 20 drops per minute.

Example: A patient is to receive 1800 mL of IV fluid over 24 hours or 75 mL per hour. The drop factor of the IV set being used is 60 gtt = 1 mL.

Solution: It was previously determined that to administer 75 mL an hour using a microdrop IV infusion set with a drop factor of 60 gtt/mL, the IV should run at the rate of 75 drops per minute.

This answer can be rapidly checked by dividing the 75 mL hourly rate of fluid by 1. The IV should be set to run at 75 drops per minute; therefore, the answer is correct.

Problem Set 18.5

Determine the drop per minute fluid rate:

1. The patient is to receive 1.5 mL of D5/W per minute. The infusion set has a drop factor of 10 gtt/mL.

   The nurse should set the drop rate at _____ gtt per minute.

2. The patient is to receive 0.75 mL of D5/1/3NS per minute. The infusion set has a drop factor of 60 gtt/mL.

   The nurse should set the drop rate at _____ gtt per minute.

3. The patient is to receive 0.5 mL of D5/1/4NS per minute. The infusion set has a drop factor of 15 gtt/mL.

   The nurse should set the drop rate at _____ gtt per minute.

4. The patient is to receive 2 mL of 100 mL of LR per minute. The infusion set has a drop factor of 20 gtt/mL.

   The nurse should set the drop rate at _____ gtt per minute.

5. The patient is to receive 1.25 mL of 30 mL of D5/W per minute. The infusion set has a drop factor of 15 gtt/mL.

   The nurse should set the drop rate at _____ gtt per minute.

Answers: **1.** 15 gtt/min   **2.** 45 gtt/min   **3.** 7.5 or 8 gtt/min   **4.** 40 gtt/min   **5.** 18.7 or 19 gtt/min

Determining Hourly Rate When the Drop Factor and the Drop Rate Are Known

The hourly rate can be determined when only the drop factor of the infusion set and the drop rate are known, by using the following formulas:

■ If the drop factor is 10 drops = 1 mL, multiply the drop rate of fluid by 6 = mL/hr

■ If the drop factor is 15 drops = 1 mL, multiply the drop rate of fluid by 4 = mL/hr

■ If the drop factor is 20 drops = 1 mL, multiply the drop rate of fluid by 3 = mL/hr

■ If the drop factor is 60 drops = 1 mL, multiply the drop rate of fluid by 1 = mL/hr

Example: A patient's IV is running at 30 gtt/min.

The infusion set being used has a drop factor of 10.

How much fluid is the patient receiving per hour?

Solution: The infusion set being used has a drop factor of 10 and the patient's IV is running at 30 gtt/min. Simply multiply the 30 gtt by 6 to determine that the patient would be receiving 180 mL of fluid per hour.

Example: A patient's IV is running at 80 gtt/min.

The infusion set being used has a drop factor of 60.

How much fluid is the patient receiving per hour?

Solution: The infusion set being used has a drop factor of 60 and the patient's IV is running at 80 gtt/min. Simply multiply the 80 gtt by 1 to determine that the patient would be receiving 80 mL of fluid per hour.

Problem Set 18.6

Determine how much fluid the patient is receiving per hour:

1. The patient's IV of D5/1/2 NS is infusing at 15 gtt per minute. The infusion set has a drop factor of 20 gtt/mL.

   The nurse recognizes that the patient will receive _____ mL/hr.

2. The patient's IV of lactated Ringer's solution is infusing at 25 gtt per minute. The infusion set has a drop factor of 15 gtt/mL.

   The nurse recognizes that the patient will receive _____ mL/hr.

3. The patient's IV D5/W is infusing at 18 gtt per minute. The infusion set has a drop factor of 10 gtt/mL.

   The nurse recognizes that the patient will receive _____ mL/hr.

4. The patient's IV D5/NS is infusing at 30 gtt per minute. The infusion set has a drop factor of 60 gtt/mL.

   The nurse recognizes that the patient will receive _____ mL/hr.

5. The patient's IV D10/NS is infusing at 8 gtt per minute. The infusion set has a drop factor of 10 gtt/mL.

   The nurse recognizes that the patient will receive _____ mL/hr.

Answers   1. 45 mL/hr   2. 100 mL/hr   3. 108 mL/hr   4. 30 mL/hr   5. 48 mL/hr

V I P

To compute the patient's fluid infusion rate, certain factors must first be determined:
- The physician's fluid orders
- Number of milliliters the patient is to receive per hour
- Number of milliliters the patient is to receive per minute
- Number of drops per minute that will equal this number of milliliters

DETERMINING TOTAL INFUSION TIME

Frequently, the physician orders the patient's fluid by a total amount and an hourly rate. In these situations, the nurse may have to determine how long it will take for the prescribed volume to infuse. This amount of time is called *total infusion time*. This problem can be set up using the familiar ratio-and-proportion method.

Example: A patient is to receive 1000 mL of D5/W to be infused at 80 mL/hr. How long should it take the IV to infuse?

Solution: One side of the proportion would be the prescribed infusion time in hours over the prescribed hourly volume in mL, and the other side would be the total infusion time in hours over the total prescribed volume to be infused in mL.

Set up the proportion:

$$\frac{\text{Prescribed infusion time in hours}}{\text{Prescribed hourly volume in mL}} = \frac{\text{Total infusion time in hours}}{\text{Total prescribed volume in mL}}$$

$$\frac{1 \text{ hour}}{80 \text{ mL}} = \frac{x \text{ hours}}{1000 \text{ mL}}$$

$$80x = 1000$$

$$x = 12.5 = 12 \text{ hours, } 30 \text{ minutes total infusion time}$$

Total infusion time can also be determined by dividing the total volume to be infused by the prescribed hourly volume in mL.

Example: A patient is to receive 1000 mL of D5/W to be infused at 80 mL/hour. How long should it take the IV to infuse?

Solution: Divide the total volume to be infused (1000) by the prescribed hourly volume in mL (80 mL).

1000 ÷ 80 = 12 hours, 30 minutes total infusion time

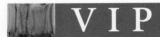

VIP

Based on the time the IV infusion or total parenteral nutrition was started, the total infusion time can be used to determine when the prescribed volume should be absorbed.

Problem Set 18.7

Determine the total infusion time:

1. D5/W 3000 mL to run at 125 mL/hour.

   Total infusion time is _____.

2. Lactated Ringer's solution 2000 mL to run at 100 mL/hour.

   Total infusion time is _____.

3. D5/1/4NS 1000 mL to run at 60 mL/hour.

   Total infusion time is _____.

4. D5/W 1500 mL to run at 75 mL/hour.

   Total infusion time is _____.

5. 1/2NS 500 mL to run at 20 mL/hour.

   Total infusion time is _____.

Answers: **1.** 24 hours **2.** 20 hours **3.** 16.67 or 16 hours, 40 minutes **4.** 20 hours **5.** 25 hours

MANUAL AND ELECTRONIC INFUSION DELIVERY DEVICES

The infusion rate of IV or TPN fluids can be set manually or electronically to ensure the administration of the infusion at the rate and amount prescribed by the physician.

Manual Infusion Devices

Manual control is achieved by use of the slide or roller clamp on the infusion set. The drops entering the drip chamber (either the macrodrip or the microdrip) are carefully counted and monitored frequently using a watch with a second hand.

Electronic Infusion Devices

Electronic infusion devices are replacing manually controlled infusion devices in most primary care situations. These electronic devices, whether classified as infusion pumps and/or controllers, allow more exact, automatic infusion of drugs, fluids, whole blood or blood components, and total parenteral nutrition solutions. Electronic infusion devices are vital in pediatric and intensive care situations because they permit the infusion of very small amounts of fluids and/or medications with precise accuracy.

Types of Devices.   In the electronic devices classified as controllers, the tubing from the infusion set was passed through a sensor that electronically monitored the flow rate. The rate depended on the force of gravity and pressure exerted on the tubing of the infusion set. These devices depended on maintaining the infusion at the proper height (gravity) as well as maintaining the patient's position. As these factors were not always easy to manage, a consistent flow rate with these devices was not always achieved and required careful monitoring.

In the electronic devices classified as infusion pumps, the pump exerted positive pressure on the tubing from the infusion set or the infusion itself, which propelled the fluid through the tubing. Because of the application of positive pressure, the infusion pumps had a greater risk of causing extensive tissue infiltration if the needle or cannula became dislodged.

Neither the electronic controllers nor the infusion pumps are currently being manufactured as separate entities. They are being replaced by a volumetric device that functions as an infusion pump and/or controller. The current electronic infusion devices utilize various mechanisms to displace fluid from the solution container to the patient. These volumetric devices can be programmed to deliver a specific volume of fluid, with or without medication, in milliliters per hour or milliliters per minute. The flow rate can be set by the user or, if the machine has a computer attached, can be calculated by the device itself based on the volume to be infused and the time period for the infusion, which are input by the nurse or user. The machine functions with a primary infusion or a secondary infusion (intravenous piggyback). See Figure 18-6 for an example. These combined devices usually contain multiple channels (two or four channels) that can function independently and have the ability to operate in any combination of pump and/or controller. Another feature is the ability to preprogram these devices for delayed start infusions, multidosing, and drug calculations.

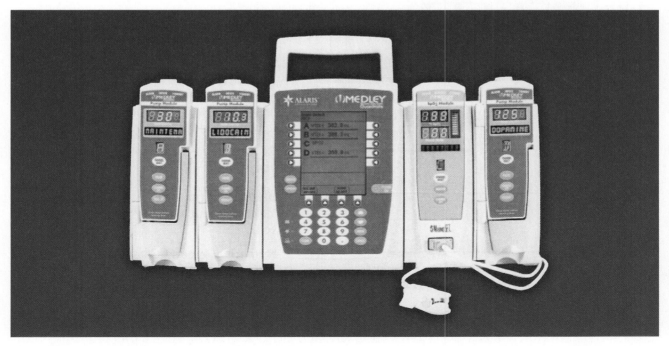

Figure 18-6   MEDLEY Medication Safety System with four channels (Reproduced with permission of Alaris Medical Systems)

Controls and indicators

Model 71XX

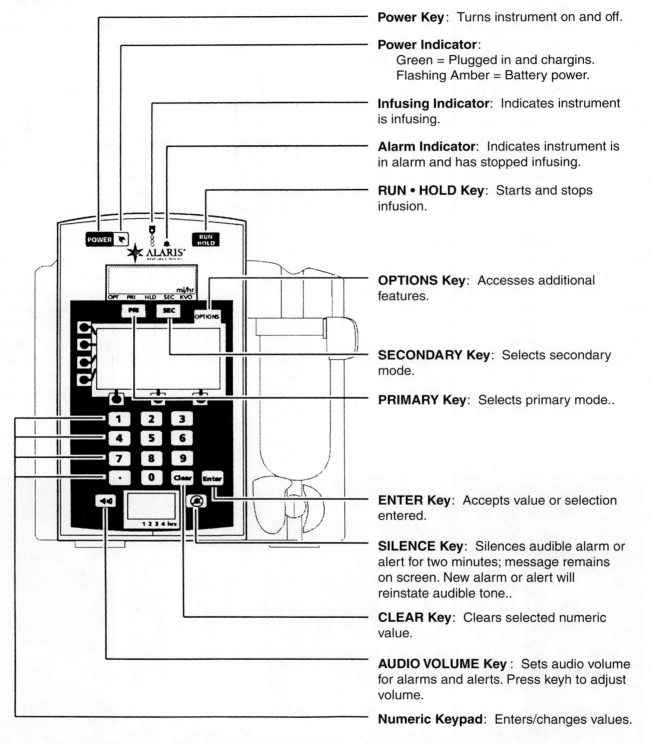

Power Key: Turns instrument on and off.

Power Indicator:
   Green = Plugged in and chargins.
   Flashing Amber = Battery power.

Infusing Indicator: Indicates instrument is infusing.

Alarm Indicator: Indicates instrument is in alarm and has stopped infusing.

RUN • HOLD Key: Starts and stops infusion.

OPTIONS Key: Accesses additional features.

SECONDARY Key: Selects secondary mode.

PRIMARY Key: Selects primary mode..

ENTER Key: Accepts value or selection entered.

SILENCE Key: Silences audible alarm or alert for two minutes; message remains on screen. New alarm or alert will reinstate audible tone..

CLEAR Key: Clears selected numeric value.

AUDIO VOLUME Key: Sets audio volume for alarms and alerts. Press keyh to adjust volume.

Numeric Keypad: Enters/changes values.

Figure 18-7   Alaris Model 71xx keypad (Reproduced with permission of Alaris Medical Systems)

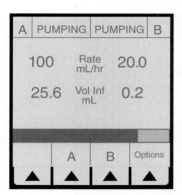

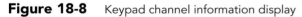

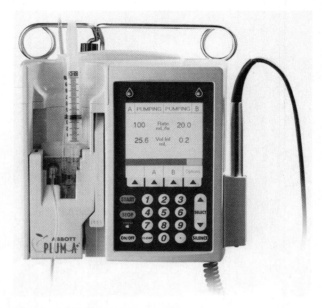

Figure 18-8 Keypad channel information display

Figure 18-9 Abbott Plum A+ volumetric infusion device (Courtesy of Abbott Laboratories)

The flow rate on these machines is set by a mL per hour (60 minutes) rate. If the infusion is ordered for a time period that is less than or more than one hour, the pump must still be set at the rate of mL per hour. Most of the time, the conversion of flow rate to the one-hour period of time is simple, but the result should still be checked by using ratio and proportion. The proportion can be set up as:

$$\frac{\text{Desired time to be set}}{\text{Prescribed time of infusion}} = \frac{\text{Desired mL per hour}}{\text{Prescribed amount to infuse}}$$

Example: The physician prescribes an infusion of 375 mL to infuse in 3 hours. How many mL per hour should the electronic pump controller be set at?

Solution: Set up the proportion:

$$\frac{\text{Desired time to be set}}{\text{Prescribed time of infusion}} = \frac{\text{Desired mL per hour}}{\text{Prescribed amount to infuse}}$$

$$\frac{60 \text{ minutes}}{180 \text{ minutes}} = \frac{x \text{ mL}}{375 \text{ mL}}$$

$$180x = 22,500$$

$$x = 125 \text{ mL per hour}$$

Although various manufacturers have different types of keypads on which the rate and volume to be infused (VTBI) are entered, the keypads are really rather similar. See Figure 18-7 for a sample keypad and Figure 18-8 for a sample channel information display.

Another type of electronic infusion device is the syringe pump, which delivers, under pressure, a preset amount of medication or fluid from a prefilled syringe that has been placed in a special chamber of the pump. These programmable pumps allow for various flow rates, especially when the desired time of infusion is less than 30 minutes. The syringe pump is especially useful in pediatric and intensive care situations. See Figure 18-9 for an example of a syringe pump.

Still another type of infusion device is the patient-controlled analgesia (PCA) pump, which is programmed to deliver a preset amount of narcotic when activated by the patient. These pumps have a tamper-resistant feature and measure the amount of analgesia activated by the patient; they also keep a record of the number of times the patient attempted unsuccessfully to administer a bolus of narcotic. Most of these pumps also permit programming for continuous administration of analgesia and for clinician-controlled administration. See Figure 18-10 for an example.

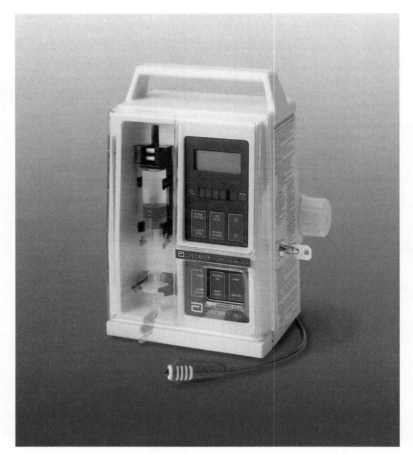

Figure 18-10   Abbott's Lifecare PCA (Patient-controlled Analgesia) Plus II Infuser (Courtesy of Abbott Laboratories)

Audio and visual alarms, which are triggered when the preset rates are not being delivered or when malfunction occurs, are featured on all these devices, but cannot be considered infallible. Even though these devices have many automatic features, it is still the responsibility of the nurse to assess the infusion site and monitor the flow rate to verify that the equipment is operating accurately.

Review Test 18.1
Intravenous Fluid Therapy and Computing Flow Rates

1. Determine the amounts of dextrose and sodium chloride in 500 mL of 10% dextrose in 0.9% saline.

    _____ grams dextrose _____ grams sodium chloride

2. Determine the amount of dextrose in 1000 mL of 5% dextrose in water.

    _____ grams dextrose

3. The physician has ordered 3000 mL of D5/W to run for 24 hours for a patient.

    The IV set available has a drop factor of 10 drops = 1 mL.

    How many mL per hour should infuse? _____ mL/hr

    How many mL per minute should infuse? _____ mL/min

    How many drops per minute delivers this amount? _____ gtt/min

4. The physician has ordered 1500 mL of D5/NS to run for 24 hours for a patient.

   The IV set delivers 60 drops per milliliter.

   How many mL per hour should infuse? _____ mL/hr

   How many mL per minute should infuse? _____ mL/min

   How many drops per minute delivers this amount? _____ gtt/min

5. The physician has ordered 2000 mL of lactated Ringer's solution IV to run for 24 hours for a 9-year-old child. The IV set delivers 20 drops per milliliter.

   How many mL per hour should infuse? _____ mL/hr

   How many mL per minute should infuse? _____ mL/min

   How many drops per minute delivers this amount? _____ gtt/min

6. The physician has ordered 1000 mL of D5/NS to run for 24 hours to keep the vein open (KVO) for a patient. The IV set has a drop factor of 10 drops per milliliter.

   How many mL per hour should infuse? _____ mL/hr

   How many mL per minute should infuse? _____ mL/min

   How many drops per minute delivers this amount? _____ gtt/min

7. The physician has ordered 75 mL per hour of a hypertonic solution for a patient receiving total parenteral nutrition. The IV set has a drop factor of 60 drops/mL.

   How many mL per hour should infuse? _____ mL/hr

   How many mL per minute should infuse? _____ mL/min

   How many drops per minute delivers this amount? _____ gtt/min

8. The physician has ordered 1500 mL of D5/NS to run at 80 mL per hour. The IV set delivers 60 drops per milliliter.

   How many mL per minute should infuse? _____ mL/min

   How many drops per minute delivers this amount? _____ gtt/min

   The total infusion time should be _____ hours.

9. The physician has ordered 1/2NS 750 mL to run at 60 mL per hour. The IV set delivers 60 drops per milliliter.

   How many mL per minute should infuse? _____ mL/min

   How many drops per minute delivers this amount? _____ gtt/min

   The total infusion time should be _____ hours.

10. The physician has ordered D10/W 1000 mL to run at 75 mL per hour. The IV set delivers 20 drops per milliliter.

   How many mL per minute should infuse? _____ mL/min

   How many drops per minute delivers this amount? _____ gtt/min

   The total infusion time should be _____ hours.

Answers   **1.** 50 grams dextrose; 4.5 grams sodium chloride   **2.** 50 grams dextrose   **3.** 125 mL per hour; 2.08 mL per minute; 20.8 or 21 drops per minute   **4.** 62.5 mL per hour; 1.04 mL per minute; 62.4 or 62 drops per minute OR, dividing the hourly amount of fluid by 1, 62.5 or 63 drops per minute   **5.** 83.3 mL per hour; 1.39 mL per minute; 27.8 or 28 drops per minute   **6.** 41.6 mL per hour; 0.69 mL per minute; 6.9 or 7 drops per minute   **7.** 75 mL per hour; 1.25 mL per minute; 75 drops per minute   **8.** 1.33 mL per minute; 79.99 or 80 drops per minute; 18.75 or 18 hours, 45 minutes   **9.** 1 mL per minute; 60 drops per minute; 12.5 or 12 hours, 30 minutes   **10.** 1.25 mL per minute; 25 drops per minute; 13.3 or 13 hours, 20 minutes

If you had fewer than three errors on Review Test 18.1, move on the next chapter. If you had four or more errors, review the material on intravenous fluid therapy and computing flow rates and complete Review Test 18.2 before continuing.

Review Test 18.2
Intravenous Fluid Therapy and Computing Flow Rates

1. Determine the amounts of dextrose and sodium chloride in 1500 mL of 5% dextrose in 0.45% saline.

   _____ grams dextrose _____ grams sodium chloride

2. Determine the amount of dextrose in 1000 mL of 20% dextrose in water.

   _____ grams dextrose

3. The physician has ordered 1000 mL of D5/W to run for 12 hours for a patient. The IV set available has a drop factor of 15 drops = 1 mL.

   How many mL per hour should infuse?   _____ mL/hr

   How many mL per minute should infuse?   _____ mL/min

   How many drops per minute delivers this amount?   _____ gtt/min

4. The physician has ordered 2500 mL of D5/NS to run for 24 hours for a patient. The IV set delivers 10 drops per milliliter.

   How many mL per hour should infuse?   _____ mL/hr

   How many mL per minute should infuse?   _____ mL/min

   How many drops per minute delivers this amount?   _____ gtt/min

5. The physician has ordered 1000 mL of lactated Ringer's solution IV to run for 24 hours for a patient. The IV set delivers 60 drops per milliliter.

   How many mL per hour should infuse?   _____ mL/hr

   How many mL per minute should infuse?   _____ mL/min

   How many drops per minute delivers this amount?   _____ gtt/min

6. The physician has ordered 500 mL of D5/NS to run for 24 hours to keep the vein open (KVO) for a patient. The IV set has a drop factor of 20 drops per milliliter.

   How many mL per hour should infuse?   _____ mL/hr

   How many mL per minute should infuse?   _____ mL/min

   How many drops per minute delivers this amount?   _____ gtt/min

7. The physician has ordered 50 mL per hour of a hypertonic solution for a patient receiving total parenteral nutrition. The IV set has a drop factor of 60 drops/mL.

   How many mL per hour should infuse?   _____ mL/hr

   How many mL per minute should infuse?   _____ mL/min

   How many drops per minute delivers this amount?   _____ gtt/min

8. The physician has ordered 1500 mL of D5/NS to run at 125 mL per hour. The IV set delivers 10 drops per milliliter.

   How many mL per minute should infuse?   _____ mL/min

   How many drops per minute delivers this amount?   _____ gtt/min

   The total infusion time should be   _____ hours.

9. The physician has ordered 1/3NS 1000 mL to run at 60 mL per hour. The IV set delivers 10 drops per milliliter.

   How many mL per minute should infuse?   _____ mL/min

   How many drops per minute delivers this amount?   _____ gtt/min

   The total infusion time should be   _____ hours.

10. The physician has ordered D10/W 1500 mL to run at 50 mL per hour. The IV set delivers 60 drops per milliliter.

    How many mL per minute should infuse? _____ mL/min

    How many drops per minute delivers this amount? _____ gtt/min

    The total infusion time should be _____ hours.

Answers: **1.** 75 grams dextrose; 6.75 grams sodium chloride **2.** 200 grams dextrose **3.** 83.3 mL per hour; 1.39 mL per minute; 20.85 or 21 drops per minute **4.** 104.16 mL per hour; 1.736 mL per minute; 17.36 or 17 drops per minute **5.** 41.67 mL per hour; 0.69 mL per minute; 41.67 or 42 drops per minute **6.** 20.83 mL per hour; 0.35 mL per minute; 6.94 or 7 drops per minute **7.** 50 mL per hour; 0.83 mL per minute; 50 drops per minute **8.** 2.08 mL per minute; 20.83 or 21 drops per minute; 12 hours **9.** 1 mL per minute; 10 drops per minute; 16.67 or 16 hours, 40 minutes **10.** 0.83 mL per minute; 50 drops per minute; 30 hours

The Review Tests on intravenous fluid therapy and computing flow rates should be repeated until fewer than three errors occur.

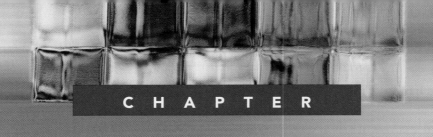

19

Computing Intravenous Medications

Learning Outcomes

After successfully completing this chapter, the learner will be able to:

- *Calculate the prescribed amount of IV medication to be added to a container of IV fluid attached to a primary line.*

- *Calculate the prescribed amount of IV medication to be added to a container of IV fluid attached to a piggyback set or a secondary infusion set.*

- *Calculate the drop rate to infuse a specified amount of intravenous fluid with medication over a specified time from a piggyback or secondary IV.*

- *Calculate the mL per hour to infuse a specified amount of intravenous fluid with medication via a volumetric infusion device over a specified period of time.*

GENERAL INFORMATION

The IV administration of medication has a rapid effect, limits the discomfort or irritation caused by some medications, and allows exact control of the amount of medication absorbed. The major hazards of IV administration are infection and rapid, severe reactions, which are more difficult to control. To limit infection, sterile technique must be used throughout the procedure. The medication should be administered slowly, the manufacturer's directions followed exactly, and the patient closely assessed during the administration. This is especially true when titrating the more potent medications used so frequently today. Any medication errors—such as incorrect drug, incorrect dosage, incorrect dilution, or incorrect speed of administration—can result in patient reactions ranging from discomfort to death. Accuracy is of the highest priority in administering IV medications, as absorption is immediate and often does not allow time for treatment. Because of the dangers involved, in most instances, when medications are added to IV fluids, an electronic device that calculates, controls, and monitors the rate of administration should be used. However, the nurse still has the responsibility for administration and the patient's response to the medication.

INTRAVENOUS MEDICATIONS

IV medications can be added to primary IV fluid containers that are already running or to new IV fluids prior to hanging (see Figure 19-1). IVs with medication are usually administered with a volumetric infusion device.

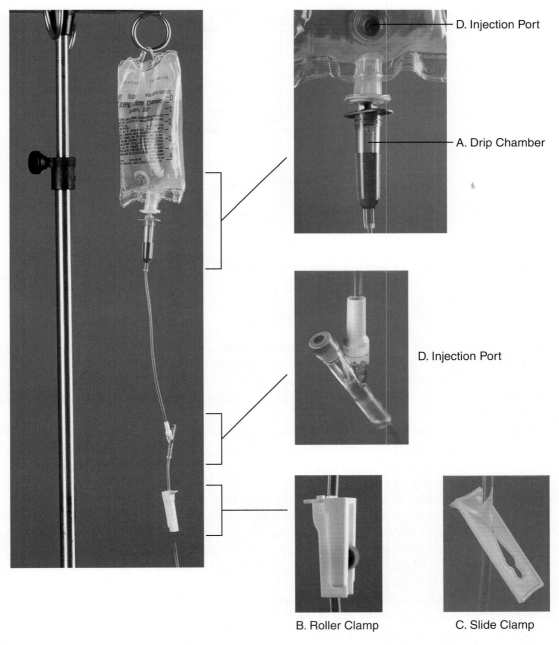

D. Injection Port

A. Drip Chamber

D. Injection Port

B. Roller Clamp

C. Slide Clamp

Figure 19-1   IV Medications can be added to primary IV fluid containers that are already running or to new IV fluids prior to hanging

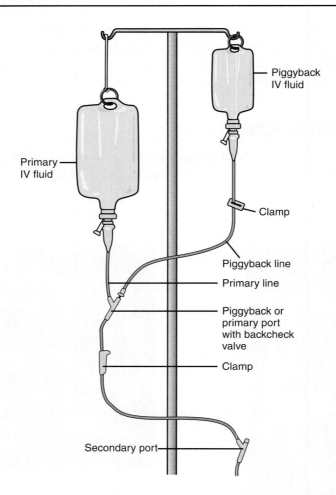

Primary
IV fluid

Piggyback
IV fluid

Clamp

Piggyback line

Primary line

Piggyback or
primary port
with backcheck
valve

Clamp

Secondary port

Figure 19-2   The piggyback line connects to the primary line via the upper or piggyback port

IV medications can be added to small-volume containers that can be attached to the primary infusion line as a piggyback line. A piggyback line can be connected to the upper port of the primary line via a short infusion set that allows it to be hung above the primary fluid container (hence the name piggyback). This setup is used for intermittent infusions of medications (see Figure 19-2). A microdrop chamber system is usually used for the piggyback infusion line.

Medications can be added to fluids that are connected to a secondary infusion line attached to the lower port of the primary line. This setup is usually run concurrently with the primary IV, and the medication may be dissolved in larger amounts of fluids than in the piggyback IV (Figure 19-3). A microdrop chamber system is most often used for the secondary infusion line.

IV medications can be added to a volume-control set (Soluset, Buretrol, Pediatrol, or Volutrol) that has a 100 to 150 mL container with either a floating valve or membrane filter at the base of the container. This set is attached to the primary infusion container as either a primary or a piggyback line and is designed to measure and allow precise control of the infusion and/or the medication (see Figure 19-4).

When administering IV medications, flush the infusion lines, if necessary, to remove air and/or incompatible fluids. Determine if the IV with the medication is to run simultaneously or if the primary line should be clamped; then start the piggyback, secondary IV, or volume-control set with the medication.

IV medications can be administered by an IV push or bolus directly into the vein. The IV bolus can be administered directly into the vein via a venipuncture, through the injection port on a primary infusion set, or through an intermittent infusion device (saline lock or heparin lock). The medication is usually administered by the nurse, the nurse specialist, or the physician (see Figure 19-5).

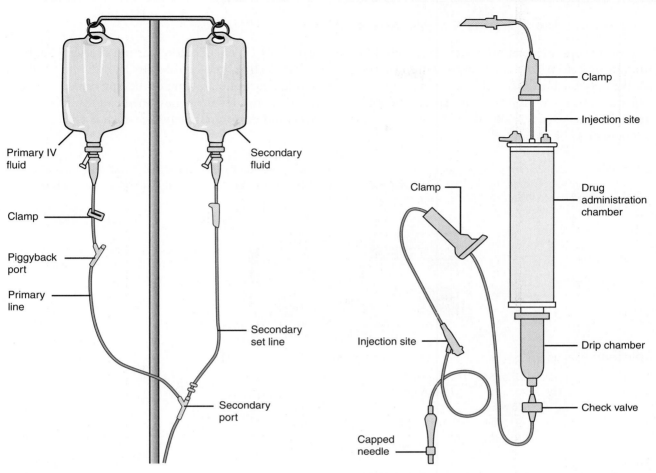

Figure 19-3 The secondary line connects to the primary line at the lower or secondary port of the primary line.

Figure 19-4 Volume-control set (Buretrol, Volutrol, or Soluset)

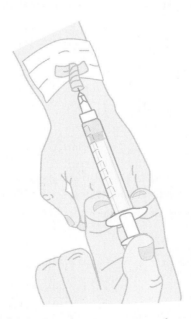

Figure 19-5 Injection of solution into the intermittent infusion device (heparin or saline lock)

Intravenous Medications Via Primary Infusions

The intravenous medications most commonly added to the primary IV, either before starting or after it has been running, are electrolytes such as potassium chloride or vitamins such as Solu-B, vitamin C, or M.V.I.-12. These are the only medications added to primary IVs, as they are often part of maintenance therapy rather than specific medications administered for specific actions or health problems. Diluting these medications in large volumes of fluid (usually 1000 mL) reduces the risk of side effects and untoward reactions, which is especially true of potassium chloride.

Example: The physician's order states: Add 25 mEq of potassium chloride to 1000 mL D5/W. Available are ampules labeled potassium chloride 40 mEq = 20 mL (see label). How much potassium chloride labeled potassium chloride 40 mEq = 20 mL should be added?

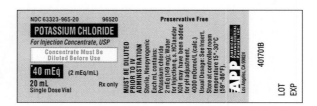

Solution: Set up the problem using ratio and proportion:

$$\frac{\text{Desired Dosage}}{\text{Have Dosage}} = \frac{\text{Desired Amount}}{\text{Have Amount}}$$

$$\frac{25 \text{ mEq}}{40 \text{ mEq}} = \frac{x \text{ mL}}{20 \text{ mL}} \qquad \text{or} \qquad \frac{25 \text{ mEq}}{2 \text{ mEq}} = \frac{x \text{ mL}}{1 \text{ mL}}$$

$$40x = 500 \qquad\qquad\qquad 2x = 25$$

$$x = 12.5 \text{ mL} \qquad\qquad\qquad x = 12.5 \text{ mL}$$

To prepare 25 mEq of potassium chloride, add 12.5 mL of potassium chloride 40 mEq = 20 mL to the patient's IV of 1000 mL D5/W, producing a total solution of 1012.5 mL.

Example: The physician's order states: Add 60 mEq of potassium chloride to 1000 mL D5/W and infuse at a rate of 2.5 mEq per hour. Available are ampules labeled potassium chloride 40 mEq = 20 mL. The infusion set has a drop factor of 60. How much potassium chloride should be added to the IV? How many mL per hour should the patient receive? How many drops per minute must infuse to deliver the required amount of drug per hour?

Solution: Set up the problem using ratio and proportion:

$$\frac{\text{Desired Dosage}}{\text{Have Dosage}} = \frac{\text{Desired Amount}}{\text{Have Amount}}$$

$$\frac{60 \text{ mEq}}{40 \text{ mEq}} = \frac{x \text{ mL}}{20 \text{ mL}}$$

$$40x = 1200$$

$$x = 30 \text{ mL}$$

To prepare 60 mEq of potassium chloride, add 30 mL of potassium chloride 40 mEq = 20 mL to the patient's IV of 1000 mL D5/W, producing a total solution of 1030 mL.

To determine how many mL per hour the patient should receive, set up the problem using ratio and proportion:

$$\frac{\text{Desired Dosage}}{\text{Have Dosage}} = \frac{\text{Desired Amount}}{\text{Have Amount}}$$

$$\frac{2.5 \text{ mEq}}{60 \text{ mEq}} = \frac{x \text{ mL}}{1030 \text{ mL}}$$

$$60x = 2575$$

$$x = 42.91 \text{ mL per hour}$$

To determine how many drops per minute must infuse to deliver the required amount of drug, divide the hourly rate by 60 and multiply by the drop factor of 60.

42.91 ÷ 60 = 0.715 mL per minute × drop factor (60) = 42.91 or 43 gtt/min

The formula which states that if the drop factor is 60 drops = 1 mL, dividing the hourly amount of fluid by 1 can also be used:

42.91 or 43 ÷ 1 = 43 gtt/min

Problem Set 19.1

1. The physician's order states: D5/W 1000 mL with potassium chloride 40 mEq to be infused at a rate of 100 mL per hour. Available are 20 mL ampules labeled potassium chloride 2 mEq/mL. The infusion set has a drop factor of 15.

   How much potassium chloride should be added? _____ mL

   What will be the total volume of the solution? _____ mL

   How many drops per minute should infuse? _____ gtt/min

2. The physician's order states: Add 20 mEq potassium chloride to 1000 mL of D5/NS, infuse at a rate of 2.5 mEq per hour. Available are 20 mL ampules labeled potassium chloride 2 mEq/mL.

   How much potassium chloride should be added? _____ mL

   What will be the total volume of the solution? _____ mL

   How many mL of the total solution contains the desired hourly amount of potassium chloride?

   _____ mL

3. The physician's order states: Add 25 mEq potassium chloride to D5/W 1000 mL, infuse over 24 hours. Available are 10 mL ampules labeled potassium chloride 20 mEq. The infusion set has a drop factor of 10.

   How much potassium chloride should be added? _____ mL

   What will be the total volume of the solution? _____ mL

   What will be the hourly rate? _____ mL

   How many drops per minute should infuse? _____ gtt/min

4. The physician's order states: Add a single dose of M.V.I.-12 to 500 mL of lactated Ringer's solution, infuse over 8 hours. Available are boxes of M.V.I.-12 that contain two 5 mL ampules labeled Vial 1 and Vial 2. The directions state use the contents of both vials for a single dose. The infusion set has a drop factor of 10.

   How much M.V.I.-12 should be added? _____ mL

   What will be the total volume of the solution? _____ mL

   What will be the hourly rate? _____ mL

   How many drops per minute should infuse? _____ gtt/min

5. The physician's order states: Add 40 mEq potassium chloride to 1 L of D5/W, infuse at a rate of 1.5 mEq per hour. Available are 20 mL ampules labeled potassium chloride 2 mEq/mL. The infusion set has a drop factor of 60.

   How much potassium chloride should be added? _____ mL

   What will be the total volume of the solution? _____ mL

   What will be the hourly rate? _____ mL

   How many drops per minute should infuse? _____ gtt/min

Answers **1.** 20 mL, 1020 mL, 25 gtt/min **2.** 10 mL, 1010 mL, 126 mL **3.** 12.5 mL, 1012.5 mL, 42.18 or 42 mL, 7 gtt/min **4.** 10 mL, 510 mL, 63.75 mL, 10.625 or 11 gtt/min **5.** 20 mL, 1020 mL, 38.25 mL, 38 gtt/min

Intravenous Medications Via Piggyback Infusions (IVPB)

The physician may order IV medications to run piggyback with IV fluids. These medications are dissolved in small-volume IV containers (either 50 or 100 mL) and are usually ordered to run for 30 minutes to 1 hour. IVPB lines can be connected to the upper port of the primary line via a short infusion set, with either a microdrip or macrodrip chamber system, that allows it to be hung above the primary IV. The primary IV is usually lowered by use of an extension hook. If the fluids and the medications are compatible, the IVPB is started. If the fluids and the IVPB medications are not compatible, the primary IV tubing must be flushed with a compatible solution before the IVPB is started. The most commonly used piggyback solution is D5/W. The drops per minute for these piggyback medications are calculated the same way as for any IV fluids and should be electronically controlled. This setup is most frequently used for the intermittent infusion of medications.

Example: The physician orders dexamethasone (Decadron) 8 mg to be added to 100 mL of D5/W as an IVPB to run for 1 hour. On hand are vials of Decadron labeled 4 mg per mL (see label). The infusion set has a drop factor of 10. How much medication should be added to the piggyback and how many drops per minute must infuse to deliver the required amount of drug in an hour?

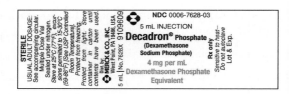

Solution: Set up the problem using ratio and proportion:

$$\frac{\text{Desired Dosage}}{\text{Have Dosage}} = \frac{\text{Desired Amount}}{\text{Have Amount}}$$

$$\frac{8 \text{ mg}}{4 \text{ mg}} = \frac{x \text{ mL}}{1 \text{ mL}}$$

$$4x = 8$$

$$x = 2 \text{ mL}$$

To prepare 8 mg of Decadron, add 2 vials of Decadron 4 mg = 1 mL to the 100 mL D5/W piggyback, producing a total solution of 102 mL.

To determine how many drops per minute must infuse to deliver the required amount of drug, divide the IVPB amount (102 mL) by 60 minutes and multiply by the drop factor of 10.

102 ÷ 60 = 1.7 mL per minute × drop factor (10) = 17 gtt/min

The formula which states that if the drop factor is 10 drops = 1 mL, dividing the hourly amount of fluid by 6 can also be used:

102 ÷ 6 = 17 gtt/min to be infused from the IVPB

Example: The physician has prescribed famotidine (Pepcid) 20 mg by IVPB hs. On hand is a 4 mL vial, which contains Pepcid 10 mg per mL (see label). The manufacturer's instruction for IVPB administration recommends that Pepcid be added to 50 mL of D5/W and infused over a 60-minute period. The drop factor of the IVPB set is 60 gtt per mL. How much medication should be added to the piggyback and how many drops per minute must infuse to deliver the required amount of drug in 60 minutes?

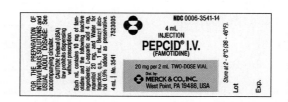

Solution: Set up the problem using ratio and proportion:

$$\frac{\text{Desired Dosage}}{\text{Have Dosage}} = \frac{\text{Desired Amount}}{\text{Have Amount}}$$

$$\frac{20 \text{ mg}}{10 \text{ mg}} = \frac{x \text{ mL}}{1 \text{ mL}}$$

$$10x = 20$$

$$x = 2 \text{ mL}$$

To prepare 20 mg of Pepcid, add 2 mL of Pepcid 10 mg = 1 mL to the 50 mL D5/W piggyback, producing a total solution of 52 mL.

To determine how many drops per minute must infuse to deliver the required amount of drug, divide the IVPB amount (52 mL) by 60 minutes and multiply by the drop factor of 60.

52 ÷ 60 = 0.87 mL per minute × drop factor (60) = 52 gtt/min

The formula which states that if the drop factor is 60 drops = 1 mL, dividing the hourly amount of fluid by 1 can also be used:

52 ÷ 1 = 52 gtt/min to be infused from the IVPB

V I P

The time and fluid required for administration of IV piggyback medications must be subtracted from the total specific fluid orders for a patient in a given time span.

Example: The physician's order states: 1000 mL of D5/W, 1000 mL of D5/NS, and 1000 mL lactated Ringer's to be infused over 24 hours; cefoxitin sodium (Mefoxin) 1 gram q6h in 100 mL of D5/W to run for 1 hour via IV piggyback. The manufacturer's instruction states that the 1 gram vial of Mefoxin should be dissolved in 10 mL of sterile water before adding to the IVPB. Both the primary and IVPB infusion sets have a drop factor of 15. How fast should the primary IV and how fast should the IVPBs with the medication infuse?

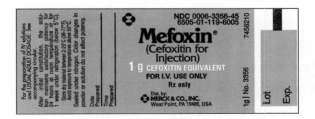

Solution: This patient will receive a total of 4 piggyback infusions daily (q6h). The 4-hour running time for the IVPB (1 hour each dose × 4 doses) and the 440 mL fluid total for the IVPB (100 mL each plus the 10 mL for the Mefoxin × 4 doses) must be subtracted from the 3000 mL of fluid for the total 24-hour period. When computing the drops per minute the primary IV should run for this patient, the figures 2560 mL (3000 mL of fluid minus the 440 mL of fluid for the IVPBs) and 20 hours (24 hours total minus the 4 hours that the IVPBs will run) should be used.

2560 mL ÷ 20 hours = 128 mL per hour

128 mL/hr ÷ 60 = 2.13 mL/min × drop factor (15) = 31.99 or 32 gtt/min

The formula which states that if the drop factor is 15 drops = 1 mL, dividing the hourly amount of fluid by 4 can also be used:

128 mL/hr ÷ 4 = 32 gtt/min for the primary IV

When computing the drops per minute the IVPBs should run for this patient,

110 mL/hr ÷ 60 = 1.83 mL/min × drop factor (15) = 27.49 or 28 gtt/min

The formula which states that if the drop factor is 15 drops = 1 mL, dividing the hourly amount of fluid by 4 can also be used:

110 mL/hr ÷ 4 = 27.5 or 28 gtt/min for the IVPBs

Problem Set 19.2

1. The physician has prescribed metoclopramide hydrochloride (Reglan) 15 mg by IVPB to run for 20 minutes. Available is a vial of Reglan labeled 10 mg = 1 mL. The manufacturer's instructions for IVPB administration state that the Reglan should be added to 50 mL of D5/W. The IVPB infusion set has a drop factor of 10.

   How much Reglan 10 mg = 1 mL should be added? _____ mL

   What will be the total volume of the IVPB solution? _____ mL

   How many drops per minute should the IVPB infuse? _____ gtt/min

2. The physician has prescribed amikacin sulfate (Amikin) 350 mg IVPB diluted in 100 mL of D5/W to be infused over 1 hour. On hand is a vial that is labeled Amikin 500 mg = 2 mL. The manufacturer's instructions agree with the physician's order. The IVPB infusion set has a drop factor of 10.

   How much Amikin 500 mg = 2 mL should be added? _____ mL

   What will be the total volume of the IVPB solution? _____ mL

   How many drops per minute should the IVPB infuse? _____ gtt/min

3. The physician's order states: cefotaxime sodium (Claforan) 1 gram, in 100 mL D5/W to run IVPB for 30 minutes q12h. Available is a vial of powdered medication labeled Claforan 2 gram. The manufacturer's directions state: Reconstitute powder with 10 mL of sterile water to yield a total solution of 11 mL where 1 mL = 180 mg of Claforan. The IVPB infusion set has a drop factor of 10.

   How much Claforan 1 mL = 180 mg should be added? _____ mL

   What will be the total volume of the IVPB solution? _____ mL

   How many drops per minute should the IVPB infuse? _____ gtt/min

4. The physician has ordered clindamycin phosphate (Cleocin) 300 mg dissolved in 50 mL of D5/W to run IVPB for 20 minutes every 8 hours for a patient who has a maximum total of 2000 mL of IV fluid for 24 hours. Available is a vial of Cleocin labeled 600 mg = 4 mL. The primary and IVPB infusion sets have drop factors of 10.

   How much Cleocin 600 mg = 4 mL should be added? _____ mL

   What will be the total volume of the IVPB solution? _____ mL

   How many drops per minute should the IVPB infuse? _____ gtt/min

   How many mL of the primary IV will be infused daily? _____ mL

   How many drops per minute should the primary IV infuse? _____ gtt/min

5. The physician has ordered cefazolin sodium (Ancef) 500 mg q6h and ampicillin sodium 500 mg q4h by IVPB. Each piggyback medication is to be added to 50 mL of D5/W and run for 1 hour. The patient is limited to a 24-hour maximum of 1500 mL of IV fluids. The vein is being kept open between the piggybacks with D5/NS. Available are two vials of powdered medication. One is labeled Ancef 500 mg with manufacturer's directions that state: Reconstitute powder with 2 mL of sterile water to yield a total solution of 2.2 mL = 500 mg. The other is labeled ampicillin sodium with manufacturer's directions that state: Reconsitute powder with 5 mL of sterile water to yield a total solution of 5 mL = 500 mg. The primary and IVPB infusion sets have drop factors of 10.

   How much Ancef 2.2 mL = 500 mg should be added? _____ mL

   What will be the total volume of the IVPB Ancef solution? _____ mL

   How many drops per minute should the Ancef IVPB infuse? _____ gtt/min

   How much ampicillin sodium 5 mL = 500 mg should be added? _____ mL

   What will be the total volume of the IVPB ampicillin sodium
   solution? _____ mL

How many drops per minute should the ampicillin sodium
IVPB infuse?   _____ gtt/min

How many mL of the primary IV will be infused daily?   _____ mL

How many drops per minute should the primary IV infuse?   _____ gtt/min

Answers **1.** 1.5 mL, 51.5 mL, 25.75 or 26 gtt/min **2.** 1.4 mL, 101.4 mL, 16.9 or 17 gtt/min **3.** 5.5 mL, 105.5 mL, 35.17 or 35 gtt/min
4. 2 mL, 52 mL, 26 gtt/min, 1844 mL, 13.36 or 13 gtt/min **5.** 2.2 mL, 52.2 mL, 8.7 or 9 gtt/min, 5 mL, 55 mL, 9.16 or 9 gtt/min, 961.2 mL, 11.44
or 11 gtt/min

Intravenous Medications Via Secondary Infusions

The physician may order medications to be added to a secondary IV and run either intermittently or continuously with the primary infusion. The infusion set from this secondary IV is connected to the lower port of the primary infusion line and the fluid is hung at the same level as the primary line. If the fluids and the medications are compatible, the secondary IV is started. If the fluids and the secondary IV are not compatible, the primary IV tubing must be flushed with a compatible solution before the secondary infusion is started. Either a micro-drop or macrodrop chamber system can be used for the secondary infusion line. The drops per minute for these secondary IV medications are calculated the same way as for any IV fluids, and administration should be electronically controlled.

Example: The physician has prescribed a continuous secondary IV of ranitidine hydrochloride (Zantac) 150 mg in 250 mL of D5/W to run at a rate of 6.25 mg of Zantac per hour. Available are 6 mL multidose vials of Zantac labeled 1 mL = 25 mg. The drop factor of the secondary infusion set is 60. How many mL of Zantac 1 mL = 25 mg should be added to the 250 mL of fluid? How many mL per hour will have to infuse to deliver the required 6.25 mg of Zantac in 1 hour? How many drops per minute will deliver this dosage?

Solution: Set up the problem using ratio and proportion:

$$\frac{\text{Desired Dosage}}{\text{Have Dosage}} = \frac{\text{Desired Amount}}{\text{Have Amount}}$$

$$\frac{150 \text{ mg}}{25 \text{ mg}} = \frac{x \text{ mL}}{1 \text{ mL}}$$

$$25x = 150$$

$$x = 6 \text{ mL}$$

To prepare 150 mg of Zantac, add 6 mL of Zantac 25 mg = 1 mL to the patient's IV of 250 mL D5/W, producing a total solution of 256 mL.

To determine how many mL per hour the patient should receive, set up the problem using the same ratio and proportion:

$$\frac{6.25 \text{ mg}}{150 \text{ mg}} = \frac{x \text{ mL}}{256 \text{ mL}}$$

$$150x = 1600$$

$$x = 10.67 \text{ or } 11 \text{ mL per hour}$$

To determine how many drops per minute must infuse to deliver the required amount of drug, divide the hourly rate by 60 and multiply by the drop factor of 60.

10.67 ÷ 60 = 0.1778 mL per minute × drop factor (60) = 10.669 or 11 gtt/min

The formula which states that if the drop factor is 60 drops = 1 mL, dividing the hourly amount of fluid by 1 can also be used:

10.67 or 11 ÷ 1 = 11 gtt/min

Example: The physician has prescribed a continuous secondary IV of cefamandole nafate (Mandol) 1 gram in 1000 mL of D5/W to run for 12 hours. Available is a 2 gram vial of powdered Mandol. The manufacturer's instruction states that each gram of the powdered Mandol should be dissolved in 10 mL of sterile water before adding to the IV. The secondary infusion set has a drop factor of 10. How many mL of Mandol 10 mL = 1 g should be added to the 1000 mL of fluid? How many mL per hour will have to infuse to deliver the required amount of Mandol in 12 hours? How many drops per minute will deliver this dosage?

Solution: Set up the problem using ratio and proportion:

$$\frac{\text{Desired Dosage}}{\text{Have Dosage}} = \frac{\text{Desired Amount}}{\text{Have Amount}}$$

$$\frac{1\text{ g}}{2\text{ g}} = \frac{x\text{ mL}}{20\text{ mL}}$$

$$2x = 20$$

$$x = 10\text{ mL}$$

To prepare 1 gram of Mandol, add 10 mL of Mandol 1 gram = 10 mL to the patient's IV of 1000 mL D5/W, producing a total solution of 1010 mL.

To determine how many mL of solution per hour the patient should receive, divide the 1010 mL of fluid per 12 hours by 12:

1010 mL ÷ 12 = 84.17 mL per hour

To determine how many drops per minute must infuse to deliver the required amount of drug, divide the hourly rate by 60 and multiply by the drop factor of 10.

84.17 ÷ 60 = 1.40 mL per minute × drop factor (10) = 14 gtt/min

The formula which states that if the drop factor is 10 drops = 1 mL, dividing the hourly amount of fluid by 6 can also be used:

84.17 ÷ 6 = 14.02 or 14 gtt/min

Problem Set 19.3

1. The physician has prescribed a continuous secondary IV of heparin sodium 25,000 units in 1000 mL of 0.9% sodium chloride to infuse at a rate of 1000 units of heparin per hour.

   How many mL per hour will have to infuse to deliver the required 1000 units of heparin in 1 hour? _____ mL/hr

2. The physician has prescribed a continuous secondary IV of penicillin G potassium 5 million units in 1000 mL of D5/W 2 times daily (for a total of 10 million units in 2000 mL) to infuse with the primary IV of lactated Ringer's solution. Available are vials labeled 5,000,000 units of penicillin G potassium with manufacturer's directions that state: Reconstitute powder with 3.2 mL of sterile water to yield a solution where 1 mL = 1,000,000 units. The infusion set has a drop factor of 15.

   How many units of penicillin G potassium should be added
   to each liter of fluid? _____ units

   What will be the total volume of the solution? _____ mL

   What will be the hourly rate? _____ mL/hr

   How many drops per minute should infuse? _____ gtt/min

3. The physician has prescribed a continuous secondary IV of cimetidine hydrochloride (Tagamet) 900 mg in 1000 mL of D5/W to infuse at a rate of 37.5 mg of Tagamet per hour for 24 hours. Available are 8 mL multidose vials labeled Tagamet 300 mg = 2 mL. The infusion set has a drop factor of 10.

   How many mL of Tagamet should be added? _____ mL

   What will be the total volume of the solution? _____ mL

   What will be the hourly rate to deliver the ordered dose
   of Tagamet? _____ mL/hr

   How many drops per minute should infuse to deliver the
   required amount of drug? _____ gtt/min

4. The physician has prescribed a secondary IV of regular insulin 50 units in 500 mL of 1/2NS to infuse at a rate of 6 units per hour. Available are multidose vials labeled 1 mL = 100 units of regular insulin. The drop factor of the secondary infusion set is 60.

How many mL of regular insulin should be added? _____ mL

What will be the hourly rate to deliver the ordered dose of
regular insulin? _____ mL/hr

How many drops per minute should infuse to deliver the
required amount of drug? _____ gtt/min

5. The physician has prescribed a secondary intravenous infusion of azithromycin for injection (Zithromax IV) 500 mg in lactated Ringer's solution 500 mL to be infused in 4 hours. Available is a vial of Zithromax 500 mg. The manufacturer's directions state: Add 4.8 mL of sterile water to yield a solution that contains 100 mg per 1 mL. The infusion set has a drop factor of 15.

How many mL of Zithromax should be added to the lactated
Ringer's solution? _____ mL

How many mg of Zithromax are in each mL of solution? _____ mg

What will be the hourly rate? _____ mL

How many drops per minute should infuse? _____ gtt

If an electronic infusion device is used, the nurse should set
the hourly rate at _____ mL

Answers   **1.** 40 mL per hour   **2.** 5,000,000 units, 1005 mL × 2 = 2010 mL, 83.75 or 84 mL/hour, 20.93 or 21 gtt/min   **3.** 6 mL, 1006 mL, 42 mL, 7 gtt/min   **4.** 0.5 mL, 60.06 or 60 mL/hr, 60 gtt/min   **5.** 5 mL, 1 mg, 125 mL per hour, 31 gtt, 125 mL

Intravenous Medications Via Volume-Controlled Infusions

The physician may order IV medications to be added to a volume-control set (Soluset, Buretrol, Pediatrol, or Volutrol). These sets have a 100 to 150 mL capacity container, calibrated in 1 mL increments, and a microdrop system with a drop factor of 60. These volume-control sets are used as either a primary or a piggyback line and are designed to measure and allow precise control of the infusion and/or the medication. These volume-control sets control the amount of fluid to infuse (fluid is limited to the capacity of the set); when they are attached to electronic delivery devices, both the volume of fluid and the time can be precisely managed. This is especially important when the patient is a child or an adult who requires strict fluid restrictions and/or prevention of circulatory overload. Volume-control sets can be used for the administration of intermittent medications or to provide a controlled hourly rate of IV fluids.

Two unique calculation factors must be considered in determining the amount of fluid to be infused and the infusion time when intermittent IV medications are ordered for administration via a volume-control set. Because of the design of the set, medication could remain in the chamber and/or tubing, and so the infusion of medication is routinely followed by a flush that is added to the chamber after the medication to ensure that the correct dosage has been delivered. The volume for this flush (15 mL for a peripheral line and 20 mL for a central line) must be added to the volume of IV fluid prescribed and must be included in the calculation of the flow rate to meet the physician's order. The other factor is the volume of the medication that contains the prescribed amount that the patient is to receive. The physician usually specifies the amount of drug and the mL of IV fluid to be used. Whether the volume of IV fluid ordered includes the volume of medication is a hospital policy, which may vary from hospital to hospital. For the purpose of consistency, all the problems in this section will subtract the medication volume from the total volume of IV fluid ordered. These special calculations can be remembered by the formula:

total volume to infuse = volume of diluent (volume of IV fluid ordered in mL − volume of medication in mL) + volume of medication in mL + 15 mL of fluid used for flush

The total volume to infuse and the prescribed time for the infusion should be used to determine the drop rate. Remember, the drop factor for controlled-volume sets is 60.

Example: The physician has prescribed gentamicin sulfate (Garamycin) 80 mg in 50 mL of D5/W to be infused in 45 minutes using an electronic infusion device. Available is a 2 mL vial labeled 1 mL = 40 mg of Garamycin. How many mL of medication will be needed? How many mL of diluent will be needed? What is the total volume to be infused? What hourly rate should be set on the electronic infusion device?

Solution: Determine the amount of medication that is to be withdrawn from the available vial of Garamycin labeled 40 mg = 1 mL.

Use ratio and proportion and determine that 2 mL = 80 mg of Garamycin, which is the prescribed amount.

Determine the volume of IV diluent needed. The physician has ordered 50 mL of diluent. The 2 mL of medication should be subtracted from this amount.

50 – 2 = 48 mL of IV diluent

Determine the total volume to be infused.

volume to infuse = volume of diluent (volume of IV fluid ordered in mL – volume of medication in mL) + volume of medication in mL + 15 mL of fluid used for flush

50 – 2 + 2 + 15 = 65 mL, which is the total volume to infuse

Determine the hourly rate to set on the electronic infusion device, using ratio and proportion:

$$\frac{\text{total volume to infuse}}{\text{time ordered in minutes}} = \frac{x \text{ mL}}{60 \text{ minutes}}$$

$$\frac{65 \text{ mL}}{45 \text{ min}} = \frac{x \text{ mL}}{60 \text{ min}}$$

$$45x = 3900$$

$$x = 86.67 \text{ or } 87 \text{ mL per hour}$$

VIP

- When administering medication via volume-controlled infusions: total volume to infuse = volume of diluent (volume of IV fluid ordered in mL – volume of medication in mL) + volume of medication in mL + 15 mL of fluid, which follows the medication and is used as a flush.
- The total volume to infuse and the prescribed time for the infusion are used to determine the drop rate.
- The drop factor for volume-controlled sets is 60.

Problem Set 19.4

1. The physician has prescribed ciprofloxacin (Cipro) 65 mg in 65 mL of D5/W via a volume-control set to be infused in 90 minutes. Available is a 20 mL multidose vial labeled 1 mL/10 mg of Cipro.

   How many mL of medication will be needed? _____ mL

   How many mL of D5/W should be added to the volume-control set? _____ mL

   What is the total volume to be infused? _____ mL

   What hourly rate should be set on the electronic infusion device? _____ mL/hr

2. The physician has prescribed tobramycin sulfate (Nebcin) 40 mg in 75 mL of D5/W via a volume-control set to be infused in 30 minutes. Available is a multidose vial labeled 1 mL/40 mg of Nebcin.

   How many mL of medication will be needed? _____ mL

   How many mL of D5/W should be added to the volume-control set? _____ mL

   What is the total volume to be infused? _____ mL

   What hourly rate should be set on the electronic infusion device? _____ mL/hr

3. The physician has prescribed amikacin sulfate (Amikin) 100 mg in 25 mL of D5/W via a volume-control set to be infused in 1 hour. Available is a multidose vial of Amikin labeled 2 mL/100 mg of Amikin.

   How many mL of medication will be needed? _____ mL

   How many mL of D5/W should be added to the volume-control set? _____ mL

   What is the total volume to be infused? _____ mL

   What hourly rate should be set on the electronic infusion device? _____ mL/hr

4. The physician has prescribed ondansetron hydrochloride (Zofran) 4 mg in 50 mL of D5/1/2NS via a volume-control set to be infused in 20 minutes. Available is a 2 mL single-dose vial labeled 1 mL/2 mg of Zofran.

   How many mL of medication will be needed? _____ mL

   How many mL of D5/W should be added to the volume-control set? _____ mL

   What is the total volume to be infused? _____ mL

   What hourly rate should be set on the electronic infusion device? _____ mL/hr

5. The physician has prescribed trimethoprim 80 mg with sulfamethoxazole 400 mg (Bactrim) 5 mL. The manufacturer's directions state that each 5 mL should be added to 125 mL of D5/W to be infused in 90 minutes. Available is a 30 mL multidose vial of Bactrim labeled trimethoprim 80 mg with sulfamethoxazole 400 mg per 5 mL.

   How many mL of medication will be needed? _____ mL

   How many mL of D5/W should be added to the volume-control set? _____ mL

   What is the total volume to be infused? _____ mL

   What hourly rate should be set on the electronic infusion device? _____ mL/hr

Answers **1.** 6.5 mL, 58.5 mL, 80 mL, 53 mL/hr **2.** 1 mL, 74 mL, 90 mL, 180 mL/hr **3.** 2 mL, 23 mL, 40 mL, 40 mL/hr **4.** 2 mL, 48 mL, 65 mL, 195 mL/hr **5.** 5 mL, 120 mL, 140 mL, 93 mL/hr

Review Test 19.1
Computing Intravenous Medications

1. The physician has written an order for 1000 mL of D5/W with ascorbic acid (vitamin C) 500 mg to run in 8 hours. The available vial is labeled 500 mg of ascorbic acid per 1 mL. The IV set has a drop factor of 10 drops = 1 mL.

   How much ascorbic acid should be added? _____ mL

   The IV should infuse at _____ gtt/min.

   The electronic infusion device should be set at _____ mL/hr.

2. The physician has ordered 45 mEq of potassium chloride IV in 1 L of D5/W to infuse at a rate of 1.5 mL per minute. The available vials are labeled potassium chloride 40 mEq = 20 mL. The IV set has a drop factor of 60 drops per 1 mL.

   How much potassium chloride should be added? _____ mL

   The IV should infuse at _____ gtt/min.

   The electronic infusion device should be set at _____ mL/hr.

3. The physician has ordered a primary IV of D5/1/3NS 3000 mL for 24 hours and cimetidine (Tagamet) 300 mg in 100 mL D5/W IVPB q6h to run for 1 hour. The available vials of Tagamet are labeled 2 mL/300 mg. The IV set has a drop factor of 10 drops = 1 mL. In the time between the piggybacks, the patient is to receive the 3000 mL of D5/1/3NS.

   How much Tagamet should be added? _____ mL

   Total volume of IVPB will be _____ mL.

    The IVPB should infuse at   _____ gtt/min.

    The piggyback electronic infusion device should be set at   _____ mL/hr.

    The primary IV should be set at   _____ gtt/min.

    The primary electronic infusion device should be set at   _____ mL/hr.

4. The physician has prescribed methyldopa (Aldomet) 375 mg q6h IVPB. Available are vials labeled Aldomet 250 mg per 5 mL. The manufacturer's instructions for IVPB administration recommend that the desired dose of Aldomet be added to 100 mL of D5/W and infused over 1 hour. The drop factor of the infusion set is 60 gtt per 1 mL. In the time between the piggybacks, the patient is to receive D5/W to KVO.

    How much Aldomet should be added?   _____ mL

    Total volume of IVPB will be   _____ mL.

    The IVPB should infuse at   _____ gtt/min.

    The electronic infusion device should be set at   _____ mL/hr.

5. The physician has ordered heparin sodium 8000 units to be added to 500 mL of isotonic sodium chloride and infused over 4 hours by secondary IV. This dilution is within the manufacturer's instructions for IV administration. The available vials of heparin contain 10,000 units per mL. The primary IV of D5/W is to resume at a KVO rate when the secondary IV is completed. The IV set has a drop factor of 60 and the IV is attached to an electronic infusion device.

    How much heparin should be added?   _____ mL

    The secondary IV should infuse at   _____ gtt/min.

    The electronic infusion device should be set at   _____ mL/hr.

6. The physician has ordered magnesium sulfate 4 grams diluted in 250 mL of D5/W and infused as a secondary IV at a rate of 2 mL/min. This dilution is within the manufacturer's instructions for IV administration. The available vials of 10% magnesium sulfate are labeled 4 g/40 mL. The IV set has a drop factor of 60 and the IV is attached to an electronic infusion device.

    How much magnesium sulfate should be added?   _____ mL

    What will be the total volume of the solution?   _____ mL

    How much magnesium sulfate is in 2 mL of the IV solution?   _____ grams

    The secondary IV should infuse at   _____ gtt/min.

    The electronic infusion device should be set at   _____ mL/hr.

7. The physician has prescribed amikacin sulfate 100 mg to be dissolved in 150 mL of D5/W via a volume-control set to infuse in 1 hour. Available is a vial labeled 1 mL/50 mg of amikacin sulfate. The Soluset has a drop factor of 60.

    How many mL of medication will be needed?   _____ mL

    How many mL of D5/W should be added to the volume-control set?   _____ mL

    What is the total volume to be infused?   _____ mL

    What hourly rate should be set on the electronic infusion device?   _____ mL/hr

8. The physician has prescribed an intravenous infusion of D5/W mL with folic acid for injection (Folvite) 5 mg to be infused in 12 hours. Available is a multidose vial of Folvite labeled 5 mg per 1 mL. The IV set has a drop factor of 10.

    How many mL of Folvite should be added to the D5/W?   _____ mL

    How many mcg of Folvite are in each mL of solution?   _____ mcg

    What will be the hourly rate?   _____ mL/hr

    How many drops per minute should infuse?   _____ gtt/min

If an electronic infusion device is used, the nurse should set
the hourly rate at _____ mL/hr.

9. The physician has prescribed famotidine (Pepcid Injection) 20 mg in 50 mL of D5/W via IVPB to be infused in 20 minutes. Available is a 4 mL multidose vial of Pepcid Injection labeled 10 mg per 1 mL. The drop factor of the infusion set is 10.

    How many Pepcid should be added to the 50 mL bag of D5/W? _____ mL

    How many drops per minute are needed to deliver 20 mg of
    Pepcid in 20 minutes? _____ gtt/min

    If an electronic infusion device is used, the nurse should set
    the hourly rate at _____ mL/hr.

10. The physician has prescribed ondansetron hydrochloride injection (Zofran Injection) 6 mg in 50 mL of D5/W via IVPB to be infused in 30 minutes. Available is a 20 mL multidose vial of Zofran labeled 2 mg in 1 mL. The drop factor of the infusion set is 15.

    How much Zofran should be added to the 50 mL bag of D5/W? _____ mL

    How many drops per minute are needed to deliver 6 mg of
    Zofran in 30 minutes? _____ gtt/min

    If an electronic infusion device is used, the nurse should set
    the hourly rate at _____ mL/hr.

Answers **1.** 1 mL, 21 gtt/min, 125 mL/hr **2.** 22.5 mL, 90 gtt/min, 90 mL/hr **3.** 2 mL, 102 mL, 17 gtt/min, 102 mL/hr, 25 gtt/min, 150 mL/hr **4.** 7.5 mL, 107.5 mL, 108 gtt/min, 108 mL/hr **5.** 0.8 mL, 125 gtt/min, 125 mL/hr **6.** 40 mL, 290 mL, 0.02759 or 0.028 g, 120 gtt/min, 120 mL/hr **7.** 2 mL, 148 mL (150 − 2), 165 mL (150 + 15 for flush), 165 mL/hr **8.** 1 mL, 5 mcg, 83 mL per hour, 14 gtts/min, 83 mL/hr **9.** 2 mL, 26 gtt/min, 156 mL/hr **10.** 3 mL, 27 gtt/min, 106 mL/hr

If you had fewer than three errors on Review Test 19.1, move on to the next chapter. If you had four or more errors, review the material on computing intravenous medications and complete Review Test 19.2 before continuing.

Review Test 19.2
Computing Intravenous Medications

1. The physician has prescribed a premixed solution of potassium chloride 20 mEq in 1000 mL of D5/NS to run intravenously at a rate of 2 mEq/hr. The infusion set delivers 60 drops per mL.

    How many mEq of drug are present in 1 mL of the premixed potassium chloride 20 mEq in 1000 mL of

    D5/NS solution? _____ mEq/mL

    How many mL of solution contain 2 mEq KCl? _____ mL

    The electronic infusion device should be set at _____ mL/hr.

2. The physician has prescribed multivitamin infusion (MVI) 5 mL to be added to 1000 mL D5/W to run intravenously at a rate of 75 mL/hr. The infusion set delivers 10 drops per mL.

    How many mL of MVI should be added? _____ mL

    What is the total volume to be infused? _____ mL

    How many drops per minute should infuse to deliver the
    required amount of drug? _____ gtt/min

    The electronic infusion device should be set at _____ mL/hr.

3. The physician has prescribed aztreonam (Azactam) 1 gram in 50 mL D5/W IVPB to run for 20 minutes. The available vials of Azactam powder are labeled 1 gram. The manufacturer's directions state that the drug should be reconstituted with 3 mL of sterile water and the entire vial added to the IV solution. The IV set has a drop factor of 60.

   How much reconstituted Azactam should be added? _____ mL

   Total volume of IVPB will be _____ mL.

   The IVPB should infuse at _____ gtt/min.

   The electronic infusion device should be set at _____ mL/hr.

4. The physician has prescribed ranitidine (Zantac) 50 mg in 50 mL D5/W IVPB to run for 15 minutes. The available vials of Zantac are labeled 50 mg/2 mL. The manufacturer's directions agree with the physician's order. The IV set has a drop factor of 10.

   How much Zantac should be added? _____ mL

   Total volume of IVPB will be _____ mL.

   The IVPB should infuse at _____ gtt/min.

   The electronic infusion device should be set at _____ mL/hr.

5. The physician has prescribed a continuous secondary infusion of Regular insulin 100 U to be added to 500 mL of 0.45% sodium chloride to run at a rate of 12 U per hour. This dilution is within the manufacturer's instructions for IV administration. The available vials of Regular insulin contain 100 units per mL. The IV set has a drop factor of 60 and the IV is attached to an electronic infusion device.

   How much Regular insulin should be added? _____ mL

   What is the total volume of solution? _____ mL

   How many units of insulin are in each mL of solution? _____ U/mL

   How many mL of solution contain 12 U of insulin? _____ mL

   The secondary IV should infuse at _____ gtt/min.

   The electronic infusion device should be set at _____ mL/hr.

6. The physician has prescribed a continuous secondary infusion of cimetidine (Tagamet) 900 mg to be added to 1000 mL of D5/W to run at a rate of 37 mg/hr. This dilution is within the manufacturer's instructions for IV administration. The available multidose vials of Tagamet are labeled 1 mL = 150 mg. The IV set has a drop factor of 60 and the IV is attached to an electronic infusion device.

   How much Tagamet should be added? _____ mL

   What is the total volume of solution? _____ mL

   How many mg of Tagamet is in each mL of solution? _____ mg/mL

   How many mL of solution contain 37 mg of Tagamet? _____ mL

   The secondary IV should infuse at _____ gtt/min.

   The electronic infusion device should be set at _____ mL/hr.

7. The physician has prescribed a continuous secondary infusion of penicillin G potassium (Pfizerpen) 15,000,000 units in D5/W 3000 mL to infuse over 24 hours. Available is a multidose vial of Pfizerpen 20,000,000 units. The manufacturer's directions state: Reconstitute with 11.5 mL of sterile water to yield a solution which contains 1,000,000 units/1 mL. The infusion set has a drop factor of 10.

   How many units of Pfizerpen should be added to each liter of fluid? _____ Units

   How many mL of the reconstituted Pfizerpen should be added to each liter? _____ mL

   What will be the hourly rate? _____ mL

How many drops per minute should infuse? _____ gtt/min

If an electronic infusion device is used, the nurse should
set the hourly rate at _____ mL/hr.

8. The physician has prescribed vancomycin hydrochloride (Vancocin) 200 mg to be dissolved in 50 mL of D5/W via a volume-control set to infuse in 1 hour. Available is a vial labeled 500 mg of Vancocin. The manufacturer's directions state that each 500 mg of Vancocin should be initially diluted with 10 mL of sterile water to yield a solution where 10 mL = 500 mg of Vancocin. The volume-control set has a drop factor of 60.

How many mL of the diluted Vancocin should be added? _____ mL

How many mL of D5/W should be added to the volume-control set? _____ mL

What is the total volume to be infused? _____ mL

What hourly rate should be set on the electronic infusion device? _____ mL/hr

9. The physician has prescribed azidothymide (Retrovir I.V.) 85 mg in 100 mL of D5/W via IVPB to infuse over 1 hour. Available is a 20 mL multidose vial labeled Retrovir 10 mg in 1 mL. The infusion set has a drop factor of 60.

How much Retrovir should be added to the 100 mL bag of
D5/W? _____ mL

What will be the total volume of the IVPB solution? _____ mL

How many drops per minute should infuse to deliver Retrovir
85 mg in 20 minutes? _____ gtt/min

If an electronic infusion device is used, the nurse should set
the hourly rate at _____ mL/hr.

10. The physician has prescribed tobramycin sulfate injection (Nebcin) 70 mg in 100 mL of D5/W via IVPB to be infused in 75 minutes. Available is a single-dose vial labeled Nebcin 80 mg in 2 mL. The drop factor of the infusion set is 60.

How much Nebcin should be added to the 100 mL bag of D5/W? _____ mL

How many drops per minute should infuse to deliver Nebcin
70 mg in 75 minutes? _____ gtt/min

If an electronic infusion device is used, the nurse should set
the hourly rate at _____ mL/hr.

Answers   **1.** 0.02 mEq/mL, 100 mL, 100 mL/hr   **2.** 5 mL, 1005 mL, 12.5 or 13 gtt/min, 75 mL/hr   **3.** 3 mL, 53 mL, 159 gtt/min, 159 mL/hr   **4.** 2 mL, 52 mL, 34.6 or 35 gtt/min, 208 mL/hr   **5.** 1 mL, 501 mL, 0.2 U/mL, 60 mL, 60 gtt/min, 60 mL/hr   **6.** 6 mL, 1006 mL, 0.89 or 0.9 mg/mL, 41.11 or 41 mL, 41 gtt/min, 41 mL/hr   **7.** 5,000,000 U, 5 mL, (125.63 mL or) 126 mL/hr, 21 gtt/min, (125.63 mL or) 126 mL/hr   **8.** 4 mL, 46 mL (50 − 4), 65 mL (50 + 15 for flush), 65 mL/hr   **9.** 8.5 mL, 108.5 or 109 mL, 109 gtt/min, 109 mL/hr   **10.** 1.75 or 1.8 mL, 82 gtt/min, 82 mL/hr

The Review Tests on computing intravenous medications should be repeated until fewer than three errors occur.

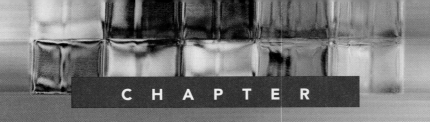

20

Intravenous Medications for Adults in Special Situations

Learning Outcomes

After successfully completing this chapter, the learner should be able to:

- *Convert weight in pounds to weight in kilograms.*
- *Calculate dosages using the patient's weight in kilograms and the manufacturer's recommended dose.*
- *Calculate dosage based on body surface area (which is expressed as square meters of body surface or m^2) estimated from the patient's height and weight by use of a nomogram or mathematical formula.*
- *Understand the importance of determining the manufacturer's recommended dose based on body weight, body surface area, and titration parameters.*
- *Recognize the importance of questioning an order that exceeds the manufacturer's recommended dose.*
- *Calculate the amount of medication to be administered in critical care situations when the medication is prescribed by flow rate (mL/hr or gtt/min) or by dosage (mg, mcg, or units/kg/hr or min) from a piggyback, secondary IV, or controlled-volume line.*
- *Recognize that some drugs are so potent that their infusions must be titrated (adjusted by concentration and administration rate) based on the patient's measurable reaction to the per-minute dosage of miniscule amounts of the drug.*

GENERAL INFORMATION

Many intravenous medications prescribed for the patient are very potent and potentially toxic. Therefore, the dosage of these drugs may be regulated according to body weight, body surface area, or physiologic response. Because the intravenous medications have a narrow therapeutic index, the nurse must be extremely accurate in calculating dosage and exercise caution when administering them. The nurse must be able to recognize the desired physiologic responses as well as early signs of toxicity.

It is highly recommended that the nurse refer to the drug insert or a current drug reference to determine the proper dosage and administration of these drugs.

Although the physician orders the medication, it is the nurse's legal responsibility to know what constitutes the usual safe dose of the medication. The nurse must make certain that an order for any dosage outside the manufacturer's recommended dosage is rechecked for accuracy before administration. It may be necessary to question the physician about orders for dosages that are outside of usual recommended amounts.

It is necessary to use an electronic infusion device to administer intravenous drugs that are highly potent with life-threatening toxic effects.

V I P

- Check the physician's order, including the amount of medication prescribed, the specific IV fluid, and the duration for administration.
- Recognize the desired physiologic response and the early signs of toxicity.
- Refer to and follow the manufacturer's instructions concerning dosage and administration.
- Question the prescribed dosage if it falls outside the usual parameters for a safe dose.
- Use an electronic infusion device to administer these intravenous medications.

WEIGHT-BASED MEDICATIONS INCLUDING HEPARIN

Calculations of Dosage Using the Body Weight Method

Today, many intravenous drugs are ordered based on the patient's body weight in kilograms. The nurse is responsible for calculating the infusion rate of the medication in mL/hr or gtt/min. The nurse is also responsible for checking to see that the prescribed dose falls within the manufacturer's recommended dose per kilogram of body weight.

To achieve the optimum physiologic response, the dosage prescribed by the physician must take into account the patient's age, weight, and gender. In addition, the physician considers the patient's metabolism, excretion, drug sensitivities, and individual idiosyncrasies.

To safely calculate intravenous drug dosages based on the patient's weight, the nurse must first convert the patient's weight in pounds to kilograms. Recall from previous material that 1 kilogram equals 2.2 pounds. The patient's weight in pounds can be converted to kilograms by dividing the number of pounds by 2.2.

Example: The physician has prescribed a secondary IV or Regular insulin 50 units in 500 mL of $\frac{1}{2}$ NS to run at a rate of 0.1 unit of Regular insulin/per kg/per hour. Available are multidose vials labeled 1 mL = 100 units of Regular insulin. The patient weights 149.6 pounds (68 kg). How many mL of the 500 mL of $\frac{1}{2}$ NS with 50 units of Regular insulin will have to infuse per hour to deliver the required unit of Regular insulin/per kg/per hour?

Solution: To determine the hourly dose the electronic infusion device for the insulin infusion should be set to deliver, multiply the patient's weight in kg by 0.1 units of insulin:

68 kg × 0.1 units = 6.8 units of Regular insulin per hour

Set up the problem using ratio and proportion to determine the mL per hour that will provide 6.8 units of Regular insulin per hour when 50 units of Regular insulin have been added to the patient's IV of 500 ml of $\frac{1}{2}$ NS:

$$\frac{\text{Desired Dosage}}{\text{Have Dosage}} = \frac{\text{Desired Amount}}{\text{Have Amount}}$$

$$\frac{6.8\,\text{U}}{50\,\text{U}} = \frac{x\ \text{mL}}{500\ \text{mL}}$$

$$50x = 3400$$

$$x = 68\ \text{mL per hour}$$

Calculation of Dosage Using the Body Weight and the Partial Thromboplastin Time (PTT)

Heparin is a medication that has proven to be most efficient when the patient's body weight and partial thromboplastin (PTT) are used to determine the actual intravenous dose. By physician's order or hospital protocol, the patient receives a loading dose of heparin by intravenous push based solely on body weight. The most commonly used loading dose is 80 units of heparin per kilogram of body weight.

After the loading dose of heparin has been administered, a continuous infusion of heparin is usually started at 18 units per kilogram per hour. The intravenous solution of heparin, in either D5/W or NS, provides either 50 units or 100 units of heparin per mL. The continuous infusion of heparin is adjusted as PTT results become available, taking into consideration the kilogram weight of the patient. The PTT laboratory test is ordered every six hours until the results indicate that a therapeutic level of heparin has been achieved. Thereafter, the PTT test is done every 24 hours.

The nurse is responsible for calculating the loading dose and the initial rate of infusion of heparin based on the physician's order or hospital protocol. The nurse also needs to adjust the continuous infusion rate based on the PTT results and the patient's weight.

A Sample Weight-Based Heparin Sliding Scale*	
PTT < 40	Rebolus with 80 units/kg Increase drip rate by 4 units/kg/hr
PTT 41–62	Rebolus with 40 units/kg Increase drip rate by 2 units/kg/hr
PTT 63–119	NO CHANGE
PTT 120–240	Reduce drip rate by 2 units/kg/hr
PTT > 240	Hold heparin infusion for 1 hour Reduce drip rate by 3 units/kg/hr

*Because PTT results vary at different laboratories, this scale, which bases action on the PTT results, varies greatly. The health care agency is responsible for establishing this scale.

At specified periodic intervals, the patient will have a PTT test done to determine if the heparin is achieving the desired effect. Based on the sliding-scale protocol, the nurse would be expected to adjust the heparin infusion rate as necessary. For example, if the results indicate a PTT of 54, the nurse would need to rebolus the patient with 40 units of heparin per kg of body weight and increase the continuous infusion drip rate by 2 units per kg of body weight per hour.

Example: The physician has prescribed weight-based heparin for a patient. As per agency protocol, the patient will receive 80 units of heparin per kilogram of body weight as a loading dose by intravenous push, followed by a continuous infusion of 18 units per kilogram per hour. The patient weighs 165 pounds. The pharmacy has provided a 250 mL bag of D5/W containing 25,000 units of heparin. The continuous infusion will be controlled by an electronic infusion device.

Solution: The nurse must first convert the patient's weight in pounds to kilograms:

165 pounds ÷ 2.2 = 75 kg

To determine the loading dose of heparin:

$$\frac{80 \text{ units}}{1 \text{kg}} = \frac{x \text{ units}}{75 \text{ units}}$$

$$x = 6000 \text{ units of heparin}$$

To determine the continuous infusion hourly rate of heparin:

$$\frac{18 \text{ units}}{1 \text{kg}} = \frac{x \text{ units}}{75 \text{ kg}}$$

x = 1350 units of heparin per hour

Set up the problem to determine the mL per hour that will provide 1350 units of heparin per hour when 25,000 units of heparin have been added to the patient's IV of 250 mL of D5/W:

$$\frac{\text{Desired Dosage}}{\text{Have Dosage}} = \frac{\text{Desired Amount}}{\text{Have Amount}}$$

$$\frac{1350 \text{ U}}{25,000 \text{ U}} = \frac{x \text{ mL}}{250 \text{ mL}}$$

25,000x = 337,500

x = 13.5 or 14 ml per hour

Problem Set 20.1

1. The nurse practitioner has prescribed a continuous IV of heparin 25,000 units in 250 mL of NS via an electronic infusion device to infuse at a rate of 18 units/kg/hour. The patient weights 110 pounds.

   How many kilograms does the patient weight? _____ kg

   How many units of heparin should the patient receive per hour? _____ units

   What hourly rate should be set on the electronic infusion device? _____ mL/hr

2. A patient is receiving 900 units per hour of heparin 25,000 units in 250 mL of NS by IV continuous infusion via an electronic infusion device. Laboratory results indicate that the patient has a partial thromboplastin (PTT) that is below 40. According to the sliding-scale protocol, the patient should receive a rebolus dose of 80 units per kg by intravenous push. The continuous IV infusion should also be increased by 4 units per kg of body weight per hour. The patient weighs 50 kg.

   How many units of heparin should the patient receive for a rebolus? _____ units

   How many additional units of heparin should the patient receive per hour? _____ units

   How many total units of heparin should the patient receive per hour? _____ units

   What will be the new hourly rate to deliver the ordered dose of heparin? _____ mL/hr

   What hourly rate should be set on the electronic infusion device to deliver the required amount of drug? _____ mL/hr

3. The physician has prescribed a continuous secondary IV of heparin 10,000 units in 500 ml D5/W to infuse at a rate of 20 units/per kg/hour. The patient weighs 38 kg.

   How many total units of heparin should the patient receive per hour? _____ units

   What will be the hourly rate to deliver the ordered dose of heparin? _____ mL/hr

   What hourly rate should be set on the electronic infusion device to deliver the required amount of drug? _____ mL/hr

4. The physician has prescribed ondansetron hydrochloride (Zofran IV) 0.15 mg per kg of body weight to be added to 50 mL of D5/W via an IV piggyback to be infused in 15 minutes. On hand is a 20 mL vial of Zofran IV which contains 2 mg per 1 mL. The patient weighs 55 kg.

   How many mg of Zofran IV will be needed? _____ mg

   How many mL will be added to the 50 mL of D5/W? _____ mL

   What hourly rate should be set on the electronic infusion device? _____ mL/hr

5. The physician has prescribed acyclovir sodium for injection (Zovirax IV) 10 mg/kg of body weight to be added to 150 mL of D5/W via IV piggyback to infuse over 1 hour. On hand are vials labeled Zovirax IV 1000 mg. The manufacturer's instructions state: To prepare the solution add 20 mL of sterile water for injection to the vial to yield a solution that contains Zovirax 50 mg/mL. The patient's weight is 176 lbs.

How many kg does the patient weigh? _____ kg

How many mg of Zovirax will be needed? _____ mg

How many mL of Zovirax should be added to the IV solution? _____ mL

What is the total volume to be infused? _____ mL

What hourly rate should be set on the electronic infusion device to deliver the required amount of drug? _____ mL/hr

Answers 1. 50 kg, 900 units, 9 mL/hr 2. 4000 units, 200 units, 1100 units (900 units + 200 units), 11 mL/hr, 11 mL/hr 3. 760 units, 38 mL/hr, 38 gtt/min 4. 8.3 mg, 4.2 mL, 217 mL/hr (216.8 mL) 5. 80 kg, 800 mg, 16 mL, 166 mL (150 mL + 16 mL), 166 mL/hr

MEDICATION DOSAGE BASED ON BODY SURFACE AREA

Calculation of the Body Surface Area

The body surface area method, using height and weight, provides a more accurate means of estimating what a safe dose would be for potent intravenous drugs than the body weight method alone.

In calculating the body surface area (BSA), the nurse uses the Adult Body Surface Area Nomogram (see Figure 20-1) by obtaining the patient's height, in centimeters or inches, and the patient's weight in kilograms or pounds. Using the nomogram, a straight line is drawn from the client's height on the height chart (a), to the client's weight on the weight chart (b). This line will intersect the chart at a point representing the body surface area (c), which is the square meters (m^2).

VIP

- Make certain you use the Adult Body Surface Area Nomogram.
- Recognize that the height scale uses centimeters or inches and the weight scale uses kilograms or pounds; make certain that the correct marking is used to draw the intersecting line.
- If the ruler is even slightly off the point, the m^2 will be incorrect.
- The calibrations on the nomogram are not of equal value and the user must determine the value of each calibration in order to accurately estimate the BSA in square meters.

Problem Set 20.2

Using the Adult Body Surface Area Nomogram, indicate the BSA in square meters (m^2).

1. The BSA for a client who is 160 cm in height and weighs 87 kg is _____ m^2.

2. The BSA for a client who is 155 cm in height and weighs 65 kg is _____ m^2.

3. The BSA for a client who is 68 in in height and weighs 160 lb is _____ m^2.

4. The BSA for a client who is 175 cm in height and weighs 105 kg is _____ m^2.

5. The BSA for a client who is 74 in in height and weighs 220 lb is _____ m^2.

Answers 1. 1.9 m^2 2. 1.65 m^2 3. 1.9 m^2 4. 2.2 m^2 5. 2.3 m^2

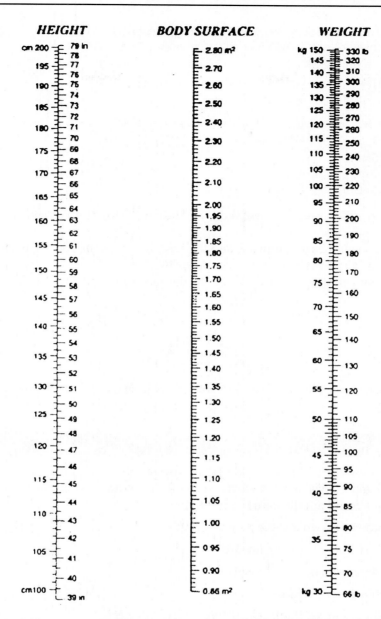

HEIGHT **BODY SURFACE** **WEIGHT**

Figure 20-1 The adult body surface area nomogram (From the formula of DuBois and DuBois, *Archives of Internal Medicine*, 17:883, 1916. Copyright 1916. American Medical Association. Reprinted by permission.)

Calculation of Dosage Using the Body Surface Area

The physician frequently applies an estimation of the patient's body surface area, calculated in square meters (m^2) based on the patient's height and weight, to a formula to determine the safe dosage of potentially dangerous medications (such as the antineoplastics). This is done when the dosage of a drug must be individualized for each person and the difference between therapeutic and toxic is tiny.

Once the BSA is known and the prescribed dose per m^2 is known, the nurse can calculate the mL of medication to be administered to the patient.

Example: The physician has prescribed IV acyclovir (Zovirax) 250 mg/m^2 every 8 hours for a patient who weigh 50 kg and is 155 cm tall. On hand is a vial labeled 500 mg in 10 mL. The total dose of the drug is to be further diluted in 100 mL of sterile water and administered over 2 hours. The BSA in square meters (m^2) is estimated to be 1.5 m^2 by using the adult nomogram.

Solution: To determine the dose, set up the proportion using the prescribed dose over 1 m² on one side and the desired dose over the patient's BSA on the other side:

$$\frac{250 \text{ mg}}{1 \text{ m}^2} = \frac{x \text{ mg}}{1.5 \text{ m}^2}$$

$$x = 375 \text{ mg}$$

To calculate how many mL are needed, using the available vial of Zovirax, which is labeled 500 mg per 10 mL, the proportion can be set up as:

$$\frac{x \text{ mL}}{10 \text{ mL}} = \frac{375 \text{ mg}}{500 \text{ mg}}$$

$$x = 7.5 \text{ mL}$$

To administer 375 mg of Zovirax, the nurse should withdraw 7.5 mL from a vial labeled Zovirax 500 mg per 10 mL.

To determine the total volume to be infused, add the 7.5 mL dose to the 100 mL of sterile water used to further dilute the medication. This provides a total volume of 107.5 mL.

To determine what hourly rate should be set on the electronic infusion device, set up the following proportion:

$$\frac{1 \text{ hr}}{2 \text{ hr}} = \frac{x \text{ mL}}{107.5 \text{ mL}}$$

$$x = 54 \text{ mL/hr}$$

To provide 375 mg of Zovirax in 100 mg of sterile water over 2 hours, the nurse should set the electronic device to 54 mL per hour.

Problem Set 20.3

1. The physician has prescribed IV doxorubicin (Adriamycin) 60 mg/m² for a patient who weighs 75 kg and is 175 cm tall. On hand is a vial labeled 10 mg per 5 mL. The total dose of the drug is to be further diluted in 50 mL of NS and administered over 2 hours.

   Using the adult nomogram, what is the patient's BSA? _____ m²

   How many mg of doxorubicin will be needed? _____ mg

   How many mL of doxorubicin will be needed? _____ mL

   What is the total volume to be infused? _____ mL

   What hourly rate should be set on the electronic infusion device? _____ mL/hr

2. The physician has prescribed dexrazoxane (Zinecard) 500 mg/m² for a patient whose BSA is 2.2 m². On hand is a vial labeled 250 mg in 25 mL. No further dilution of this drug is required before administration. The drug is to be administered over 15 minutes.

   Using the adult nomogram, what is the patient's BSA? _____ m²

   How many mg of Zinecard will be needed? _____ mg

   How many mL of Zinecard will be needed? _____ mL

   What is the total volume to be infused? _____ mL

   What hourly rate should be set on the electronic infusion device? _____ mL/hr

3. The physician has prescribed interferon alpha 2b (Intron A) 20,000,000 units/m² for a patient who weighs 65 kg and is 170 cm tall. On hand is a vial labeled 25 million units in 10 mL. The total dose of the drug is to be further diluted in 100 mL of NS and administered over 20 minutes.

   Using the adult nomogram, what is the patient's BSA? _____ m²

   How many units of Intron A will be needed? _____ U

   How many mL of Intron A will be needed? _____ mL

What is the total volume to be infused? _____ mL

What hourly rate should be set on the electronic infusion device? _____ mL/hr

4. The physician has prescribed zidovudine (Retrovir) 100 mg/m^2 for a patient who weighs 40 kg and is 140 cm tall. On hand is a vial labeled 200 mg in 20 mL. The total dose of the drug is to be further diluted in 50 mL of D5/W and administered over 1 hour.

   Using the adult nomogram, what is the patient's BSA? _____ m^2

   How many mg of Retrovir will be needed? _____ mg

   How many mL of Retrovir will be needed? _____ mL

   What is the total volume to be infused? _____ mL

   What hourly rate should be set on the electronic infusion device? _____ mL/hr

5. The physician has prescribed allopurinol (Alloprim) 300 mg/m^2 for a patient whose BSA is 2 m^2. On hand is a vial labeled 500 mg in 20 mL. The total dose of the drug is to be further diluted in 100 mL D5/W and administered over 30 minutes.

   How many mg of Alloprim will be needed? _____ mg

   How many mL of Alloprim will be needed? _____ mL

   What is the total volume to be infused? _____ mL

   What hourly rate should be set on the electronic infusion device? _____ mL/hr

Answers **1.** 1.8 m^2, 108 mg, 54 mL, 104 mL, 52 mL/hr **2.** 2.2 m^2, 1100 mg, 110 mL, 110 mL, 440 mL/hr **3.** 1.8 m^2, 36,000,000 units, 14.4 mL, 114.4 mL, 343 mL/hr **4.** 1.2 m^2, 120 mg, 12 mL, 62 mL, 62 mL/hr **5.** 600 mg, 24 mL, 124 mL, 248 mL/hr

CRITICAL CARE INTRAVENOUS MEDICATIONS AND TITRATION

All intensive care units use potent, life-saving intravenous drugs that are prescribed by the physician either by flow rate (mL per hour or gtt per minute) or by dosage (mg, mcg, units/kg/min or hour). Infusions containing these medications should only be administered with an electronic infusion device programmed in mL/hr using microdrop tubing with a drop factor of 60. Because microdrop tubing must always be used, and because micro-drop tubing has a drop factor of 60, the gtt/min rate is multiplied by 1 to determine the mL/hr rate.

Because many of these drugs are so potent and have a narrow therapeutic index, infusions such as dopamine, pitocin, nitroprusside, and so on, are titrated (adjusted by concentration and administration rate) based on the patient's measurable reaction to the per minute dosage of medication. These medications are usually prescribed by a range of dosage with the lower level first set and the infusion adjusted upward until the desired measurable response is obtained. The upper level is not exceeded without a change in the order, even if the measurable results are not obtained. Patients receiving any of these drugs require close, continuous monitoring.

The nurse can become confused when confronted with this method of prescribing because it requires computing the amount of medication to be delivered by the minute and the rate of flow that is required to deliver this per-minute amount. The three most important points to follow when computing this type of order are:

■ Check the physician's order indicating the amount of medication, the specified IV fluid, and the amount of medication to be given in a specified time period.

■ Refer to and follow the manufacturer's instructions.

■ Use an electronic infusion device to regulate delivery of the medication.

Example: The physician has ordered a prediluted solution of theophylline 500 mg in 250 mL D5/W to be infused at a rate of 750 µg per minute for the patient. The IV administration set delivers 60 gtt/mL. How many mL per hour will deliver this dosage?

Solution: Based on the physician's order and the manufacturer's instructions, determine how much drug is present in 1 mL of the theophylline 500 mg in 250 mL D5/W solution.

Set up the problem using ratio and proportion to determine the mg per mL strength of solution:

$$\frac{1\ mL}{250\ mL} = \frac{x\ mg}{500\ mg}$$

$$250x = 500$$

$$x = 2\ mg\ of\ theophylline\ per\ mL$$

Therefore, a solution of 1 mL of the prediluted theophylline 500 mg in 250 mL D5/W contains 2 mg of theophylline per mL.

Then convert the desired dose and the available dose to the same unit of measure. In this situation, convert 2 mg to micrograms. This can be done by moving the decimal point three places to the right. Therefore, 2 mg equal 2000 µg or mcg of theophylline.

Since 1 mL of the solution is equal to 2000 µg of theophylline, determine how many milliliters are equal to 750 µg of the drug by using the proportion:

$$\frac{750\ \mu g}{2000\ \mu g} = \frac{x\ mL}{1\ mL}$$

$$2000x = 750$$

$$x = 0.375\ mL\ equals\ 750\ \mu g\ of\ theophylline$$

To compute mL/hr, you multiply 0.375 mL, the amount the patient should receive per minute, by 60 minutes to determine the mL/hr rate. Therefore, the infusion rate on the electronic infusion device should be set to deliver 22.5 mL/hr, which will deliver 750 µg of theophylline per minute.

The mL/hr can also be determined by using the proportion:

$$\frac{60\ minutes}{1\ minute} = \frac{x\ mL}{0.375\ mL}$$

$$x = 22.5\ mL\ /\ hr$$

Example: The physician has ordered dopamine hydrochloride (Intropin) 200 mg in 250 mL of D5/W to be administered at a rate of 5 µg/kg/minute to be infused until the systolic blood pressure is greater than 110 mmHg. The IV administration set delivers 60 gtt/mL. How many mL per hour will deliver this dosage?

Solution: The manufacturer's instructions state to dilute one 5 mL/200 mg ampule of Intropin in 250 mL of D5/W. Determine how much drug is present in 1 mL of the dopamine hydrochloride 200 mg in 250 mL D5/W solution.

Set up the problem using ratio and proportion to determine the mg per mL of solution:

$$\frac{1\ mL}{250\ mL} = \frac{x\ mg}{200\ mg}$$

$$250x = 200$$

$$x = 0.8\ mg\ of\ dopamine\ hydrochloride\ per\ mL$$

Therefore, a 5 mL/200 mg ampule of dopamine hydrochloride in 250 mL D5/W contains 0.8 mg of dopamine hydrochloride per mL.

Then convert the desired dose and the available dose to the same unit of measure. In this situation, convert 0.8 mg to micrograms. This can be done by moving the decimal point three places to the right. Therefore, 0.8 mg equal 800 µg or mcg of dopamine hydrochloride and 1 mL contains 800 µg.

The patient weighs 80 kg and the physician's order states that the patient is to receive 5 µg/kg/min. How many µg per minute should this patient receive?

$$\frac{80\ kg}{1\ kg} = \frac{x\ \mu g}{5\ \mu g}$$

$$x = 400\ \mu g\ /\ min$$

Since 1 mL of the solution is equal to 800 µg of dopamine hydrochloride, determine how many milliliters are equal to 400 µg of the drug by using the proportion:

$$\frac{400\ \mu g}{800\ \mu g} = \frac{x\ mL}{1\ mL}$$

$$800x = 400$$

$$x = 0.5\ mL\ contains\ 400\ \mu g$$

To compute mL/hr, you multiply 0.5 mL, the amount the patient should receive per minute, by 60 minutes to determine the mL/hr rate. Therefore, the infusion rate on the electronic infusion device should be set to deliver 30 mL/hr, which will deliver 400 µg of dopamine hydrochloride per minute.

The mL/hr can also be determined by using the proportion:

$$\frac{60\ minutes}{1\ minute} = \frac{x\ mL}{0.5\ mL}$$

$$x = 30\ mL\ /\ hr$$

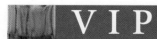

VIP

- ■ The concentration of the medication in the IV fluid and the flow rate of the IV fluid determine the rate of medication to the patient.

- ■ The concentration of medication is stated in mg or mg/mL or amount of medication per volume of fluid.

- ■ The dose is stated in mg or mg/min or amount of medication per specified time.

- ■ The flow rate is stated in mL/min or volume per specified time.

- ■ An electronic infusion device must be used to deliver these medications by intravenous drip.

Problem Set 20.4

1. The physician has ordered procainamide hydrochloride (Pronestyl) IV, titrated to control dysrhythmia at a rate of 1500 µg per minute. The available vial contains 1000 mg per 2 mL. The physician's order and the manufacturer's directions recommend that 1000 mg of the drug be added to 500 mL of D5/W. The infusion set delivers 60 drops per 1 mL.

   How many mL of Pronestyl should the nurse add to the 500 mL D5/W? _____ mL

   How many mg of drug are present in 1 mL of the Pronestyl 1000 mg in 500 mL of D5/W solution? _____ mg/mL

   Convert this value to µg/mL. _____ µg/mL

   How many mL per minute must infuse to deliver the prescribed amount of the drug? _____ mL/min

   How many mL per hour should the electronic infusion device be set to deliver? _____ mL/hr

2. The physician has prescribed isoproterenol hydrochloride (Isuprel) 5 µg per minute by intravenous infusion. The physician's order and the manufacturer's instructions recommend that 2 mg of Isuprel be added to 500 mL of D5/W. The infusion set delivers 60 drops per 1 mL. The available vial of Isuprel contains 1 mg per 5 mL.

   How many mL of Isuprel should the nurse add to the 500 mL D5/W? _____ mL

   How many mg of drug are present in 1 mL of the Isuprel 2 mg in 500 mL of D5/W solution? _____ mg/mL

Convert this value to µg/mL. _____ µg/mL

How many mL per minute must infuse to deliver the prescribed
amount of the drug? _____ mL/min

How many mL per hour should the electronic infusion device be
set to deliver? _____ mL/hr

3. The physician has ordered amiodarone hydrochloride (Cordarone Intravenous) 900 mg to be added to
500 mL of D5/W and run intravenously at a rate of 1 mg/min for 6 hours. The manufacturer's directions
agree with the physician's order. The available 3 mL vials of Cordarone Intravenous contain 50 mg per 1
mL. The infusion set delivers 60 drops per 1 mL.

How many mL of Cordarone Intravenous should the nurse add to
the 500 mL D5/W? _____ mL

How many mg of drug are present in 1 mL of the Cordarone
Intravenous 900 mg in 500 mL of D5/W solution? _____ mg/mL

How many mL per minute must infuse to deliver the prescribed
amount of the drug? _____ mL/min

How many mL per hour should the electronic infusion device
be set to deliver? _____ mL/hr

4. The physician has ordered dobutamine hydrochloride (Dobutrex) 250 mg to be added to 500 mL of
D5/W and run intravenously at a rate of 5 mcg/kg/min. The manufacturer's directions agree with the
physician's order. The available 20 mL vials of Dobutrex contain 250 mg. The infusion set delivers 60
drops per 1 mL. The patient weighs 65 kg.

How many mL of Dobutrex should the nurse add to the
500 mL D5/W? _____ mL

Based on weight, how many µg/min of Dobutrex should
this patient receive? _____ µg/min

How many mg of drug are present in 1 mL of the Dobutrex
250 mg in 500 mL of D5/W solution? _____ mg/mL

Convert this value to µg/mL. _____ µg/mL

How many mL per minute must infuse to deliver the prescribed
amount of the drug? _____ mL/min

How many mL per hour should the electronic infusion device
be set to deliver? _____ mL/hr

5. The physician has ordered dopamine hydrochloride (Intropin) 200 mg to be added to 250 mL of D5/W
and run intravenously at a rate of 5 mcg/kg/min until the patient's systolic blood pressure is greater than
110 mmHg. The manufacturer's directions agree with the physician's order. The available 5 mL vials of
Intropin contain 200 mg. The infusion set delivers 60 drops per 1 mL. The patient weighs 80 kg.

How many mL of Intropin should the nurse add to the
250 mL D5/W? _____ mL

Based on weight, how many mcg/min of Intropin should
this patient receive? _____ mcg/min

How many mg of drug are present in 1 mL of the Intropin
200 mg in 250 mL of D5/W solution? _____ mg/mL

Convert this value to mcg/mL. _____ mcg/mL

How many mL per minute must infuse to deliver the prescribed
amount of the drug? _____ mL/min

How many mL per hour should the electronic infusion device be
set to deliver? _____ mL/hr

Answers **1.** 2 mL, 2 mg/1 mL, 2000 µg/mL, 0.75 mL/min = 1500 µg, 45 mL/hr **2.** 10 mL, 0.004 mg/mL, 4 mcg/mL, 1.25 mL/min = 5 mcg, 75 mL/hr **3.** 18 mL, 1.8 mg/mL, 0.56 mL/min = 1 mg, 33.6 mL/hr **4.** 20 mL, 325 µg/min, 0.5 mg/mL, 500 µg/mL, 0.65 mL/min = 325 µg, 39 mL/hr **5.** 5 mL, 400 mcg/min, 0.8 mg/mL, 800 mcg/mL, 0.5 mL/min = 400 mcg, 30 mL/hr

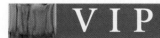

V I P

When administering prescribed IV medications:

- Always confirm the compatibility of the medication and IV solution; check drug label for appropriateness for IV use.

- Follow manufacturer's direction for diluting; if these directions differ from the physician's order, check with the physician.

- Ensure that the drug is adequately mixed.

- Attach a medication label to the IV container or volume-control set.

- Flush the primary line if necessary; determine if medication is to run simultaneously or if the primary line should be clamped; start the piggyback or secondary set with medication; set at appropriate rate.

- If a heparin or saline lock (intermittent infusion device) is being used, flush the lock with the ordered heparin flush or saline solution to maintain patency; follow hospital protocol.

- Monitor patient's response to the medication during and following its administration.

Review Test 20.1
Computing Intravenous Medications for Adults in Special Situations

1. The physician has prescribed a loading dose of metronidozole hydrochloride sterile (Flagyl IV) 15 mg/kg of body weight to be added to 100 mL of D5/W and infused over 1 hour using an electronic infusion device. On hand is a single-dose vial labeled Flagyl IV 500 mg. The manufacturer's instructions for reconstitution state: To prepare the solution add 4.4 mL of sterile water for injection to the 500 mg vial, mix thoroughly. The resulting withdrawal volume is approximately 5.0 mL to yield an approximate concentration of 100 mg/mL. The patient's weight is 60 kg.

   How many mg of medication will be needed? _____ mg

   How many vials will be needed? _____ vials

   How many mL of Flagyl should be added to the 100 mL bag of D5/W? _____ mL

   What is the total volume to be infused? _____ mL

   What hourly rate should be set on the electronic infusion device? _____ mL/hr

2. The physician has prescribed a continuous secondary IV of heparin 10,000 units in 500 mL of D5/W to infuse at a rate of 20 units/per kg/hour using an electronic infusion device. The patient weighs 38 kg.

   How many units of heparin should the patient receive per hour? _____ U

   What will be the hourly rate to deliver the ordered dose of heparin? _____ mL/hr

   What hourly rate should be set on the electronic infusion device? _____ mL/hr

3. The physician has prescribed a continuous IV of heparin 25,000 units in 250 mL of D5/W to infuse via an electronic infusion device at a rate of 18 units/kg/hour. The patient weighs 220 pounds.

   How many kilograms does the patient weigh? _____ kg

How many units of heparin should the patient receive per hour? _____ U

What hourly rate should be set on the electronic infusion device? _____ mL/hr

4. A patient is receiving 1800 units per hour of heparin 25,000 units in 250 mL of D5/W by continuous IV infusion via an electronic infusion device. Lab results indicate that the patient has a partial thromboplastin time (PTT) of 54. According to sliding-scale protocol, the patient should receive a rebolus of 40 units per kg intravenous push. The continuous IV infusion should also be increased by 2 units per kg of body weight per hour. The patient weighs 100 kg.

How many units of heparin should the patient receive for a rebolus? _____ U

How many additional units of heparin should the patient receive per hour? _____ U

How many total units of heparin should the patient receive per hour? _____ U

What hourly rate should be set on the electronic infusion device now? _____ mL/hr

5. The physician has prescribed folinic acid (leucovorin) 10 mg/m^2 for a patient who weighs 60 kg and is 167 cm tall. On hand is a vial labeled 10 mg/mL. The total dose of the drug is to be further diluted in 100 mL of LR and administered over 20 minutes.

Using the adult nomogram, what is the patient's BSA? _____ m^2

How many mg of folinic acid will be needed? _____ mg

How many mL of folinic acid will be needed? _____ mL

What is the total volume to be infused? _____ mL

What hourly rate should be set on the electronic infusion device? _____ mL/hr

6. The physician has prescribed edetate calcium disodium (calcium EDTA) 1000 mg/m^2 for a patient who weighs 82 kg and is 182 cm tall. On hand is a vial labeled 1 g in 5 mL. The total dose of the drug is to be further diluted in 500 mL of NS and administered over 8 hours.

Using the adult nomogram, what is the patient's BSA? _____ m^2

How many mg of calcium EDTA will be needed? _____ mg

How many mL of calcium EDTA will be needed? _____ mL

What is the total volume to be infused? _____ mL

What hourly rate should be set on the electronic infusion device? _____ mL/hr

7. The physician has prescribed paclitaxel (Taxol) 170 mg/m^2 for a patient who weighs 72 kg and is 168 cm tall. On hand is a vial labeled 150 mg in 25 mL. The total dose of the drug is to be further diluted in 180 mL of D5/NS and administered over 3 hours.

Using the adult nomogram, what is the patient's BSA? _____ m^2

How many mg of Taxol will be needed? _____ mg

How many mL of Taxol will be needed? _____ mL

What is the total volume to be infused? _____ mL

What hourly rate should be set on the electronic infusion device? _____ mL/hr

8. The physician has prescribed a premixed solution of nitroglycerin 25 mg in 250 mL D5/W to be titrated at a rate of 5 mcg per minute, and to be increased in increments of 5 mcg per minute at 5- to 10-minute intervals until angina subsides. The manufacturer's directions agree with the physician's order. The infusion set is attached to an electronic infusion device.

How many mcg of drug are present in 1 mL of the premixed nitroglycerin 25 mg in 250 mL of D5/W solution? _____ mcg/mL

How many mL of the premixed solution contain 5 mcg of nitroglycerin? _____ mL

How many mL per hour should the electronic infusion device be set to deliver? _____ mL/hr

9. The physician has ordered oxytocin (Pitocin) 10 units to be added to 1000 mL of D5/NS to run intravenously at a rate of 1 mU/min for the first 20 minutes and to be increased in increments of 1 mU/min at 20-minute intervals until regular contractions are established. The manufacturer's directions agree with the physician's orders. The available vials of Pitocin contain 10 U per 1 mL. The IV is attached to an electronic infusion device.

   How many mL of Pitocin should the nurse add to the 1000 mL of D5/NS?   _____ mL

   How many units of drug are present in 1 mL of the Pitocin 10 U in 1,000 mL of D5/NS solution?   _____ U/mL

   Change these U/mL to mU/mL (milliunits)   _____ mU/mL

   How many mL per minute must infuse to deliver the prescribed amount of the drug?   _____ mL/min

   How many mL per hour should the electronic infusion device be set to deliver?   _____ mL/hr

10. The physician has ordered diltiazem (Cardizem) 125 mg to be added to 100 mL of D5/W and run intravenously at a rate of 5 mg/hr and titrated for dysrhythmia control. The manufacturer's directions agree with the physician's order. The available vials of Cardizem contain 25 mg per 5 ml.

    How many mL of Cardizem should be added?   _____ mL

    How many mg of drug are present in 1 mL of the Cardizem 125 mg in 100 mL of D5/W solution?   _____ mg

    How many mL per hour must infuse to deliver 5 mg/hr of drug? _____ mL/hr

    How many mL per hour should the electronic infusion device be set to deliver?   _____ mL/hr

Answers   **1.** 900 mg, 2 vials, 9 mL, 109 mL, 109 mL/hr   **2.** 760 U, 38 mL/hr, 38 mL/hr   **3.** 100 kg, 1800 U, 18 mL/hr   **4.** 4000 U, 200 U, 2000 U (1800 units + 200 units), 20 mL/hr   **5.** 1.7 m², 17 mg, 1.7 mL, 101.7 mL or 102 mL, 305 mL/hr or 306 mL/hr   **6.** 2 m², 2000 mg, 10 mL, 510 mL, 64 mL/hr   **7.** 1.2 m², 204 mg, 34 mL, 214 mL, 71 mL/hr   **8.** 100 mcg/mL, 0.05 mL, 3 mL/hr   **9.** 1 mL, 0.01 U/mL, 10 mU/mL, 0.1 mL/min, 6 mL/hr   **10.** 25 mL, 1 mg, 5 mL/hr, 5 mL/hr

If you had fewer than three errors on Review Test 20.1, move on to the next chapter. If you had four or more errors, review the material on computing intravenous medications for adults in special situations and complete Review Test 20.2 before continuing.

Review Test 20.2
Computing Intravenous Medications for Adults in Special Situations

1. The physician has prescribed cyclosporine for injection (Sandimmune) 5 mg/kg of body weight to be added to 100 mL of D5/W via IV piggyback to be infused over 2 hours. Available are 5 mL vials labeled Sandimmune Injection 50 mg/mL. The patient weighs 165 lbs.

   What is the patients weight in kg?   _____ kg

   How many mg of medication should the patient receive?   _____ mg

   How many vials of Sandimmune will be needed?   _____ vials

   How many mL of Sandimmune should be added to the 100 mL bag of D5/W?   _____ mL

   What is the total volume to be infused?   _____ mL

   What hourly rate should be set on the electronic infusion device?   _____ mL/hr

2. The physician has prescribed granisetron hydrochloride (Kytril) 10 mcg/kg of body weight to be added to 50 mL of D5/W via an IVPB to infuse over 15 minutes using an electronic infusion device. Available is a vial labeled Kytril 1 mL/1 mg. The patient weighs 50 kg.

    How many mcg of medication should the patient receive? _____ mcg

    How many mL of Kytril should be added to the 50 mL bag of D5/W? _____ mL

    What is the total volume to be infused? _____ mL

    What hourly rate should be set on the electronic infusion device? _____ mL/hr

3. The physician has prescribed a continuous IV of heparin 25,000 units in 250 mL of D5/W to infuse via an electronic infusion device at a rate of 18 units/kg/hour. The patient weighs 165 pounds.

    How many kilograms does the patient weigh? _____ kg

    How many units of heparin should the patient receive per hour? _____ units

    What hourly rate should be set on the electronic infusion device? _____ mL/hr

4. A patient is receiving 1200 units per hour of heparin 25,000 units in 250 mL of D5/W by continuous IV infusion via an electronic infusion device. The patient has a PTT of 142. According to sliding-scale protocol, the heparin infusion should be decreased by 2 units per kg of body weight per hour. The patient weighs 75 kg.

    How many units should the heparin be decreased per hour? _____ units

    How many total units of heparin should the patient receive per hour? _____ units

    What new hourly rate should be set on the electronic infusion device? _____ mL/hr

5. The physician has prescribed fluorouracil (5FU) 425 mg/m^2 for a patient whose BSA is 2.2. On hand is a vial labeled 500 mg in 10 mL. The total dose of the drug is to be further diluted in 250 mL of D5/W and administered over 6 hours.

    How many mg of 5FU will be needed? _____ mg

    How many mL of 5FU will be needed? _____ mL

    What is the total volume to be infused? _____ mL

    What hourly rate should be set on the electronic infusion device? _____ mL/hr

6. The physician has prescribed vincristine (Oncovin) 1.4 mg/m^2 for a patient who weighs 60 kg and is 165 cm tall. On hand is a vial labeled 5 mg in 5 mL. The total dose of the drug is to be further diluted in 50 mL of NS and administered over 30 minutes.

    Using the adult nomogram, what is the patient's BSA? _____ m^2

    How many mg of Oncovin will be needed? _____ mg

    How many mL of Oncovin will be needed? _____ mL

    What is the total volume to be infused? _____ mL

    What hourly rate should be set on the electronic infusion device? _____ mL/hr

7. The physician has prescribed cisplatin (Platinol) 100 mg/m^2 for a patient who weighs 85 kg and is 170 cm tall. On hand is a vial labeled 50 mg in 50 mL. The total dose of the drug is to be further diluted in 2000 mL of D5/0.3% NaCl and administered over 8 hours.

    Using the adult nomogram, what is the patient's BSA? _____ m^2

    How many mg of Platinol will be needed? _____ mg

    How many mL of Platinol will be needed? _____ mL

    What is the total volume to be infused? _____ mL

    What hourly rate should be set on the electronic infusion device? _____ mL/hr

8. The physician has prescribed 400 mg of dopamine HCl (Intropin) to be diluted in 250 mL of D5/W and administered at a rate of 100 mcg per minute; the manufacturer's directions agree. Available are 5 mL vials labeled Intropin 400 mg/5 mL. The IV infusion is attached to an electronic infusion device.

   How many mg of Intropin 400 mg/5 mL should the nurse add to the 250 mL D5/W? _____ mg

   How many mg of drug are present in 1 mL of the Intropin 400 mg in 250 mL of D5/W solution? _____ mg/mL

   Convert this value to mcg/mL _____ mcg/mL

   How many mL per hour should the electronic infusion device be set to deliver? _____ mL/hr

9. The physician has ordered procainamide hydrochloride (Pronestyl) 0.5 g to be added to 500 mL of D5/W to be given at a rate of 5 mg/min to control arrhythmia. The available vial is labeled Pronestyl 500 mg/1 mL. The IV infusion is attached to an electronic infusion device.

   How many mL of Pronestyl 500 mg/1 mL should be added to the 500 mL of D5/W? _____ mL

   How many mg of drug are present in 1 mL of the Pronestyl 0.5 g in 500 mL of D5/W solution? _____ mg/mL

   How many mL per minute must infuse to deliver the prescribed amount of the drug? _____ mL/min

   How many mL per hour should the electronic infusion device be set to deliver? _____ mL/hr

10. The physician has prescribed a prediluted solution of theophylline 800 mg in 250 mL D5/W to run intravenously at a rate of 0.8 mg/kg/hr. The manufacturer's directions agree with the physician's order. The patient weighs 198 pounds. The infusion set is attached to an electronic infusion device.

    What is the patient's weight in kg? _____ kg

    How many mg of drug are present in 1 mL of the prediluted theophylline 800 mg in 250 mL D5/W solution? _____ mg/mL

    How many mg per hour should the patient who weighs 198 pounds receive? _____ mg/hr

    How many mL per hour should the electronic infusion device be set to deliver? _____ mL/hr

Answers **1.** 75 kg, 375 mg, 1½ vials (2 vials), 7.5 mL, 108 mL, 54 mL/hr **2.** 500 mcg, 0.5 mL, 50.5 or 51 mL, 204 mL/hr **3.** 75 kg, 1350 units, 14 mL/hr **4.** 150 units, 1050 units, 11 mL/hr **5.** 935 mg, 18.7 mL, 268.7 mL, 45 mL/hr **6.** 1.7 m², 2.4 mg, 2.4 mL, 52.4 mL, 105 mL/hr **7.** 2 m², 200 mg, 200 mL, 2200 mL, 275 mL/hr **8.** 5 mL, 1.6 mg/mL, 1,600 mcg/mL, 3.75 mL/hr **9.** 1 mL, 1 mg/mL, 4 mL/min, 240 mL/hr **10.** 90 kg, 3.2 mg/mL, 72 mg/hr, 22.5 mL/hr

The Review Tests on computing intravenous medications for adults in special situations should be repeated until fewer than three errors occur.

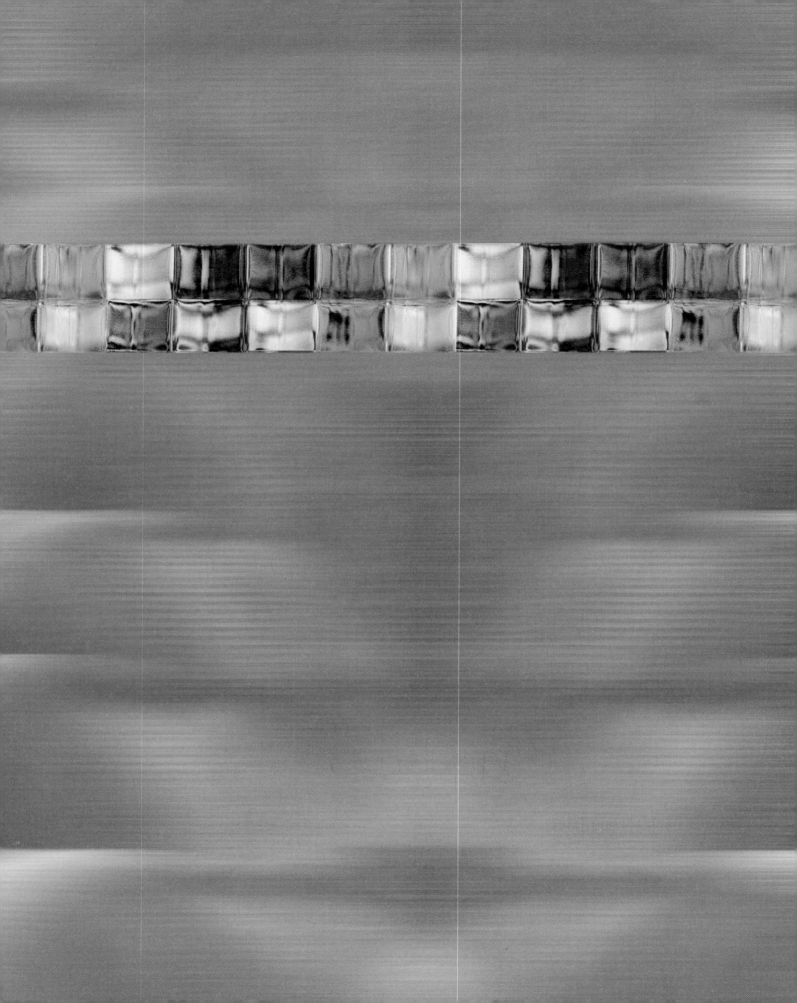

Unit 6

Medication Dosages for Infants and Children

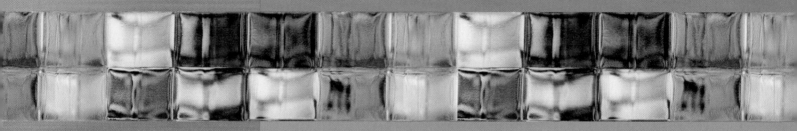

Chapter 21
Computing Dosage for Infants and Children

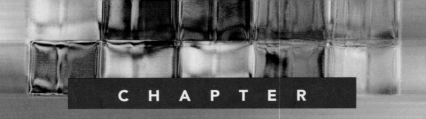

21

Computing Dosage for Infants and Children

Learning Outcomes

After successfully completing this chapter, the learner should be able to:

- *Convert weight in pounds to weight in kilograms, or weight in kilograms to weight in pounds.*
- *Calculate pediatric dosage using the child's weight in kilograms and the manufacturer's recommended daily dose based on the weight in kilograms.*
- *Calculate pediatric dosage based on body surface area (which is expressed as square meters of body surface or m^2) estimated from the patient's height and weight by use of the Pediatric Body Surface Area nomogram or mathematical formulas.*
- *Understand the importance of determining the manufacturer's recommended daily dose based on weight in kg or estimated m^2.*
- *Recognize the importance of questioning any order that exceeds the manufacturer's recommended daily dose.*

GENERAL INFORMATION

Infants and children should not receive the same amount of medication that is considered within the safe range of dosage for adults. Even minor mistakes in administering medication to an infant or child can be extremely serious because of differences in their ability to absorb, distribute, metabolize, and excrete substances such as drugs.

Although the physician prescribes medications, it is the nurse's legal responsibility to know what constitutes the usual dosage of a medication and whether that medication can be used for an infant, child, or adult. The nurse must make certain that an order for any dosage outside the manufacturer's recommended range is rechecked for accuracy, regardless of the route of administration.

In the past, a number of rules were developed to determine pediatric dosage. The only methods considered safe today are those based on the recommended amount of drug per kilogram or pound of body weight and the recommended amount of drug per estimated square meter (m^2) of body surface. These methods are used to determine oral and parenteral (IM, SQ, or IV) dosages.

Because pediatric dosage must be accurate, rounding off to the next whole number is not acceptable and is not permitted. Decimal amounts must remain decimal amounts and the proper syringes must be used to permit accurate administration of the correct amount.

CALCULATION OF DOSAGE USING THE BODY WEIGHT METHOD

Today, most drug books and drug manufacturers provide the recommended pediatric dosage based on kilograms of body weight, and many physicians prescribe medications for pediatric patients in this manner. The nurse is responsible for calculating the daily dose, and is also responsible for checking to see that the prescribed dose falls within the manufacturer's recommended daily dose per kilogram of body weight. The physician's order is usually written as a total daily dose divided into a specific number of doses per day.

To safely fill an order of this type, the nurse must first determine the child's weight in pounds and then convert this weight in pounds to kilograms. Recall from Chapter 13 that 1 kilogram equals 2.2 pounds; thus, the child's weight in pounds can be converted to kilograms by dividing the number of pounds by 2.2. If the weight is given in grams, it can be converted to kilograms by dividing by 1000.

Calculation Alert

1 kilogram (kg) = 1000 grams (g)   1 kilogram (kg) = 2.2 pounds (lb)
   To convert lb to kg: divide the number of lb by 2.2.
   To convert kg to lb: multiply the number of kg by 2.2.

Example: The physician's order for a child states: Ibuprofen 40 mg per kg in four divided doses daily. The nurse checks the drug book and finds that the recommended daily dose is 16 to 40 mg/kg/day in divided doses q6–8 hours. With the prescribed dose falling within the recommended dose range, the nurse must then determine the child's weight in pounds and convert the pounds to kilograms.

Solution: After determining that the child weighs 44 pounds, the nurse converts this weight to kilograms:
44 lb ÷ 2.2 kg = 20 kg

To determine the daily dose, set up the proportion using the prescribed dose over 1 kg on one side and the desired dose over the child's weight in kilograms on the other:

$$\frac{40 \text{ mg}}{1 \text{ kg}} = \frac{x \text{ mg}}{20 \text{ kg}}$$

x = 800 mg per day in 4 divided doses or 200 mg per dose

Using 200 mg ibuprofen tablets, the child should receive 1 tablet q6h.

Example: The physician has prescribed tobramycin (Nebcin) injection 7.5 mg per kg of body weight per day to be administered in divided doses q8h, IM, for a 9-month-old. The manufacturer's recommended daily pediatric dose is 7.5 mg/kg/day in divided doses q6–8 hours. With the prescribed dose falling within the recommended dose range, the nurse must then determine the child's weight in pounds and convert the pounds to kilograms.

The drug on hand is labeled:

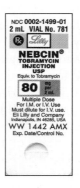

Solution: After determining that the child weighs 19 pounds, the nurse converts this weight to kilograms: 19 lb ÷ 2.2 kg = 8.64 kg

To determine the daily dose, set up the proportion using the prescribed dose over 1 kg on one side and the desired dose over the child's weight in kilograms on the other:

$$\frac{7.5 \text{ mg}}{1 \text{ kg}} = \frac{x \text{ mg}}{8.64 \text{ kg}}$$

x = 64.8 or 65 mg per day in 3 divided doses or 22 mg per dose

Using the available vial of Nebcin injection, which is labeled 80 mg per 2 mL, the proportion can be set up as:

$$\frac{22 \text{ mg}}{80 \text{ mg}} = \frac{x \text{ mL}}{2 \text{ mL}}$$

80x = 44

x = 0.55 mL

To provide 22 mg of Nebcin, the nurse should administer 0.55 mL from a vial labeled Nebcin injection 80 mg per 2 mL.

Example: The physician orders a maintenance dose of 0.075 mg of digoxin elixir q12h by mouth for a 33-pound, 18-month-old. In checking the manufacturer's recommended dosage, the nurse finds that the maintenance dose for children under 2 years of age is 0.01 to 0.02 mg per kg of body weight daily in divided doses q12h. The bottle available is labeled Digoxin Elixer 50 µg per mL.

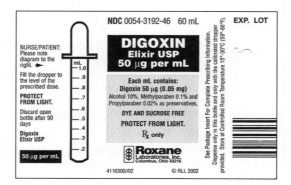

Solution: To determine if the order is within the recommended daily dosage, the nurse converts the child's weight of 33 pounds to kg: 33 lb ÷ 2.2 kg = 15 kg

The nurse then multiplies 15 kg by the recommended dose of 0.01 to 0.02 mg/kg of body weight daily and finds that the physician's order for a total daily dose of 0.15 mg (0.075 mg × 2 doses) is within the recommended dose of 0.15 to 0.3 mg for a child of this weight. Using the available bottle of Digoxin elixir 50 µg (0.05 mg) = 1 mL, the proportion can be set up as:

$$\frac{0.075 \text{ mg}}{0.05 \text{ mg}} = \frac{x \text{ mL}}{1 \text{ mL}}$$
$$0.05x = 0.075$$
$$x = 1.5 \text{ mL}$$

To provide 0.075 mg of digoxin, the nurse should administer 1.5 mL of Digoxin elixir labeled 0.05 mg = 1 mL.

Example: The physician orders gentamicin sulfate 40 mg, to be dissolved in 50 mL of NS to infuse in 2 hours, for a 7-year-old who weighs 44 pounds. Available is a vial of gentamicin labeled:

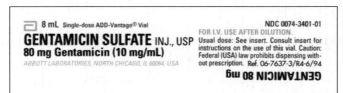

Solution: Checking the drug book, the nurse finds that the manufacturer's recommended initial pediatric dose for gentamicin is 2 to 2.5 mg per kg. To determine if the physician's order is within the recommended dosage, the nurse converts the child's weight of 44 pounds to kg: 44 lb ÷ 2.2 kg = 20 kg

The nurse computes that the initial dose could be as high as 40 to 50 mg, and therefore an order for 40 mg is within the recommended range for a child of this weight.

Using the available strength gentamicin 10 mg/mL, the proportion can be set up as:

$$\frac{40 \text{ mg}}{10 \text{ mg}} = \frac{x \text{ mL}}{1 \text{ mL}}$$
$$10x = 40$$
$$x = 4 \text{ mL}$$

To provide 40 mg of gentamicin, the nurse should add 4 mL of gentamicin labeled 10 mg = 1 mL to a 50 mL bag of normal saline.

Example: The physician has prescribed cefamandole nafate (Mandol) 50 mg/kg of body weight per day in four equally divided doses by IM injection for a 10-year-old who weighs 75 pounds. On hand is a vial of powdered Mandol labeled:

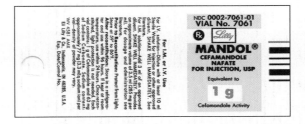

Solution: The nurse determines that the child weighs 75 lb or 34 kg. Using the physician's order of 50 mg/kg, the nurse determines that the child should receive:

34 kg × 50 mg = 1700 mg in four equally divided doses or 425 mg q6h

The nurse determines that this amount is within the manufacturer's recommended child's dosage of 50 to 150 mg/kg/24 hr in divided doses q4 to 8 hours.

To reconstitute the drug, the manufacturer recommends that the Mandol be diluted with 3 mL of sterile water for injection to yield a solution that contains 285 mg/1 mL.

Using the available strength Mandol 285 mg/1 mL, the proportion can be set up as:

$$\frac{425 \text{ mg}}{285 \text{ mg}} = \frac{x \text{ mL}}{1 \text{ mL}}$$
$$285x = 425$$
$$x = 1.5 \text{ mL}$$

To provide 425 mg of Mandol, the nurse should administer 1.5 mL of the drug that has been reconstituted to provide 285 mg/1 mL.

Problem Set 21.1

1. The physician orders prednisone 0.15 mg/kg/day by mouth for a 14-year-old patient who weighs 110 lb. The nurse checks the drug book and finds that the manufacturer's recommended dose for prednisone is 0.1 to 0.15 mg/kg/day. On hand are tablets labeled 2.5 mg. The nurse, after determining the patient's weight to be _____ kg, should administer _____ tablets.

2. The physician orders amoxicillin (Amoxil) oral suspension 20 mg/kg/day in three divided doses by mouth for a 4-year-old who weighs 33 lb. The nurse checks the drug book and finds that the manufacturer's recommended dose for amoxicillin is 20 to 40 mg/kg/day in three divided doses q8h. On hand is a bottle of oral suspension labeled 125 mg per 5 mL. The nurse, after determining the child's weight to be _____ kg, should administer _____ mL q8h.

3. The anesthesiologist orders hydroxyzine hydrochloride (Vistaril) 0.5 mg/lb IM stat for a 10-year-old who weighs 35 kg. The nurse checks the drug book and finds that the manufacturer's recommended dose for Vistaril is 0.5 mg/lb/day. On hand is a multidose vial labeled 25 mg per mL. The nurse, after determining the child's weight to be _____ lb, should administer _____ mL.

4. The physician orders cefazolin sodium (Ancef) 30 mg/kg/day in 3 divided doses IM for a 9-month-old who weighs 22 lb. The nurse checks the drug book and finds that the manufacturer's recommended dose for Ancef is 25 to 50 mg/kg/day in three divided doses. On hand is a vial of powdered Ancef labeled 500 mg. To reconstitute the drug, the manufacturer recommends that the Ancef be diluted with 2 mL of sterile water for injection to yield a solution of 2.2 mL that contains 225 mg/1 mL. The nurse, after determining the child's weight to be _____ kg, should administer _____ mL q8h.

5. The physician has prescribed a loading dose of dexamethasone sodium phosphate (Decadron phosphate) 72 mg IV to be added to D5/W 50 mL for a child. The 11-year-old child weighs 36 kg. The manufacturer's recommended dose is 3 mg/kg of body weight. On hand is a multidose vial of Decadron phosphate labeled 24 mg/1 mL. The nurse should add _____ mL of Decadron phosphate to the 50 mL bag of D5/W.

Answers   1. 50 kg; 3 tablets   2. 15 kg; 4 mL/q8h   3. 77 lb; 1.5 mL   4. 10 kg; 0.44 or 0.45 mL/q8h   5. 3 mL

V I P

The nurse should check with the physician any time the total daily prescribed dose for any patient, particularly a child, does not fall within the range of the manufacturer's recommended daily dose for a given medication.

CALCULATION OF DOSAGE USING THE BODY SURFACE AREA (BSA) METHOD

Medications are the shared responsibility of the ordering physician and the nurse that carries out the order. The nurse does not prescribe the dosage, but must check the physician's order to make certain that the prescribed dose falls within the manufacturer's recommended daily dose. The physician frequently applies an estimation of the child's body surface calculated in square meters (m^2) based on the child's height and weight to a formula to determine the safe dosage of certain potentially dangerous medications (such as antineoplastics), where the dosage of the drug must be individualized for each person and the difference between therapeutic and toxic levels is minute. The body surface area (BSA) method, using the height and weight, provides a more accurate means of estimating what a safe dose would be for these medications for infants, children, or adults than does using the body weight method alone.

The body surface area in square meters (m^2) can be estimated by using the Pediatric Body Surface Area nomogram (Figure 21-1). If a straight line is drawn from the client's height in either inches or centimeters marked on the height column (a) to the client's weight in either pounds or kilograms marked on the weight column (c), the intersecting mark on the body surface column (b) will provide the estimated body surface area in square meters.

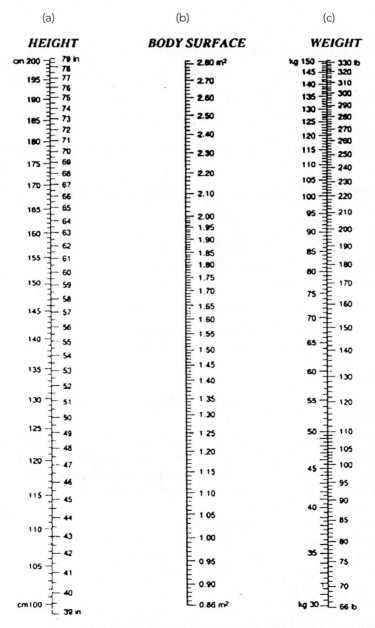

Figure 21-1 Pediatric body surface area nomogram (From the formula of DuBois and DuBois, *Archives of Internal Medicine*, 17:863, 1916. Copyright 1916, American Medical Association. Reprinted by permission)

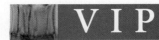

V I P

- If the ruler is even slightly off in either the height or weight columns, the m² will be incorrect.
- Carefully check the nomogram to see what value the markings and calibrations represent.
- The calibrations on the nomogram are not of equal value; the user must determine the value of each calibration to accurately estimate the BSA in square meters.

Problem Set 21.2

Using the Pediatric Body Surface Area nomogram (Figure 21-1), indicate the BSA in square meters (m²).

1. The BSA for a newborn who is 20 inches in height and weighs 7 pounds is _____ m².

2. The BSA for an 18-month-old who is 83 cm in height and weighs 12 kg is _____ m².

3. The BSA for a 6-year-old who is 45 inches in height and weighs 45 pounds is _____ m².

4. The BSA for a 12-year-old who is 150 cm in height and weighs 40 kg is _____ m².

5. The BSA for a 15-year-old who is 67 inches in height and weighs 150 pounds is _____ m².

Answers   **1.** 0.22 m²   **2.** 0.54 m²   **3.** 0.81 m²   **4.** 1.3 m²   **5.** 1.84 m²

DETERMINING ESTIMATED SAFE DOSAGES BASED ON BODY SURFACE AREA

Two formulas are used to estimate safe dosage based on the body surface area:

1. To determine the estimated child's dose, use the child's body surface area (m²) multiplied by the recommended average dose per m²:

    Surface area of child (m²) × Average dose per m² = Estimated child's dose

2. To determine the estimated child's dose, use the child's body surface area (m²) divided by the mean body surface area of an adult (for which m² has an accepted value of 1.7) multiplied by the recommended average adult dose.

$$\frac{\text{Body surface area of child (m}^2)}{\text{Mean body surface area of adult (1.7)}} \times \text{Average adult dose} = \text{Estimated child's dose}$$

The choice of formula is dictated by the way the recommended dose is presented by the manufacturer. If the manufacturer's recommended dose is written using the average dose per m², the first formula should be used. If the manufacturer's recommended dose is written using the average adult dose per adult mean body surface area (1.7), the second formula should be used. It should be noted that the second formula, using the average adult dose and the adult mean body surface area, is rarely used because it compares the child to the adult and assumes that the child is just like the adult. It also assumes that the child's dose is proportionally related to the adult dose. In addition, it assumes that the adult's mean body surface area (1.7) describes most adults and provides a safe standard for dosage of drugs that really require individualized computation for safety.

The formula *surface area of child (m²) × Average dose per 1 m² = Estimated child's dose* can be written in the more familiar ratio-and-proportion format.

One side of the proportion would be the average dose and the 1 m². The other side would be the estimated child's dose (the unknown) and the child's BSA m² from the nomogram:

$$\frac{\text{Recommended average dose}}{1 \text{ m}^2} = \frac{\text{Child's dose (the unknown)}}{\text{Child's BSA m}^2}$$

For consistency, this formula, written as a proportion, will be used for these problems.

Example: The physician has prescribed doxorubicin (Adriamycin) 39 mg once a day for 3 days IV for a 12-year-old who weighs 40 kg and is 150 cm tall.

Solution:

The nurse, needing to check if this dose falls within the safe range for Adriamycin, finds the manufacturer's recommended average dose to be 30 mg/m². Using a pediatric nomogram, the nurse determines that this child's BSA is 1.3 m² and sets up the proportion:

$$\frac{\text{Recommended average dose}}{1\ m^2} = \frac{\text{Child's dose (the unknown)}}{\text{Child's BSA } m^2}$$

$$\frac{30\ mg}{1\ m^2} = \frac{x\ mg}{1.3\ m^2}$$

$$x = 39\ mg$$

The nurse evaluates that the prescribed dose is a safe dose for this child.

The next step would be to determine how much drug should be administered to provide this dose. On hand are 10 mg/10 mL vials labeled 2 mg per mL (see label).

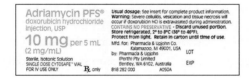

Using the available vials of Adriamycin, which are labeled 2 mg per mL, the proportion can be set up as:

$$\frac{39\ mg}{2\ mg} = \frac{x\ mL}{1\ mL}$$

$$2x = 39$$

$$x = 19.5\ mL$$

To provide 39 mg of Adriamycin, the nurse should administer 19.5 mL from vials labeled Adriamycin 2 mg per 1 mL.

Example: The physician has prescribed dexamethasone (Decadron) 1 mg every 6 hours IV for a 6-month-old who weighs 15 lb and is 25 inches tall.

Solution: The nurse, needing to check if this dose falls within the safe range for Decadron, finds that the manufacturer's recommended average child's dose is 3 mg/m² every 6 hours. Using a pediatric nomogram, the nurse determines this infant's BSA is 0.35 m² and sets up the proportion:

$$\frac{\text{Recommended average dose}}{1\ m^2} = \frac{\text{Child's dose (x)}}{\text{Child's BSA } m^2}$$

$$\frac{3\ mg}{1\ m^2} = \frac{x\ mg}{0.35\ m^2}$$

$$x = 1.05\ mg\ \text{every 6 hours}$$

The nurse evaluates that the prescribed dose is a safe dose for this child.

The next step is to determine how much drug should be administered to provide this dose. On hand is a 5 mL vial of Decadron labeled 4 mg per mL (see label).

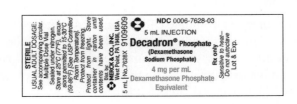

Using the available vial of Decadron, which is labeled 4 mg per mL, the proportion can be set up as:

$$\frac{1 \text{ mg}}{4 \text{ mg}} = \frac{x \text{ mL}}{1 \text{ mL}}$$
$$4x = 1$$
$$x = 0.25 \text{ mL}$$

To provide 0.25 mg of Decadron, the nurse should administer 0.25 mL from a multidose vial labeled Decadron 4 mg per mL.

Example: The physician has prescribed cyproheptadine HCl syrup (Periactin Syrup) 1.7 mg, three times a day, for a 6-year-old who weighs 16 kg and is 102 cm tall.

Solution: The nurse, needing to check if this dose falls within the safe range for Periactin, finds that the manufacturer's recommended average dose is 8 mg/m² daily. Using a pediatric nomogram, the nurse determines this child's BSA is 0.67 m² and sets up the proportion:

$$\frac{\text{Recommended average dose}}{1 \text{ m}^2} = \frac{\text{Child's dose } (x)}{\text{Child's BSA m}^2}$$
$$\frac{8 \text{ mg}}{1 \text{ m}^2} = \frac{x \text{ mg}}{0.67 \text{ m}^2}$$
$$x = 5.36 \text{ mg daily in three divided doses or } 1.79 \text{ or}$$
$$1.8 \text{ mg per single dose}$$

The nurse evaluates that the prescribed dose is a safe dose for this child.

The next step would be to determine how much drug should be administered to provide this dose. On hand is a bottle of Periactin Syrup labeled 2 mg per 5 mL.

Using the available bottle of Periactin Syrup, which is labeled 2 mg per 5 mL, the proportion can be set up as:

$$\frac{1.8 \text{ mg}}{2 \text{ mg}} = \frac{x \text{ mL}}{5 \text{ mL}}$$
$$2x = 9$$
$$x = 4.5 \text{ mL per dose}$$

To provide 1.8 mg of Periactin Syrup, the nurse should administer 4.5 mL from a multidose bottle labeled Periactin Syrup 2 mg per 5 mL.

Problem Set 21.3

1. The physician has prescribed leucovorin calcium (Wellcovorin) tablets 15 mg by mouth q6h for a 15-year-old whose BSA is 1.5 m². The nurse, needing to check if this dose falls within the safe range for leucovorin calcium, finds that the manufacturer's recommended average dose is 10 mg per m² every 6 hours.

   After setting up the proportion, the nurse evaluates that this:

   Is a safe dose and administers the medication. (a) _____

   Is an unsafe dose and questions the physician. (b) _____

2. The physician has prescribed prednisone 80 mg daily by mouth for an 8-year-old with leukemia whose BSA is 0.95 m². The nurse, needing to check if this dose falls within the safe range for prednisone, finds that the manufacturer's recommended average dose is 60 mg per m² daily. After setting up the proportion, the nurse evaluates that this:

   Is a safe dose and administers the medication. (a) _____

   Is an unsafe dose and questions the physician. (b) _____

3. The physician has prescribed bleomycin sulfate (Blenoxane) 14 units twice weekly by injection for a 14-year-old whose BSA is 1.4 m². The nurse, needing to check if this dose falls within the safe range for bleomycin sulfate, finds that the manufacturer's recommended average dose is 10 to 20 units per m² twice weekly. After setting up the proportion using the lowest number of the manufacturer's recommended average dose, the nurse evaluates that this:

Is a safe dose and administers the medication.   (a) _____

Is an unsafe dose and questions the physician.   (b) _____

4. The physician has prescribed an initial dose of lomustine capsules (CeeNU) 220 mg orally for a 10-year-old whose BSA is 1.15 m². The nurse, needing to check if this dose falls within the safe range for lomustine, finds that the manufacturer's recommended average dose is 130 mg per m² initially. After setting up the proportion, the nurse evaluates that this:

Is a safe dose and administers the medication.   (a) _____

Is an unsafe dose and questions the physician.   (b) _____

5. The physician has prescribed quinidine sulfate 150 mg orally q6h for a 6-year-old whose BSA is 0.7 m². The nurse, needing to check if this dose falls within the safe range for quinidine sulfate, finds that the manufacturer's recommended average dose for pediatric use is 900 mg per m² daily in three to five divided doses. After setting up the proportion, the nurse evaluates that this:

Is a safe dose and administers the medication.   (a) _____

Is an unsafe dose and questions the physician.   (b) _____

Answers   1. a   2. b   3. a   4. b   5. a

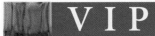

VIP

To determine the estimated child's dose, use the child's body surface area (m²) multiplied by the recommended average dose per m²:

Surface area of child (m²) × Average dose per m² = Estimated child's dose

This formula can be converted to the more familiar proportion format:

$$\frac{\text{Recommended average dose}}{1 \text{ m}^2} = \frac{\text{Child's dose (the unknown)}}{\text{Child's BSA m}^2}$$

Review Test 21.1
Computing Dosage for Infants and Children

1. The physician has prescribed gentamicin sulfate (Garamycin) 9 mg IM q12h for a 5-day-old who weighs 8 lb. The nurse, needing to check if this dose falls within the safe range for gentamicin sulfate, finds that the manufacturer's recommended dose is 2.5 mg per kg q12h. On hand is a vial labeled Pediatric Injectable Garamycin 1 mL/10 mg. The nurse evaluates that this:

Is a safe dose and administers   (a) _____ mL.

Is an unsafe dose and questions the physician.   (b) _____

2. The physician has prescribed a maintenance oral dose of sulfasalazine (Azulfidine) 30 mg/kg per day in divided doses q6h for a 10-year-old who weighs 72.6 pounds. The nurse, needing to check if this dose falls within the safe range for sulfasalazine, finds that the manufacturer's recommended maintenance dose for pediatric use is 30 mg per kg daily in four divided doses. On hand is a bottle of scored tablets labeled Azulfidine 500 mg. The nurse evaluates that this:

Is a safe dose and administers   (a) _____ tablet(s).

Is an unsafe dose and questions the physician.   (b) _____

3. The physician has prescribed vancomycin HCl pulvules (Vancocin) 250 mg q6h for an 8-year-old who weighs 25 kg. The nurse, needing to check if this dose falls within the safe range for vancomycin, finds that the manufacturer's recommended dose is 40 mg per kg daily in three or four divided doses. On hand is a bottle labeled Vancocin pulvules 125 mg. The nurse evaluates that this:

   Is a safe dose and administers   (a) _____ pulvule(s).

   Is an unsafe dose and questions the physician.   (b) _____

4. The physician has prescribed propranolol HCl (Inderal) orally 1 mg per kg daily in two divided doses for a 13-year-old who weighs 99 lb. The nurse, needing to check if this dose falls within the safe range for Inderal, finds that the manufacturer's recommended beginning pediatric dose is 0.5 mg per kg twice a day. On hand is a bottle labeled Inderal tablets 10 mg. The nurse evaluates that this:

   Is a safe dose and administers   (a) _____ tablet(s).

   Is an unsafe dose and questions the physician.   (b) _____

5. The physician has prescribed rifampin (Rifadin) 750 mg daily by mouth for a 12-year-old who weighs 82.5 pounds (37.5 kg). The nurse, needing to check if this dose falls within the safe range for Rifadin, finds that the manufacturer's recommended single daily dose is 10 to 20 mg per kg not to exceed 600 mg per day. On hand are two bottles of the drug, one labeled Rifadin tablets 150 mg and the other labeled Rifadin tablets 300 mg. The nurse evaluates that this:

   Is a safe dose and administers   (a) _____ tablet(s).

   Is an unsafe dose and questions the physician.   (b) _____

6. Using the pediatric nomogram (Figure 21-1), determine the BSA in m^2 for a 3-month-old who weighs 14 lb and is 24 inches tall.   _____ m^2

7. Using the pediatric nomogram (Figure 21-1), determine the BSA in m^2 for an 8-year-old who weighs 25 kg and is 126 cm tall.   _____ m^2

8. Using the pediatric nomogram (Figure 21-1), determine the BSA in m^2 for a 4-year-old of normal height and weight who weighs 36 lb.   _____ m^2

9. The physician has prescribed tripelennamine hydrochloride tablets (PBZ) 25 mg orally q4h for a 12-year-old whose BSA is 1.15 m^2. The nurse, needing to check if this dose falls within the safe range for PBZ, finds that the manufacturer's recommended child's dose is 150 mg/m^2 per day in four to six divided doses. On hand are bottles of the drug containing scored tablets labeled PBZ tablets 25 mg. The nurse evaluates that this:

   Is a safe dose and administers   (a) _____ tablet(s).

   Is an unsafe dose and questions the physician.   (b) _____

10. The physician has prescribed asparaginase (Elspar) 6000 IU IM every third day for 9 doses for a 9-year-old whose BSA is 0.91 m^2. The nurse, needing to check if this dose falls within the safe range for Elspar, finds that the manufacturer's recommended child's dose is 6000 mg/m^2 every three days. On hand is a 10,000 IU vial of powdered drug with directions to add 2 mL of sodium chloride for injection to yield a total solution of 10,000 IU/2 mL. The nurse evaluates that this:

    Is a safe dose and administers   (a) _____ mL.

    Is an unsafe dose and questions the physician.   (b) _____

Answers   **1.** a; 0.9 mL (9 mg)   **2.** a; $\frac{1}{2}$ tablet (250 [248] mg)   **3.** a; 2 pulvules (250 mg)   **4.** a; 2 tablets (22.5 mg)
5. b; the 750 mg prescribed dose is within the manufacturer's recommended dose but exceeds the 600 mg per day recommended maximum, so the physician should be questioned about this order   **6.** 0.34 m^2 **7.** 0.92 m^2 **8.** 0.68 m^2 **9.** a; 1 tablet (25 mg)   **10.** b; the dose recommended by the manufacturer would be 5400 IU every 3 days, not the 6000 IU prescribed; the physician should be questioned about this order

---

If you had fewer than three errors on Review Test 21.1, move on to the next chapter. If you had four or more errors, review the material on computing dosage for infants and children and complete Review Test 21.2 before continuing.

Review Test 21.2
Computing Dosage for Infants and Children

1. The physician has prescribed amikacin sulfate (Amikin injectable) 275 mg IM q12h for an 11-year-old who weighs 83 lb (37.7 kg). The nurse, needing to check if this dose falls within the safe range for Amikin, finds that the manufacturer's recommended dose is 7.5 mg per kg twice a day. On hand are single-dose vials labeled Amikin injectable 500 mg per 2 mL. The nurse evaluates that this:

    Is a safe dose and administers   (a) _____ mL.

    Is an unsafe dose and questions the physician.   (b) _____

2. The physician has prescribed tobramycin sulfate injection (Nebcin) 50 mg IM q8h for an 8-year-old who weighs 51 lb (23 kg). The nurse, needing to check if this dose falls within the safe range for Nebcin, finds that the manufacturer's recommended child's dose is 2 to 2.5 mg per kg every 8 hours. On hand are single-dose vials labeled Nebcin 80 mg per 2 mL. The nurse evaluates that this:

    Is a safe dose and administers   (a) _____ mL.

    Is an unsafe dose and questions the physician.   (b) _____

3. The physician has prescribed vancomycin hydrochloride (Vancocin) 500 mg orally q6h for a 13-year-old who weighs 110 lb (50 kg). The nurse, needing to check if this dose falls within the safe range for Vancocin, finds that the manufacturer's recommended child's dose is 40 mg per kg in three or four divided doses for seven to ten days, not to exceed 2 g per day. On hand is a bottle of oral solution labeled Vancocin solution 500 mg per 6 mL. The nurse evaluates that this:

    Is a safe dose and administers   (a) _____ mL.

    Is an unsafe dose and questions the physician.   (b) _____

4. The physician has prescribed clindamycin palmitrate hydrochloride oral solution (Cleocin Pediatric) 45 mg orally q8h for a $1\frac{1}{2}$-year-old who weighs 28 lb (12.7 kg). The nurse, needing to check if this dose falls within the safe range for Cleocin Pediatric, finds that the manufacturer's recommended dose is 8 to 12 mg per kg per day in three or four divided doses. On hand is a bottle of oral solution labeled Cleocin Pediatric 75 mg/5 mL. The nurse evaluates that this:

    Is a safe dose and administers   (a) _____ mL.

    Is an unsafe dose and questions the physician.   (b) _____

5. The physician has prescribed digoxin elixir (Lanoxin Pediatric Elixir) 120 μg orally q8h for a 1-year-old who weighs 22 lb (10 kg). The nurse, needing to check if this dose falls within the safe range for Lanoxin Pediatric, finds that the manufacturer's recommended loading dose is 35 to 60 μg per day in three divided doses. On hand is a bottle labeled Lanoxin Pediatric Elixir 50 mcg/mL. The nurse evaluates that this:

    Is a safe dose and administers   (a) _____ mL.

    Is an unsafe dose and questions the physician.   (b) _____

6. Using the pediatric nomogram (Figure 21.1), determine the BSA in m^2 for a 4-month-old who weighs 15 lb and is 25 inches tall.   _____ m^2

7. Using the pediatric nomogram (Figure 21.1), determine the BSA in m^2 for a 3-year-old who weighs 11 kg and is 80 cm tall.   _____ m^2

8. The physician has prescribed interferon gamma-1b (Actimmune) 68 mcg by SC injection three times a week for a 14-year-old whose BSA is 1.35 m^2. The nurse, needing to check if this dose falls within the safe range for Actimmune, finds that the manufacturer's recommended dose is 50 $μg/m^2$ 3x a week. On hand are single-dose vials of the drug labeled Actimmune 100 mcg/0.5 mL. The nurse evaluates that this:

    Is a safe dose and administers   (a) _____ mL.

    Is an unsafe dose and questions the physician.   (b) _____

9. The physician has prescribed methotrexate (Methotrexate LPF) 24 mg twice a week IM as a maintenance dose for a 6-year-old whose BSA is 0.8 m². The nurse, needing to check if this dose falls within the safe range for Methotrexate LPF, finds that the manufacturer's recommended maintenance dose for a child is 30 mg/m² twice weekly. On hand are single-dose vials of the drug labeled Methotrexate LPF 25 mg/1 mL. The nurse evaluates that this:

   Is a safe dose and administers (a) _____ mL.

   Is an unsafe dose and questions the physician. (b) _____

10. The physician has prescribed prednisone 70 mg daily by mouth for a 10-year-old whose BSA is 1.2 m². The nurse, needing to check if this dose falls within the safe range for prednisone, finds that the manufacturer's recommended induction dose is 60 mg/m² daily. On hand are two bottles of scored tablets of the drug, one labeled prednisone 10 mg, and one labeled prednisone 50 mg. The nurse evaluates that this:

   Is a safe dose and administers (a) _____ tablets.

   Is an unsafe dose and questions the physician. (b) _____

Answers 1. a; 1.1 mL (275 mg) 2. a; 1.25 mL (50 mg) 3. a; 6 mL (500 mg) 4. a; 3 mL (45 mg) 5. a; 2.4 mL (120 µg) 6. 0.36 m²
7. 0.5 m² 8. a; 0.34 mL (68 µg) 9. a; 0.96 mL (24 mg) 10. a; 1 tablet 50 mg and 2 tablets 10 mg (70 mg)

   The Review Tests on computing dosage for infants and children should be repeated until fewer than three errors occur.

Unit

7

Alternative Methods of Calculating Dosage

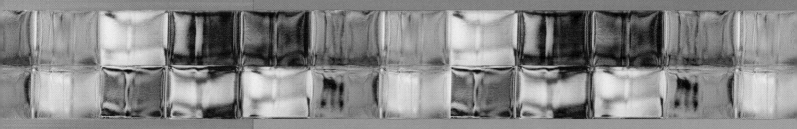

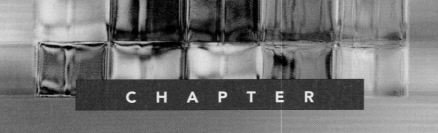

22

Using the Formula Method

Learning Outcomes

After successfully completing this chapter, the learner should be able to:

- *Set up the formula for computing medication dosage and label all terms.*
- *Convert the available medication to the desired dose.*
- *Calculate the amount of medication to be poured or injected to administer a desired dose.*

GENERAL INFORMATION

The nurse is responsible for giving the correct medication in the correct dosage, at the correct time, by the correct route, to the correct patient, but the method used to compute the correct dose is the nurse's choice. Although this book uses the ratio-and-proportion method throughout, there is also a formula method that some nurses find easier to use for some calculations.

Frequently, the nurse who must administer medications does not find the exact dosage of drug that has been ordered. In such instances, the nurse must compute the amount to be administered, remembering that the calculated dosage must never differ by more than 10% from the prescribed dosage and should be the same if possible.

SETTING UP THE FORMULA

The first step in computing medication dosage, regardless of the method used, is to make certain the strength of the drug ordered and the strength of the drug available are in the same unit of measure. If necessary, conversion to a single unit must be carried out. Once this is done, the problem can be set up using the formula:

$$\frac{D}{H} \times Q = x$$

The answer or the unknown, most commonly signified by the letter x, is usually placed on the right side of the formula preceded by an equal sign.

In this formula, the D represents the desired dosage of the drug to be administered. The H represents the dosage of the drug available. The D and H must always be in the same unit of measure. The Q represents the number of tablets, capsules, milliliters, minims, and so on, that contains the available dosage. The x represents the number of tablets, capsules, milliliters, minims, and so on that the desired dose will be contained in (the amount to be administered). The Q and x must always be in the same unit of measure. Make certain all the terms in the formula are labeled with the correct units of measure.

$$\frac{\text{Desired}}{\text{Have}} \times \text{Quantity} = x$$

Example: A patient is to receive alprazolam (Xanax) 0.5 mg by mouth. Available is a bottle of tablets labeled 0.25 mg (see label). How much medication should the patient receive?

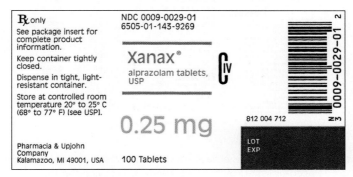

Solution: Because the desired dosage and the available dosage are in the same unit of measure, no conversion is necessary in this problem. Being certain to label all terms, set up the problem using the formula:

$$\frac{\text{Desired}}{\text{Have}} \times Q = x$$

$$\frac{0.5 \text{ mg}}{0.25 \text{ mg}} \times 1 \text{ tablet} = x \text{ tablets}$$

$$\frac{\overset{2}{\cancel{0.50}}}{\underset{1}{\cancel{0.25}}} \times 1 = x = 2$$

x = 2 tablets

To administer alprazolam (Xanax) 0.5 mg, the patient should receive 2 tablets of Xanax labeled 0.25 mg.

Example: A patient is to receive nitroglycerin tablets (Nitrostat) 0.6 mg sublingually. Nitrostat is available in 0.3 mg tablets (see label). How many 0.3 mg tablets should the patient receive?

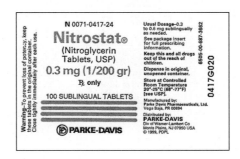

Solution: Because the desired dosage and the available dosage are in the same unit of measure, no conversion is necessary in this problem. Being certain to label all terms, set up the problem using the formula:

$$\frac{\text{Desired}}{\text{Have}} \times Q = x$$

$$\frac{0.6 \text{ mg}}{0.3 \text{ mg}} \times 1 \text{ tablet} = x \text{ tablets}$$

$$\frac{\overset{2}{\cancel{0.6}}}{\underset{1}{\cancel{0.3}}} \times 1 = x = 2$$

$$x = 2 \text{ tablets}$$

To administer 0.6 mg of Nitrostat, the nurse should give the patient 2 tablets of 0.3 mg strength.

Example: A patient is to receive amoxicillin oral suspension (Amoxil) 0.25 g by mouth. Available is a bottle labeled Amoxil 125 mg per 5 mL (see label). How many mL should the patient receive?

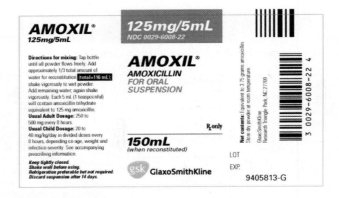

Solution: Proceed by first converting the dosage desired, 0.25 g, and the dosage available, 125 mg, to one unit of measure. This can be accomplished by moving the decimal place three places to the right, changing 0.25 g to 250 mg. Being certain to label all terms, set up the problem using the formula:

$$\frac{\text{Desired}}{\text{Have}} \times Q = x$$

$$\frac{250 \text{ mg}}{125 \text{ mg}} \times 5 \text{ mL} = x \text{ mL}$$

$$\frac{\overset{2}{\cancel{250}}}{\underset{1}{\cancel{125}}} \times 5 = x = 10$$

$$x = 10 \text{ mL}$$

To administer amoxicillin 0.25 mg, the patient should receive 10 mL of Amoxil labeled 125 mg per 5 mL.

Example: A patient is to receive heparin sodium 850 units by injection. The multidose vial is labeled 1000 units per mL (see heparin sodium label). How much medication should the patient receive?

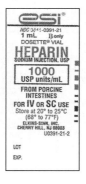

Solution: Because the desired dosage and the available dosage are in the same unit of measure, no conversion is necessary in this problem. Being certain to label all terms, set up the problem using the formula:

$$\frac{\text{Desired}}{\text{Have}} \times Q = x$$

$$\frac{850 \text{ units}}{1000 \text{ units}} \times 1 \text{ mL} = x \text{ mL}$$

$$\frac{\overset{17}{\cancel{850}}}{\underset{20}{\cancel{1000}}} \times 1 = x$$

$$x = 0.85 \text{ mL}$$

To administer heparin sodium 850 units subcutaneously from a multidose vial labeled 1000 units =1 mL, the nurse would withdraw and inject 0.85 mL.

Mark the tuberculin syringe in Figure 22-1 to show the required dose.

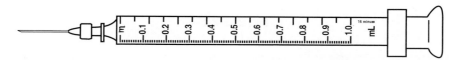

Figure 22-1

The syringe should look like Figure 22-2:

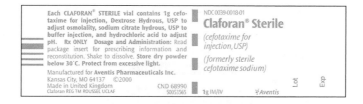

Figure 22-2

Example: A patient is to receive cefotaxime sodium (Claforan) 575 mg IM for injection. The vial of powdered medication is labeled Claforan 1 gram. The package insert states: for IM injection, add 3 mL of sterile water to produce an approximate volume of 3.4 mL containing 300 mg of drug per mL.

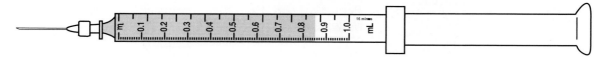

Solution: Because the desired dosage and the available dosage are in the same unit of measure, no conversion is necessary in this problem. Being certain to label all terms, set up the problem using the formula:

$$\frac{\text{Desired}}{\text{Have}} \times Q = x$$

$$\frac{575 \text{ mg}}{1000 \text{ mg}} \times 3.4 \text{ mL} = \frac{1955}{1000}$$

$$\frac{1955}{1000} = 1.95 \text{ or } 2.0 \text{ mL}$$

To administer Claforan 575 mg IM from a 1 gram vial of powdered Claforan to which 3 mL of sterile water has been added, the nurse would withdraw and inject 1.95 or 2 mL of solution.

Mark the syringe in Figure 22-3 to show the required dose.

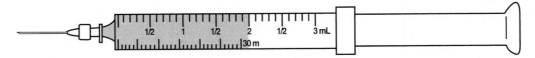

Figure 22-3

The syringe should look like Figure 22-4:

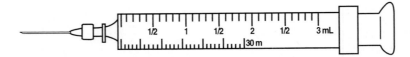

Figure 22-4

Problem Set 22.1

1. A patient is to receive triazolam (Halcion) tablets 250 mcg. The drug on hand is labeled:

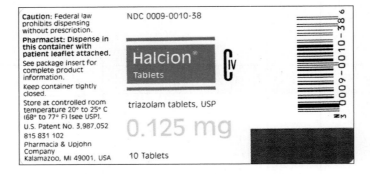

The nurse should administer _____ tablets.

2. A patient is to receive lithium citrate (lithium syrup) orally 300 mg by mouth every 4 hours. The drug on hand is labeled:

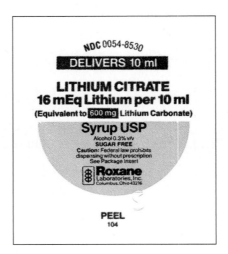

The nurse should administer _____ mL.

3. A patient is to receive Depo-Medrol 30 mg by injection. The vial on hand is labeled:

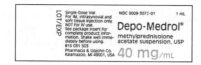

The nurse should withdraw and administer _____ mL.

Mark the syringe in Figure 22-5 to show the required dose.

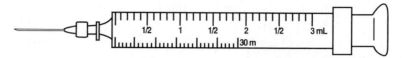

Figure 22-5

4. A patient is to receive tobramycin sulfate (Nebcin) 50 mg by injection. The drug on hand is labeled:

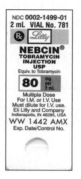

The nurse should withdraw and administer _____ mL.

Mark the syringe in Figure 22-6 to show the required dose.

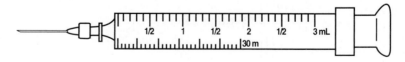

Figure 22-6

5. A patient is to receive 65 mg of hydroxyzine hydrochloride (Vistaril) by injection. The drug on hand is labeled:

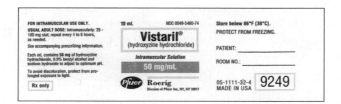

The nurse should withdraw and administer _____ mL.

Mark the syringe in Figure 22-7 to show the required dose.

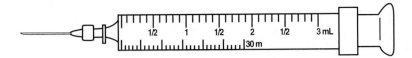

Figure 22-7

Answers **1.** To provide 250 mcg of the drug, the patient should receive 2 tablets from the bottle labeled triazolam (Halcion) tablets 0.125 mg per tablet. **2.** To provide 300 mg of the drug, the patient should receive 5 mL from the 10 mL patient cup labeled lithium citrate syrup 16 mEq per 10 mL. **3.** To provide 30 mg of the drug by injection, the patient should receive 0.75 mL from a vial labeled Depo-Medrol 4o mg per mL. The syringe should look like Figure 22-8.

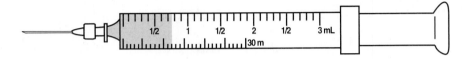

Figure 22-8

4. To provide 50 mg of the drug by injection, the patient should receive 1.25 mL from a multidose vial labeled tobramycin sulfate (Nebcin) 80 mg per 2 mL. The syringe should look like Figure 22-9.

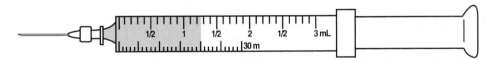

Figure 22-9

5. To provide 65 mg of hydroxyzine hydrochloride (Vistaril) by injection, the patient should receive 1.3 mL from a vial labeled Vistaril 50 mg per mL. The syringe should look like Figure 22-10.

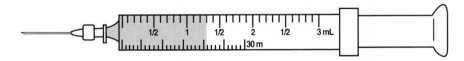

Figure 22-10

VIP

- The nurse is responsible for giving the correct medication, in the correct dosage, at the correct time, by the correct route, to the correct patient—but the method used to compute the correct dose is the nurse's choice.

- The first step in computing medication dosage, regardless of the method used, is to make certain the strength of the drug ordered and the strength of the drug available are in the same unit of measure. If necessary, conversion to a single unit of measure must be carried out.

- Computing uncomplicated dosages can be achieved by using the formula:

$$\frac{D}{H} \times Q = x$$

This formula does not replace the ratio-and-proportion method, which must still be used for solving advanced, more complex clinical calculations.

Review Test 22.1
Using the Formula Method

It is important that you use the formula method in solving these problems.

1. The patient is to receive meclofenamate sodium (Meclomen) 0.2 g orally. On hand is a bottle of tablets labeled: Meclomen 100 mg.

   The nurse should administer _____ tablet(s).

2. The patient is to receive phenobarbital $\frac{3}{4}$ grains by mouth. On hand is a bottle of tablets labeled: Phenobarbital 15 mg.

   The nurse should administer _____ tablet(s).

3. The patient is to receive cloxacillin sodium oral solution (Tegopen) 500 mg. On hand is a bottle of solution labeled: Tegopen 125 mg per 5 mL.

   The nurse should administer _____ mL.

4. The patient is to receive clorazepete dipotassium (Tranxene) 15 mg by mouth. On hand is a bottle of tablets labeled: Tranxene 7.5 mg.

   The nurse should administer _____ tablet(s).

5. The patient is to receive ergonovine maleate (Ergotrate Maleate) 200 mcg by injection. On hand is an ampule labeled: Ergotrate Maleate 0.2 mg per 1 mL.

   The nurse should administer _____ mL.

6. The patient is to receive cefazolin sodium (Ancef) 250 mg IM. On hand is a vial of powdered medication labeled: Ancef 500 mg with directions for reconstitution that state "For IM use, add 2 mL of sterile water to provide a total solution of 2.2 mL (225 mg of Ancef per mL)."

   The nurse should administer _____ mL.

7. The patient is to receive dexamethasone phosphate (Decadron) 5 mg IM. On hand is a multidose vial labeled: Decadron 4 mg/mL.

   The nurse should administer _____ mL.

8. The patient is to receive Humulin R Insulin 35 units by injection. On hand is a multidose vial labeled: Humulin R Insulin 100 units per mL.

   The nurse should administer _____ mL.

9. The patient is to receive heparin sodium 8000 units by injection. On hand is a multidose vial labeled: Heparin Sodium 10,000 units per mL.

   The nurse, using a tuberculin syringe, should administer _____ mL.

10. The patient is to receive hydromorphone hydrochloride (Dilaudid) gr 1/30 by injection. On hand is an ampule labeled: Dilaudid 3 mg per mL.

    The nurse should administer _____ mL.

Answers   **1.** 2 tablets   **2.** 3 tablets   **3.** 20 mL   **4.** 2 tablets   **5.** 1 mL   **6.** 1.1 mL   **7.** 1.25 mL   **8.** 0.35 mL   **9.** 0.8 mL
10. 0.66 or 0.7 mL

If you had fewer than three errors on Review Test 22.1, move on to the next chapter. If you had four or more errors, review the material on using the formula method and complete Review Test 22.2 before continuing.

Review Test 22.2
Using the Formula Method

It is important that you use the formula method in solving these problems.

1. The patient is to receive acyclovir suspension (Zovirax) 0.8 g by mouth. On hand is a bottle labeled: Zovirax 200 mg per 5 mL.

   The nurse should administer _____ mL.

2. The patient is to receive epoetin alfa (Epogen) 1400 units by injection. On hand are single-dose ampules labeled: Epogen 2000 units per mL.

   The nurse should administer _____ mL.

3. The patient is to receive azathioprime (Imuran) 125 mg by mouth. On hand is a bottle of tablets labeled: Imuran tablets 50 mg.

   The nurse should administer _____ tablet(s).

4. The patient is to receive valproic acid syrup (Depakene) 0.75 g by mouth. On hand is a bottle of syrup labeled: Depakene 250 mg per 5 mL.

   The nurse should administer _____ mL.

5. The patient is to receive codeine sulfate 1 grain by mouth. On hand are tablets labeled: codeine sulfate tablets 30 mg.

   The nurse should administer _____ tablet(s).

6. The patient is to receive isoniazid (INH) (Nydrazid) 270 mg IM. On hand is a multidose vial labeled: Nydrazid 100 mg/1 mL.

   The nurse should administer _____ mL.

7. The patient is to receive ceftriazone sodium (Rocephin) 0.75 g IM. On hand is a vial of powdered medication labeled: Rocephin 1 g with directions for reconstitution that state "Add 3.6 mL of sterile diluent to produce a solution, which provides 250 mg of Rocephin per mL."

   The nurse should administer _____ mL.

8. The patient is to receive phenytoin sodium (Dilantin) 150 mg IM. On hand is a multidose vial labeled: Dilantin 50 mg per 1 mL.

   The nurse should administer _____ mL.

9. The patient is to receive penicillin G potassium 400,000 units IM. On hand is a vial of powdered medication labeled: Penicillin G Potassium 1,000,000 units with directions for reconstitution that state "Add 1.6 mL of sterile diluent to produce a solution, which provides 500,000 units of Penicillin G Potassium per mL."

   The nurse should administer _____ mL.

10. The patient is to receive digoxin (Lanoxin) 125 mcg IM. On hand is a single-dose vial labeled: Lanoxin 0.5 mg per 2 mL.

    The nurse should administer _____ mL.

Answers   1. 20 mL   2. 0.7 mL   3. $2\frac{1}{2}$ tablets   4. 15 mL   5. 2 tablets   6. 2.7 mL   7. 3 mL   8. 3 mL   9. 0.8 mL   10. 0.5 mL

The Review Tests on using the formula method should be repeated until fewer than three errors occur.

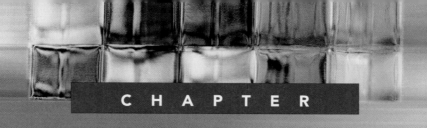

23

Using Dimensional Analysis

Learning Outcomes

After successfully completing this chapter, the learner should be able to:

- *Set up the dimensional analysis equation for computing medication dosage and label all factors.*
- *Use cancellation to reduce the number of dimensions (units of measure).*
- *Determine the correct unit and amount to be administered.*

GENERAL INFORMATION

Although this book focuses on the ratio-and-proportion method throughout, there are alternative methods, such as the formula method presented in Chapter 22 and the dimensional analysis method presented in this chapter.

Dimensional analysis (DA) uses a series of ratios that are called *factors*. It focuses on dimensions (dimensions are units of measure such as mL, capsules, drops, tablets, etc.) rather than numbers.

SETTING UP THE DIMENSIONAL EQUATION

To use this method, the problem must be carefully read and a decision reached as to the desired dimension or unit of measure that is to be determined (mL, capsules, drops, tablets, etc.)

Ratios or factors are entered into the equation by analyzing the dimensions and adding numbers from the problem, or known conversions. A factor may be a prescriber's order, the strength of the medication available, or a known conversion between units of measure from the systems of measurement. These factors are expressed as common fractions and placed in the DA equation.

Cancellation of these dimensions, after they have been set up as a series or ratios or factors, is then performed. Using cancellation of the dimensions, the desired dimension can be determined.

Example: A patient is to receive cephalexin (Keflex) 500 mg. Available is a bottle of Keflex capsules labeled 250 mg capsules. How many capsules should the patient receive?

Solution: To solve this problem using ratio and proportion:

$$\frac{\text{Desired Dose}}{\text{Have Dose}} = \frac{\text{Desired Amount}}{\text{Have Amount}}$$

$$\frac{500 \text{ mg}}{250 \text{ mg}} = \frac{x \text{ capsule}}{1 \text{ capsule}}$$

$$250x = 2 \text{ capsules}$$

Solution: To solve the same problem using dimensional analysis:

The desired dimension must be determined first. By analysis, it can be determined that in this problem the desired dimension is the number of capsules the patient should receive.

Capsules and milligrams are the only two dimensions in this problem. Thus, there are two complete factors in this problem:

250 mg in 1 capsule

500 mg in an unknown number of capsules

The number of capsules that contain the prescribed amount is the unknown.

The first item in the DA equation is the unknown dimension, followed by an equal sign. This must always be determined first.

capsule =

The first factor or ratio can be determined by going back to the problem and identifying capsules as a unit of measure whose strength is 250 mg.

$$\text{capsule} = \frac{1 \text{ capsule}}{250 \text{ mg}}$$

After a multipication sign, the next factor must be added. The numerator of this factor must match the denominator of the previous factor. Again, going back to the problem, 500 mg can be identified as the strength or amount of drug to be administered.

$$\text{capsule} = \frac{1 \text{ capsule}}{250 \text{ mg}} \times 500 \text{ mg}$$

The numerator of one factor must always be the same as the denominator of the previous factor so that the principle of cancellation may be used.

$$\text{capsule} = \frac{1 \text{ capsule}}{\cancel{250} \text{ mg}} \times \cancel{500}^{\,2} \text{ mg} = 2 \text{ capsules}$$

V I P

- A dimension is simply a unit of measure, such as tablets, mL, drops, grams, and the like.
- A factor is the amount and form of the drug over the strength of the drug.
- In dimensional analysis, the focus is on units of measure rather than numbers.
- In dimensional analysis, the first step is to determine the desired dimension.
- The factors in the dimensional analysis equation are determined by analyzing information in the problem or using known conversions of units of measure from the systems of measurement.
- Make certain that the problem is correctly set up and that all terms are labeled. No method of computation will correctly solve problems unless the terms or factors are set up and labeled correctly.

Example: A patient is to receive 40 mg of furosemide (Lasix) by mouth. On hand are Lasix 20 mg tablets. How many 20 mg tablets must the patient receive?

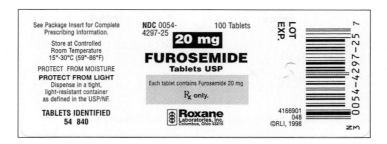

Solution: First, identify the unit of measure to be determined. This is the desired dimension. In this instance the unit of measure is tablets. Place this unit of measure to the left, followed by an equal (=) sign.

Tablets =

Following the equal sign, place the starting factor, which is the dosage strength available. In this problem, this would be 1 tablet that is 20 mg.

$$\text{tablet} = \frac{1 \text{ tablet}}{20 \text{ mg}}$$

Add the next factor, which is the physician's order. In this instance, the order is for 40 mg.

$$\text{tablet} = \frac{1 \text{ tablet}}{20 \text{ mg}} \times 40 \text{ mg}$$

The next step is to cancel like units of measure in the denominator of one factor with the unit of measure in the adjacent factor. This cancellation can occur only when the units of measure match. If there is no matching unit of measure, the factors have been entered into the problem incorrectly.

$$\text{tablet} = \frac{1 \text{ tablet}}{20 \text{ \cancel{mg}}} \times 40 \text{ \cancel{mg}}$$

The answer can then be calculated by multiplying the string of denominators and the string of numerators, then reducing the resulting fraction to its lowest terms. This answer must be labeled with the unit of measure you started out to determine.

$$\text{tablet} = \frac{1 \text{ tablet}}{20} \times 40 = 2$$

To provide 40 mg of Lasix, the nurse should administer 2 tablets of Lasix labeled 20 mg per tablet.

Example: A patient is to receive digoxin (Lanoxin) 0.25 mg by mouth. Available is a container labeled Lanoxin 125 mcg tablets. How much medication should the patient receive?

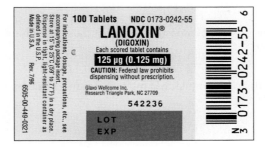

Solution: First, identify the dimension (unit of measurement) that must be determined. In this example it is tablets. Write "tablets," then an equal sign.

Tablets =

Next, locate a factor in the problem that has tablets as a dimension and enter the factor into the equation with tablets in the numerator position.

$$\text{tablets} = \frac{1 \text{ tablet}}{125 \text{ mcg}}$$

Because the drug is ordered in mg and is available in mcg, a known conversion factor must be included in this equation. In this case, 1000 mcg in 1 mg is included.

$$\text{tablets} = \frac{1 \text{ tablet}}{125 \text{ mcg}} \times \frac{1000 \text{ mcg}}{1 \text{ mg}}$$

The last factor to be placed in the equation is the dose ordered for this patient. The dimensional analysis equation should now look like this:

$$\text{tablets} = \frac{1 \text{ tablet}}{125 \text{ mcg}} \times \frac{1000 \text{ mcg}}{1 \text{ mg}} \times 0.25 \text{ mg}$$

Cancel the similar dimensions in the numerators and the denominators.

$$\text{tablets} = \frac{1 \text{ tablet}}{125 \text{ mcg}} \times \frac{1000 \text{ mcg}}{1 \text{ mg}} \times 0.25 \text{ mg}$$

Finally, compute the dose.

$$\frac{1 \times 1000 \times 0.25}{125} = \frac{250}{125} = 2 \text{ tablets}$$

To provide 0.25 mg of Lanoxin, the nurse should administer 2 tablets of Lanoxin labeled 125 mcg per tablet.

Example: A patient is to receive theophylline anhydrous (Elixophyllin Elixir) 110 mg by mouth. Available is a bottle labeled Elixophyllin Elixir 80 mg/15 mL. How many mL of medication should the patient receive?

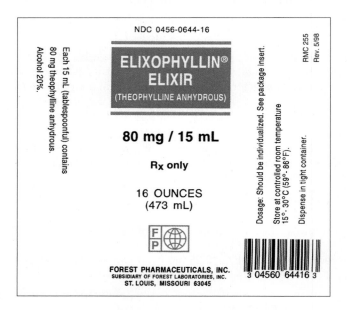

Solution: First, identify the dimension (unit of measurement) that must be determined. In this example, it is mL. Write "mL," then an equal sign.

mL =

Next, locate a factor in the problem that has mL as a dimension and enter the factor into the equation with mL in the numerator position.

$$\text{mL} = \frac{15 \text{ mL}}{80 \text{ mg}}$$

The factor to be placed in the last equation is the dose ordered for this patient. The dimensional analysis equation should now look like this:

$$\text{mL} = \frac{15 \text{ mL}}{80 \text{ mg}} \times 110 \text{ mg}$$

Cancel the similar dimensions in the numerator and the denominator.

$$\text{mL} = \frac{15 \text{ mL}}{80 \text{ mg}} \times 110 \text{ mg}$$

Finally, compute the dose.

$$\frac{15 \times 110}{80} = \frac{1650}{80} = 20.6 \text{ mL}$$

To provide 110 mg of Elixophyllin, the nurse should administer 20.6 mL of Elixophyllin labeled 80 mg per 15 mL.

Example: A patient is to receive cefotaxime (Claforan) 750 mg IM. Available is a vial labeled Claforan 1 g. The package insert states: "reconstitute with 3 mL of an appropriate diluent to yield a withdrawal volume of 3.4 mL where each mL will contain Claforan 330 mg." How many mL of medication should the patient receive?

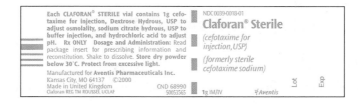

Solution: First, identify the dimension (unit of measurement) that must be determined. In this example it is mL. Write "mL," then an equal sign.

mL =

Next, locate a factor in the problem that has mL as a dimension and enter the factor into the equation with mL in the numerator position.

$$mL = \frac{1 \text{ mL}}{330 \text{ mg}}$$

The last factor to be placed in the equation is the dose ordered for this patient. The dimensional analysis equation should now look like this:

$$mL = \frac{1 \text{ mL}}{330 \text{ mg}} \times 750 \text{ mg}$$

Cancel the similar dimensions in the numerator and the denominator.

$$mL = \frac{1 \text{ mL}}{330 \cancel{\text{ mg}}} \times 750 \cancel{\text{ mg}}$$

Finally, compute the dose.

$$\frac{1 \times 75\cancel{0}}{33\cancel{0}} = \frac{75\cancel{0}}{33\cancel{0}} = 2.27 \text{ or } 2.3$$

To provide 750 mg of Claforan, the nurse should administer 2.27 or 2.3 mL of Claforan labeled 330 mg per mL.

Problem Set 23.1

1. A patient is to receive erythromycin ethylsuccinate oral suspension (EryPed) 0.4 g. Available is a bottle labeled EryPed 200 mg/5 mL.

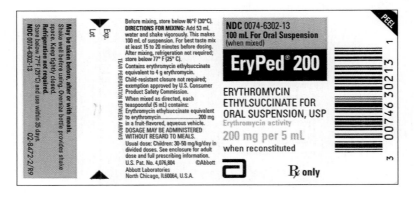

The nurse should administer _____ mL.

2. A patient is to receive cyclosporine (Neoral) 175 mg by mouth. Available are capsules labeled Neoral 25 mg capsules.

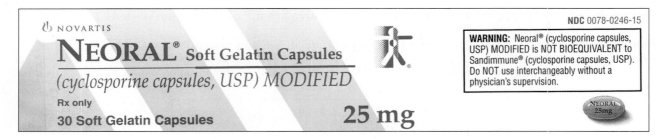

The nurse should administer _____ capsules.

3. A patient is to receive furosemide 80 mg by mouth. Available is a container with tablets labeled furosemide 20 mg.

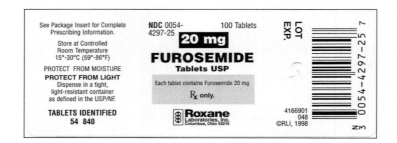

The nurse should administer _____ tablets.

4. A patient is to receive penicillin G potassium (Pfizerpen) 600,000 units by IM injection. Available is a vial of powdered medication labeled Pfizerpen 1,000,000 units. The directions state: "Reconstitute with 4 mL of Sterile Water to provide a solution which contains 250,000 units/mL.

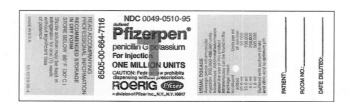

The nurse should withdraw and administer _____ mL.

5. A patient is to receive 65 μg (mcg) of fentanyl citrate by injection. The drug on hand is labeled Fentanyl Citrate Injection 250 mcg/5mL, 50 mcg/mL.

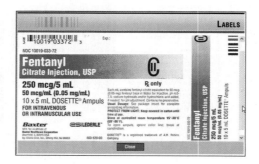

The nurse should withdraw and administer _____ mL.

Review Test 23.1
Dimensional Analysis

1. A patient is to receive nitroglycerin (Nitrostat) 600 mcg sublingually. Available is a container labeled Nitrostat 0.3 mg tablets.

   The nurse should administer _____ tablets.

2. A patient is to receive verapamil hydrochloride extended release tablets (Covera HS) 480 mg by mouth at bedtime. Available is a bottle labeled Covera HS 240 mg.

   The nurse should administer _____ tablets.

3. The patient is to receive potassium chloride 10% oral solution 30 mEq by mouth. Available are containers labeled potassium chloride 20 mEq per 15 mL.

   The nurse should administer _____ mL.

4. The patient is to receive cefdinir (Omnicef) oral suspension 400 mg by mouth. Available is a bottle labeled Omnicef 125 mg/5 mL.

   The nurse should administer _____ mL.

5. The patient is to receive metoprolol tartrate (Lopressor) 25 mg by mouth. Available is a container labeled Lopressor 50 mg tablets.

   The nurse should administer _____ tablets.

6. A patient is to receive diphenhydramine hydrochloride (Benadryl) liquid medication 50 mg. Available is a bottle labeled Benadryl 12.5 mg/5 mL.

   The nurse should administer _____ mL.

7. The patient is to receive penicillin G benzathine (Bicillin LA) 450,000 units by IM injection. Available is a 10 mL multidose vial labeled Bicillin LA 300,000 units/1 mL.

   The nurse should administer _____ mL.

8. A patient is to receive naloxone HCl (Narcan) 0.3 mg by IM injection. Available is a multidose vial labeled Narcan HCl 0.4 mg/1 mL.

   The nurse should administer _____ mL.

9. A patient is to receive ceftazidine (Tazicef) 500 mg by IM injection. The vial of powdered medication on hand is labeled Tazicef 1 gram. The directions state: "Reconstitute with 3 mL of sterile water to yield an approximate volume of 3.6 mL."

   The nurse should administer _____ mL.

10. A patient is to receive furosemide (Lasix) 20 mg by IM injection. The multidose vial on hand is labeled Lasix 40 mg/4 mL.

    The nurse should administer _____ mL.

Answers: **1.** 2 tablets **2.** 2 tablets **3.** 22.5 mL **4.** 16 mL **5.** $\frac{1}{2}$ tablet **6.** 20 mL **7.** 1.5 mL **8.** 0.75 mL or 0.8 mL **9.** 1.8 mL **10.** 2 mL

If you had fewer than three errors on Review Test 23.1, move on to the next chapter. If you had four or more errors, review the material on dimensional analysis and complete Review Test 23.2 before continuing.

Review Test 23.2
Dimensional Analysis

1. A patient is to receive zidovudine (Retrovir) syrup 200 mg by mouth. Available is a bottle labeled Retrovir syrup 50 mg per 5 mL.

    The nurse should administer _____ mL.

2. A patient is to receive azithromycin (Zithromax) oral suspension 1 g by mouth. Available is a bottle labeled Zithromax Oral Suspension 200 mg/5 mL.

    The nurse should administer _____ mL.

3. A patient is to receive a loading dose of amiodarone (Cordarone) 800 mg by mouth. Available are tablets labeled Cordarone 200 mg.

    The nurse should administer _____ tablets.

4. A patient is to receive acyclovir (Zovirax) 600 mg by mouth. Available are capsules labeled Zovirax 200 mg.

    The nurse should administer _____ capsules.

5. A patient is to receive levothyroxine sodium (Synthroid) 0.2 mg by mouth. Available are tablets labeled Synthroid 100 mcg.

    The nurse should administer _____ tablets.

6. A patient is to receive epinephrine 0.25 mg by SQ injection. Available are ampules labeled epinephrine 1 mg per mL.

    The nurse should administer _____ mL.

7. A patient is to receive ticarillin (Ticar) 730 mg by injection. The vial of powdered medication available is labeled Ticar 1 g. The directions state: "For IM solution add 2 mL of sterile diluent and shake well to provide an approximate volume of 2.6 mL."

    The nurse should administer _____ mL.

8. A patient is to receive digoxin (Lanoxin) 0.125 mg by IM injection. The vial of medication available is labeled Lanoxin 500 mcg/2 mL.

    The nurse should administer _____ mL.

9. A patient is to receive cefuroxime sodium (Kefurox) 0.5 g by IM injection. The vial of powdered medication available is labeled Kefurox 750 mg. The directions state: "For IM solution add 3.6 mL of sterile water to provide an approximate volume of 3.6 mL."

    The nurse should administer _____ mL.

10. A patient is to receive clindamycin phosphate (Cleocin phosphate) 250 mg by IM injection. The multidose vial available is labeled Cleocin Phosphate 150 mg/mL.

    The nurse should administer _____ mL.

Answers: **1.** 20 mL. **2.** 25 mL **3.** 4 tablets **4.** 3 capsules **5.** 2 tablets **6.** 0.25 mL **7.** 1.89 or 1.9 mL **8.** 0.5 mL **9.** 2.4 mL **10.** 1.67 or 1.7 mL

The Review Tests on dimensional analysis should be repeated until fewer than three errors occur.

Unit 8

Application and Review

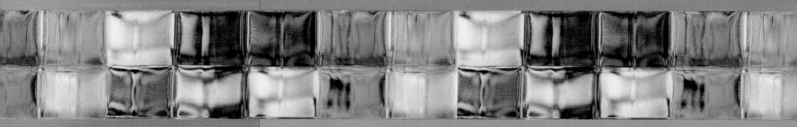

Chapter 24

Medication Orders and Medication Records Applied
to Clinical Situations

Chapter 25

Posttest in Computations of Drugs and Solutions

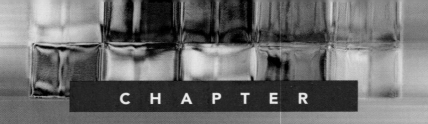

24

Medication Orders and Medication Records Applied to Clinical Situations

Learning Outcomes

After successfully completing this chapter, the learner should be able to:

- *Interpret the physician's order and recognize the necessary legal components.*
- *Transcribe the physician's order accurately on the patient's medication record and Kardex (if a Kardex system is being used).*
- *Identify the common components that are essential for all medication records.*
- *Understand the importance of documenting the administration of, or failure to administer, a prescribed medication.*
- *Recognize the importance of questioning any physician's order that is incomplete or varies from the manufacturer's recommended dosage.*
- *Recognize the importance of signing for any medication administered as soon as possible after the administration.*

GENERAL INFORMATION

Although hospital records concerned with medications may vary in style, their purpose and legality are rather consistent. The physician's order may be written on a separate physician's order sheet, it may be part of a patient's progress record, or it may be a part of any other form the hospital designates. The hospital has the legal responsibility for designating the form to be used for the physician's order, but it is the nurse who is responsible for determining that a legal order exists and that the medication records being used in the particular institution have all the necessary legal documentation.

Hospital records concerned with medications include, but are not limited to:

■ Physician's order: Some type of physician's order sheet on which a physician writes, signs, and dates an order for a specific patient; the order includes the name of the drug (generic or trade), the amount to be given, the time, the route of administration, and the duration of the order if applicable.

■ Medication record: Some type of medication record that is used to document the administration of the prescribed medication by the nurse. Although these records may vary by category (STAT or PRN, standing orders, insulin administration, IV medications, and so forth), they will in one form or another include the patient's name and hospital number, the name (generic or trade) of the medication, the amount administered, the date and time administered, the route of administration (in some hospitals the site of administration is also documented), and the nurse's initial and signature.

■ Kardex or Medex: A Kardex, Medex, medication administration record (MAR), or some other form of quick reference to the patient's medication and treatments. The use of such a record is a variable and its legality is questionable. In some institutions, the unit secretary copies the physician's order onto the Kardex and the nurse verifies the order, countersigns it, makes certain that the patient is not allergic to the prescribed medication, and writes the order on the medication record used for patients in that particular institution.

See Figures 24-2 to 24-16 for samples of some of the wide variety of records used in the area of medication.

Many health care agencies use the 24-hour clock (also known as military time) for documentation in charting rather than the standard clock. The 24-hour clock (Figure 24-1) avoids the need to use a.m. or p.m. designations and reduces medication errors because all times are written as four-digit numbers.

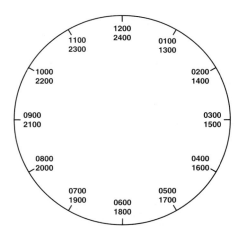

Figure 24-1 The 24-hour clock

Comparison of Standard and 24-Hour Time					
Standard	**24-hour**	**Standard**	**24-hour**	**Standard**	**24-hour**
7:00 a.m.	0700	3:00 p.m.	1500	11:00 p.m.	2300
8:00 a.m.	0800	4:00 p.m.	1600	Midnight	2400
9:00 a.m.	0900	5:00 p.m.	1700	1:00 a.m.	0100
10:00 a.m.	1000	6:00 p.m.	1800	2:00 a.m.	0200
11:00 a.m.	1100	7:00 p.m.	1900	3:00 a.m.	0300
noon	1200	8:00 p.m.	2000	4:00 a.m.	0400
1:00 p.m.	1300	9:00 p.m.	2100	5:00 a.m.	0500
2:00 p.m.	1400	10:00 p.m.	2200	6:00 a.m.	0600

| | | NORTH SHORE - LONG ISLAND JEWISH HEALTH SYSTEM | |
| | | DIRECT DOCTOR ORDER SHEET | |

DRUG ALLERGIES: **PLEASE PRINT - DO NOT USE LABEL**

WEIGHT:
HEIGHT:

DATE & TIME	PROB NO.	ORDERS (BEFORE WRITING ORDERS BE SURE THERE IS A YELLOW COPY) →	SIGNATURE

FORM NO. 536963-1

PATIENT'S CHART

Figure 24-2 Doctor order sheet

		LONG ISLAND JEWISH MEDICAL CENTER PROGRESS NOTES	
		Format of Sample Entry:	
Date	**Problem No.**	Subjective Objective Assessment Plan	Signature, Title, Dept.

DATE/ TIME	PROB NO.	

PROGRESS NOTES

FORM NO. 536198

NOTE: NUMBER EACH PAGE ➝

Figure 24-3 Progress notes

North Shore - Long Island Jewish Health System
MEDICATION RECORD

PLACE ALLERGY STICKER HERE

DATE OF ORDER	DATE OF EXP	MEDICATION DOSE ROUTE FREQUENCY	DATE:	DATE:	DATE:	DATE:	DATE:	DATE:	DATE:
			time/init						
init		med dose							
init		rte freq							
init									
init									
init									
init									
init									
init									
init									
init									
init									
init									
init									
init									
init									
init									
init									
init									
init									
init									
init									
init									
init									
init									
init									
init									
init									
init									

SIGNATURE	INIT				

(OVER)

Figure 24-4 Medication record

NORTH SHORE - LONG ISLAND JEWISH HEALTH SYSTEM
STAT-PRN MEDICATION RECORD

PLACE ALLERGY STICKER HERE

DATE OF ORDER	DATE OF EXP	MEDICATION DOSE ROUTE FREQUENCY	DATE:	DATE:	DATE:	DATE:	DATE:	DATE:	DATE:
			time/init						
init		med dose							
init		rte freq							
init									
init									
init									
init									
init									
init									
init									
init									
init									
init									
init									
init									
init									
init									
init									
init									
init									
init									
init									
init									
init									
init									
init									
init									

SIGNATURE		INIT						

LIJ-HMC #522777   (OVER)

Figure 24-5 STAT-PRN medication record

NORTH SHORE - LONG ISLAND JEWISH HEALTH SYSTEM

IV MEDICATION DRIP RECORD

☐ IV MEDICATION DRIP
   -CONTINUOUS MED DRIPS
   -COMBINATION BOLUS/DRIP MEDS
☐ CHEMOTHERAPY PROTOCOL
   -USE ONE COLUMN FOR BOLUS MEDS
   -USE A SEPARATE COLUMN FOR EACH
                    CONTINUOUS DRIP

RECORD AT THE BEGINNING OF EACH SHIFT & ANY CHANGES MADE DURING THE SHIFT

DATE	TIME	INIT	MEDICATION	DATE	TIME	INIT	MEDICATION

SIGNATURE	INIT	SIGNATURE	INIT	SIGNATURE	INIT

FORM NO. 22465 2/90

(OVER)

Figure 24-6 IV/chemotherapy record

NORTH SHORE - LONG ISLAND JEWISH HEALTH SYSTEM

**DOCTOR'S CHEMOTHERAPY
ORDER SHEET**

Page   of   pages

DRUG
ALLERGIES:

PATIENT CLINICAL INFORMATION (MUST COMPLETE):

DIAGNOSIS: _____

HEIGHT: _____ inches   WEIGHT: _____ pounds

USE BALLPOINT PEN AND PRESS FIRMLY

CYCLE #: _____   PROTOCOL/REGIMEN: _____
                             (e.g. CALGB, CHOP, GOG, ABVD, or specific reference)

BODY SURFACE AREA (M^2) _____

NON-CHEMOTHERAPY ORDERS:

	PRE-CHEMO HYDRATION ORDERS:
DATE:	

	PRE-MEDICATIONS (including anti-emetic therapy and orders for associated medications as indicated)
	i.e. Leucovorin, Metoclopramide, Lorazepam, Dexamethasone, Diphenhydramine, Methylprednisolone, Allopurinol
DATE:	

	POST-CHEMO HYDRATION ORDERS:
DATE:	

CHEMOTHERAPY ORDERS:

DRUG	DOSE (mg/M^2)	DOSE TO BE GIVEN	FLUID (indicate soltn. & volume)	ROUTE	RATE OF INFUSION	FREQUENCY/ DURATION OF THERAPY	START DATES OF ADMIN. OF EACH DOSE

_____ DATE

_____ AM/PM TIME

BEEPER # _____

_____ MD/PA/NP
                (Signature)

_____ MD

Figure 24-7 Doctor's chemotherapy order sheet

KARDEX FORM

ALLERGIES: ☐ NO ☐ YES

SPECIAL
CONSIDERATIONS:

ADM DATE	AGE	REL	COND:		HO:
DIAGNOSIS:					
OP DATE	OPERATION:				
MED HX:					
SURG HX:					
NOTES:					
D/C PLAN: ☐ HOME ☐ OTHER:			HELP AVAIL:		

DATE	TREATMENTS

DATE ORD	DATE DONE	TEST/CONSULTS

DATE	DIET

DATE	ACTIVITY

DATE ORD	UP DATE	NURSING DIAGNOSES/PROBLEMS
		ACTIVITIES OF DAILY LIVING

11/86

Figure 24-8A Kardex

ALLERGIES: ☐ NO   ☐ YES

STANDING MEDICATIONS

ORD DATE	INIT	REORD DATE	INIT	MEDICATION DOSAGE ROUTE FREQ	TIMES	DC DATE	INIT

PRN MEDICATIONS

ORD DATE	INIT	REORD DATE	INIT	MEDICATION DOSAGE ROUTE FREQ	TIMES	DC DATE	INIT

Figure 24-8B Kardex

ST FRANCIS HOSPITAL
Roslyn, New York

MEDICATION ADMINISTRATION RECORD

ADDRESSOGRAPH BELOW ☛

REFER TO:
- ☐ RESPIRATORY FLOW SHEET
- ☐ INSULIN MAR
- ☐ HEPARIN FLOW SHEET
- ☐ PCA RECORD
- ☐ EPIDURAL RECORD

PAGE # OF

YEAR

Code to Chart Unadministered Meds:

HELD - See Patient Progress Notes
REF - Refused - See Patient Progress Notes
D/C - Discontinue Drug Use

SEE REVERSE SIDE FOR INJECTION SITE CODES

RECOPIED DATE

RECOPIED BY

REVIEWED BY

DIAGNOSIS

OPERATIVE PROCEDURE AND DATE

ALLERGIES:
☐ NONE

DATE ORD / INITIAL	EXP DATE	SCHEDULED MEDS DOSE - FREQ - ROUTE	HOUR / SITE	DATE	DATE	DATE	DATE	DATE	DATE	DATE	DATE	DATE
Medication Instruction Sheet Given												
Medication Instruction Sheet Given												
Medication Instruction Sheet Given												
Medication Instruction Sheet Given												
Medication Instruction Sheet Given												
Medication Instruction Sheet Given												
Medication Instruction Sheet Given												

INITIAL	SIGNATURE/TITLE	INITIAL	SIGNATURE/TITLE	INITIAL	SIGNATURE/TITLE

FORM # 80080 REV. 3/28/97 MADISON BUSINESS SYSTEMS

Figure 24-9A Medication administration record

ORD. DATE/ INIT.	MEDICATION - DOSAGE - ROUTE	TO BE GIVEN		NURSE INIT.
		DATE	TIME SITE	

SINGLE ORDERS - PRE-OP - STAT ORDERS

ADDRESSOGRAPH BELOW ➧

INJECTION SITE CODE
A = BUTTOCK RUOQ
B = BUTTOCK LUOQ
C = DELTOID R
D = DELTOID L
E = THIGH R LAT
F = THIGH L LAT
G = ILIAC CREST R
H = ILIAC CREST L

PRN MEDICATION ORDERS

ORD. DATE/ INIT.	EXP. DATE	MEDICATION - DOSAGE FREQUENCY - ROUTE OF ADM.	PRN MEDICATIONS													
			DATE													
			TIME													
			SITE													
			INIT													
			DATE													
			TIME													
			SITE													
			INIT													
			DATE													
			TIME													
			SITE													
			INIT													
			DATE													
			TIME													
			SITE													
			INIT													
			DATE													
			TIME													
			SITE													
			INIT													
			DATE													
			TIME													
			SITE													
			INIT													
			DATE													
			TIME													
			SITE													
			INIT													

St. Francis Hospital - MEDICATION ADMINISTRATION RECORD

Figure 24-9B Medication administration record

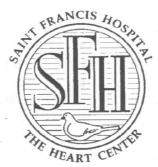

St. Francis Hospital
ROSLYN, NEW YORK

Diabetic Flow Record

1. PATIENT EDUCATION
- Initiate the Diabetic Patient Education Record.
- Provide Literature "Balance your Act".

2. ASSESSMENT
- Monitor Patient q2h for the first 12 hours after the initial dose of insulin for signs and symptoms of hypoglycemia or insulin shock.
- Monitor the Blood Glucose, Serum and Finger Stick Results.
- Continuously Monitor for Signs and Symptoms of Hypo and Hyperglycemia.

3. TRANSITION MANAGEMENT
- Contact Care Manager to plan a home care visit for new onset insulin dependent diabetics.
- Assure patient access to a home meter and instructions.
- Review medications, administration and side effects.
- Provide out-patient educational programs and support groups.

COMMENTS: _____

_____

_____

_____

_____

_____

_____

Figure 24-10A Diabetic flow record

ST FRANCIS HOSPITAL
Roslyn, New York

ADDRESSOGRAPH BELOW ➡

INSULIN ADMINISTRATION AND DIABETIC RECORD

BEDISDE BLOOD GLUCOSE METER ORDERS:	PAGE #	
☐ PERFOM LAB BACK-UP FOR RESULTS <60 OR >400		
☐ NO LAB BACK-UP	RECOPIED BY	REVIEWED BY
☐ BMP QD		

SPECIAL INSTRUCTIONS:

SLIDING SCALES: Date and initial the scale according to physicians order.   *USE REGULAR INSULIN*

STANDARD		ALTERNATIVE		MODIFIED	
DATE FREQUENCY of BBGM		DATE FREQUENCY of BBGM		DATE FREQUENCY of BBGM	
INITIAL		INITIAL		INITIAL	
Route:_____		Route:_____		Route:_____	
Blood Glucose	**Units**	**Blood Glucose**	**Units**	**Blood Glucose**	**Units**
200 – 250 mg/dl	2 units	150 – 200 mg/dl	2 units	_____mg/dl	_____units
251 – 300 mg/dl	4 units	200 – 250 mg/dl	4 units	_____mg/dl	_____units
301 – 350 mg/dl	6 units	251 – 300 mg/dl	6 units	_____mg/dl	_____units
351 – 400 mg/dl	8 units	301 – 350 mg/dl	8 units	_____mg/dl	_____units
> 400 mg/dl	Call MD	351 – 400 mg/dl	10 units	_____mg/dl	_____units
		> 400 mg/dl	Call MD	> 400 mg/dl	Call MD

DATE / INITIALS	SINGLE - STAT - PRE - OP INSULIN ORDERS	DATE / TIME TO BE GIVEN	INITIALS	DATE / INITIALS	INSULIN DRIP CONCENTRATION

AM DAILY INSULIN ORDERS			PM DAILY INSULIN ORDERS		
ORDER DATE / INITIALS	INSULIN Type - Dose - Route	TIME TO BE GIVEN	ORDER DATE / INITIALS	INSULIN Type - Dose - Route	TIME TO BE GIVEN

Figure 24-10B Diabetic flow record

St. Francis Hospital
ROSLYN, NEW YORK

INSULIN / MEDICATION ADMINISRTATION RECORD

ADDRESSOGRAPH BELOW

BEDSIDE BLOOD GLUCOSE RESULTS <60 OR >400:
1-Assess / Treat Patient
2-Call Physician, and
3-Perfom Lab Back-up

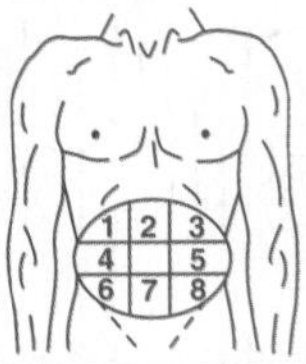

INJECTION SITE CODE:
C = DELTOID R
D = DELTOID L
E = THIGH R LAT
F = THIGH L LAT

BLOOD GLUCOSE RESULTS				MEDICATIONS ADMINISTERED				
DATE	TIME	METER RESULT	SERUM RESULT	MEDICATION	DOSE	SITE / ROUTE	INIT	TIME

Figure 24-10C Diabetic flow record

St. Francis Hospital - ROSLYN, NEW YORK
INITIALS - SIGNATURE VERIFICATION

INITIAL	SIGNATURE / TITLE	INITIAL	SIGNATURE / TITLE

Figure 24-10D Diabetic flow record

USE BALLPOINT PEN - PRESS FIRMLY

St. Francis Hospital
ROSLYN, NEW YORK

PHYSICIAN ORDER RECORD

DOCTOR: PLEASE PRINT NAME & I.D. # AFTER EACH ORDER. ALSO, PLEASE SIGN OFF ON ALL TELEPHONE AND P.A. ORDERS	
DATE / TIME	

Figure 24-11 Physician order record

ST FRANCIS HOSPITAL
Roslyn, NY

NURSING CARE PLAN
KARDEX

ADMISSION DATE / UNIT TRANSFERS (date / unit):

ADMITTING DIAGNOSIS (and or most current diagnosis)

STATUS:
☐ DNR   ☐ HEALTH CARE PROXY

SURGICAL PROCEDURES / DATE

PATIENT SAFETY:
RISK LEVEL   ☐ I   ☐ II   ☐ III   ☐ IV
☐ RESTRAINTS   ☐ POSEY VEST

ACTIVITY: ☐ BEDREST   ☐ BRP   ☐ OOB

TRANSFER: ☐ ASSIST   ☐ HOYER

PRIOR MEDICAL HISTORY

DISABILITY OR LIMITATIONS:
Vision: ☐ Glasses   ☐ Contact lenses   ☐ Blind
Hearing: ☐ Deaf   ☐ HOH   ☐ Hearing aid
Dentures: ☐ Upper   ☐ Lower

VITAL SIGNS:	**CARDIAC MONITORING:**	**PACEMAKERS:**	**NUTRITION:**
☐ Q SHIFT	☐ TRANSPORT WITH	☐ PERMANENT	☐ WEIGHT Q _____
		type _____	☐ DIET _____
☐ Q 4HR	☐ TRANSPORT WITHOUT	rate _____	
		☐ TEMPORARY ☐ on ☐ off	☐ I&O ☐ FLUID RESTRICTION
☐ PRN	☐ TREATMENT ORDERS	MA _____	☐ NGT ☐ PEG
		rate _____	☐ FEEDING
☐		☐ AICD ☐ on ☐ off	☐ FOLEY
		rate _____	☐ DRAINAGE

CONSULTATIONS (PHYSICIAN / DATE / SERVICE)

TREATMENTS

LAB STUDIES (PENDING) [DATE / STUDY]

TESTS (PENDING)   [DATE / TEST]

IV THERAPY (DATE LINE INSERTED / SOLUTION)
☐ PERIPHERAL
☐ ARTERIAL
☐ SUBCLAVIAN
☐ SWAN GANZ
☐ RIJ
☐ MULTILUMEN
☐ PCA
☐ EPIDURAL

RESPIRATORY THERAPY
☐ TREATMENTS
☐ O2 _____
☐ VENTILATOR SETTINGS
   mode _____
   rate _____
   FIO2 _____
   TV _____
☐ CPT
☐ INCENTIVE SPIROMETER
☐ ET TUBE   size ____   date ____
☐ TRACH   size ____   date ____
☐ CHEST TUBES

PATIENT TEACHING: (DATE)
☐ CARDIAC MEDICAL
☐ DIABETES
☐ POST OP

DISCHARGE PLANNING:
☐ CASE WORKER

PLANS:
☐ HOME
☐ REHAB
☐ NSG HOME

Figure 24-12 Nursing care plan Kardex

USE BALLPOINT PEN - PRESS FIRMLY

St. Francis Hospital
ROSLYN, NEW YORK

PHYSICIAN'S ORDERS

HEPARIN THERAPY

DOCTOR: PLEASE SIGN OFF ON ALL TELEPHONE AND P.A. ORDERS

DATE / TIME	
	1.) Heparin _____ units IV push (initial bolus)
	2.) IV infusion heparin 25,000 units / 250cc D₅W
	(100 units = 1cc)
	run at _____ units / hour and _____ cc /hr.
	3.) Check first aPPT in 6 hours and then follow nomogram below.
	4.) Record all aPPT results and heparin adjustments on the Heparin Flow Sheet.
	5.) **GOAL OF THERAPY = THERAPEUTIC aPPT OF 50 - 75**
	6.) Notify MD for more than _____ consecutive out of range aPPTs.

PHYSICIAN'S SIGNATURE ➤

NOMOGRAM

	aPPT	IV Bolus Of Heparin	Hold Drip (Minutes)	Drip Rate Change / hr.	Repeat aPPT in:
	<35	3,000 units	0 min	+ 200 units = + 2cc / hr	6 hrs
	35 – 49	1,000 units	0 min	+ 100 units = 1cc / hr	6 hrs
GOAL OF THERAPY	**50 – 75**	0 units	0 min	0 units = 0cc	next AM
	76 – 85	0 units	0 min	− 100 units = 1cc / hr	next AM
	86 – 100	0 units	0 min	− 100 units = 1cc / hr	6 hrs
	101 – 120	0 units	30 min	− 200 units = 2cc / hr	6 hrs
	> 120	0 units	60 min	− 200 units = 2cc / hr	4 hrs

Figure 24-13 Physician's orders, heparin therapy

St. Francis Hospital
ROSLYN, NEW YORK

HEPARIN FLOW SHEET

INFUSION STARTED: DATE: _____ TIME: _____

INITIAL RATE: _____cc / hr and _____Units / hr

Date / Time Drawn	aPPT (Seconds)	Heparin Bolus (Units)	Heparin Stop Time	Heparin Start Time	Heparin Rate (cc / hr & Units / hr)	Repeat aPPT Time

GOAL OF THERAPY = THERAPEUTIC aPPT OF 50 – 75

NOMOGRAM

aPPT	IV Bolus Of Heparin	Hold Drip (Minutes)	Drip Rate Change / hr.	Repeat aPPT in:
<35	3,000 units	0 min	+ 200 units = + 2cc / hr	6 hrs
35 – 49	1,000 units	0 min	+ 100 units = 1cc / hr	6 hrs
50 – 75	0 units	0 min	0 units = 0cc	next AM
76 – 85	0 units	0 min	− 100 units = 1cc / hr	next AM
86 – 100	0 units	0 min	− 100 units = 1cc / hr	6 hrs
101 – 120	0 units	30 min	− 200 units = 2cc / hr	6 hrs
> 120	0 units	60 min	− 200 units = 2cc / hr	4 hrs

Figure 24-14   Heparin flow sheet

MEDICATION RECORD - INDIVIDUAL ORDERS
(single orders; stat, prn and preop. orders)

PAGE _____   WEIGHT _____

KNOWN
ALLERGIES _____

Addressograph

DATE			Fri.	Sat.	Sun.	Mon.	Tues.	Wed.	Thurs.
Date Order	Renew Date	Medication; Dosage; Route; Frequency; Physician; Nurse	Time Initial	Time Initial	Time Initial	Time Initial	Time Initial	Time Initial	Time Initial

PROGRESS NOTES:

_____
_____
_____
_____
_____
_____

In.	Signature/Title	In.	Signature/Title	In.	Signature/Title

Figure 24-15 Medication record—Individual orders

MEDICATION RECORD - STANDING ORDERS

PAGE _____   WEIGHT _____

KNOWN
ALLERGIES _____   Addressograph

DATE			Fri.	Sat.	Sun.	Mon.	Tues.	Wed.	Thurs.
Date Order	Renew Date	Medication; Dosage; Route; Frequency; Physician; Nurse	Time Initial	Time Initial	Time Initial	Time Initial	Time Initial	Time Initial	Time Initial

In.	Signature/Title	In.	Signature/Title	In.	Signature/Title	In.	Signature/Title

Figure 24-16 Medication record—Standing orders

APPLICATION TO CLINICAL SITUATIONS

Following are examples of critical situations and the forms used for medication records.

Example: The physician's order for a patient who just had surgery is:

Santiago, Juan   Age 37
268479

NORTH SHORE - LONG ISLAND JEWISH HEALTH SYSTEM
DIRECT DOCTOR ORDER SHEET
DRUG ALLERGIES: **PLEASE PRINT - DO NOT USE LABEL**
WEIGHT: *135 lbs*
HEIGHT: *5' + 7"*

DATE & TIME	PROB NO.	ORDERS (BEFORE WRITING ORDERS BE SURE THERE IS A YELLOW COPY) →	SIGNATURE
2/20/xx 10^{AM}		Demerol 50 mg Im q4h prn for pain	A. Murphy

At 10:00 p.m. the patient complains of pain that is unrelieved by other measures. After checking the order and the medication record, the nurse administers 50 mg of Demerol IM and makes the following notations on the patient's PRN medication record and progress notes. (The Demerol must also be recorded on the narcotic or controlled drug record, because it is a narcotic.)

Santiago, Juan   Age 37
268479

LONG ISLAND JEWISH MEDICAL CENTER PROGRESS NOTES			
		Format of Sample Entry:	
Date		**Problem No.**	
		Subjective Objective Assessment Plan	Signature, Title, Dept.

PROGRESS NOTES

DATE/ TIME	PROB NO.		
2/20/xx 10^{PM}		Restless and complaining of abdominal pain. Comfort measures did not relieve pain. Demerol 50 mg 1M given at 10:00^{PM}	Shirley Schmidt RN

Santiago, Juan   Age 37
268479

NORTH SHORE - LONG ISLAND JEWISH HEALTH SYSTEM
MEDICATION RECORD

PLACE ALLERGY STICKER HERE

DATE OF ORDER	DATE OF EXP	MEDICATION DOSE ROUTE FREQUENCY	DATE:	DATE:	DATE:	DATE:	DATE:	DATE:	DATE:
2/20/xx init *NCO*	2/22/xx	med *Demerol IM 50 mg* dose	time/init *3ᴾᴹ LS*						
init		rte *IM* *q4h prn* freq	*10ᴾᴹ SS*						
init		*for pain*							

SIGNATURE	INIT								
Lilly Schnider RN	*LS*								
Shirley Schmidt	*SS*								

LIJ-HMC #522777   (OVER)

Example: The physician's orders for a patient admitted with hypothyroidism and obesity are:

USE BALLPOINT PEN - PRESS FIRMLY

St. Francis Hospital
ROSLYN, NEW YORK

Tischer, Elizabeth   Age 25
#125306

PHYSICIAN ORDER RECORD

DOCTOR: PLEASE PRINT NAME & I.D. # AFTER EACH ORDER.
ALSO, PLEASE SIGN OFF ON ALL TELEPHONE AND P.A. ORDERS

DATE / TIME	
2/11/xx	*Cytomel 25 mcg po qd*
	Colace 100 mg po bid
	Ampicillin 1 g IVPB q6h
	ASA 650 mg po q4h prn for headache
	Chest x-ray
	2000 calorie diet
	OOB c̄ assistance
	E Chan MD

On the day after admission, the notations on this patient's medication record and Kardex would be:

ST FRANCIS HOSPITAL
Roslyn, New York

MEDICATION ADMINISTRATION RECORD

ADDRESSOGRAPH BELOW ➦

Tischer, Elizabeth   Age 25
#125306

REFER TO:
☐ RESPIRATORY FLOW SHEET
☐ INSULIN MAR
☐ HEPARIN FLOW SHEET
☐ PCA RECORD
☐ EPIDURAL RECORD

PAGE #		
1	OF	**1**
YEAR **20xx**		

RECOPIED DATE	DIAGNOSIS Hypothyroidism, Pneumonia
RECOPIED BY	OPERATIVE PROCEDURE AND DATE
REVIEWED BY	ALLERGIES: ☒ NONE

Code to Chart Unadministered Meds:

HELD - See Patient Progress Notes
REF - Refused - See Patient Progress Notes
D/C - Discontinue Drug Use

SEE REVERSE SIDE FOR INJECTION SITE CODES

DATE ORD / INITIAL	EXP DATE	SCHEDULED MEDS DOSE - FREQ - ROUTE	HOUR / SITE	DATE 2/11	DATE 2/12	DATE 2/13	DATE 2/14	DATE 2/15	DATE 2/16	DATE 2/17	DATE 2/18	DATE 2/19
2/11 MY		Cytomel 25 mcg po od	10ᴬᴹ	✕	LM							
		Medication Instruction Sheet Given										
2/11 MY		Colace 100 mg po bid	10ᴬᴹ 6ᴾᴹ	✕ MY	LM							
		Medication Instruction Sheet Given										
2/11 MY		Ampicillin 1 g IVPB q6h	6ᴬᴹ 12ᴺ 6ᴾᴹ 12ᴹ	✕ ✕ MY TSJ	TSJ LM AG							
		Medication Instruction Sheet Given										
		Medication Instruction Sheet Given										
		Medication Instruction Sheet Given										
		Medication Instruction Sheet Given										
		Medication Instruction Sheet Given										

INITIAL	SIGNATURE/TITLE	INITIAL	SIGNATURE/TITLE	INITIAL	SIGNATURE/TITLE
MY	Margaret Yang RN	TSJ	Tariq S. Johnson RN		
AG	Anna Garcia RN				
LM	Lisa Molinari RN				

FORM # 80080 REV. 3/28/97 MADISON BUSINESS SYSTEMS

Tischer, Elizabeth Age 25
#125306

ALLERGIES: ☒ NO ☐ YES

STANDING MEDICATIONS

ORD DATE	INIT	REORD DATE	INIT	MEDICATION	DOSAGE	ROUTE	FREQ	TIMES	DC DATE	INIT
2-11	JG			Cytomel	25 mcg	po	od	10ᴬᴹ		
2-11	JG			Colace	100 mg	po	bid	10ᴬᴹ 6ᴾᴹ		
2-11	JG			Ampicillin	1 g	IVPB	q6h	6ᴬᴹ 12ᴾᴹ 6ᴾᴹ 12ᴬᴹ		

PRN MEDICATIONS

ORD DATE	INIT	REORD DATE	INIT	MEDICATION	DOSAGE	ROUTE	FREQ	TIMES	DC DATE	INIT
2-11	JG			ASA for headache	650 mg	po q4h	prn			

Example: The physician's orders for a patient admitted with coronary artery disease and diabetes mellitus are:

USE BALLPOINT PEN - PRESS FIRMLY

St. Francis Hospital
ROSLYN, NEW YORK

PHYSICIAN ORDER RECORD

Blake, Stanley   Age 68
#1253478

DATE / TIME	**DOCTOR: PLEASE PRINT NAME & I.D. # AFTER EACH ORDER. ALSO, PLEASE SIGN OFF ON ALL TELEPHONE AND P.A. ORDERS**
2/27/xx	Zestril 10 mg qd po
6ᴾᴹ	Digoxin 0.125 mg qod po for pulse ↑ 60
	Novolin N 25 U qd @ 7ᴬᴹ SC
	Daily blood sugar by lab
	Coumadin 5 mg qd
	Daily prothrombin time / INR
	Lasix 40 mg stat IM
	R Tobias MD

These orders would be transferred to the appropriate records as follows:

ST FRANCIS HOSPITAL
Roslyn, New York

MEDICATION ADMINISTRATION RECORD

REFER TO:
☐ RESPIRATORY FLOW SHEET
☐ INSULIN MAR
☐ HEPARIN FLOW SHEET
☐ PCA RECORD
☐ EPIDURAL RECORD

| PAGE # 2 OF 2 |
| YEAR 20xx |

ADDRESSOGRAPH BELOW ➡

Blake, Stanley Age 68
#1253478

Code to Chart Unadministered Meds:	RECOPIED DATE	DIAGNOSIS *Coronary Artery Disease, Diabetes, Mellitus*
HELD - See Patient Progress Notes	RECOPIED BY	OPERATIVE PROCEDURE AND DATE
REF - Refused - See Patient Progress Notes		
D/C - Discontinue Drug Use	REVIEWED BY	
		ALLERGIES: ☒ NONE

SEE REVERSE SIDE FOR INJECTION SITE CODES

DATE ORD / INITIAL	EXP DATE	SCHEDULED MEDS DOSE - FREQ - ROUTE	HOUR / SITE	DATE 2/28	DATE 3/1	DATE 3/2	DATE 3/3	DATE 3/4	DATE 3/5	DATE 3/6	DATE 3/7	DATE 3/8
2/27 RS		Zestril 10 mg qd po	10AM	RS	JOB	JOB	RS					
Medication Instruction Sheet Given												
2/27 RS		Digoxin 0.125 mg qod po for pulse over 60	10AM Pulse	RS 68	✕ ✕	JOB 70	✕ ✕		✕ ✕		✕ ✕	
Medication Instruction Sheet Given												
2/27 RS		Coumadin 5 mg qd	10AM	RS	JOB	JOB	RS					
Medication Instruction Sheet Given												
Medication Instruction Sheet Given												
Medication Instruction Sheet Given												
Medication Instruction Sheet Given												
Medication Instruction Sheet Given												

INITIAL	SIGNATURE/TITLE	INITIAL	SIGNATURE/TITLE	INITIAL	SIGNATURE/TITLE
RS	Ryan Sorenson RN				
JOB	Jane O'Brien RN				

FORM # 80080 REV. 3/28/97 MADISON BUSINESS SYSTEMS

SINGLE ORDERS - PRE-OP - STAT ORDERS				
ORD. DATE/ INIT.	MEDICATION - DOSAGE - ROUTE	TO BE GIVEN DATE	TO BE GIVEN TIME / SITE	NURSE INIT.
2/27 / RT	Lasix 40 mg IM stat	2/27	6:30PM / B	TSJ

ADDRESSOGRAPH BELOW

Blake, Stanley Age 68
#1253478

INJECTION SITE CODE
A = BUTTOCK RUOQ
B = BUTTOCK LUOQ
C = DELTOID R
D = DELTOID L
E = THIGH R LAT
F = THIGH L LAT
G = ILIAC CREST R
H = ILIAC CREST L

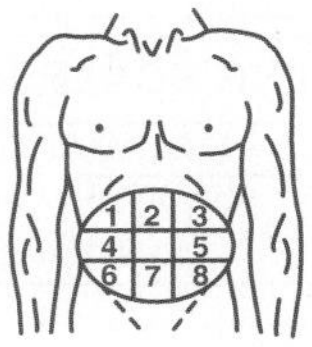

PRN MEDICATION ORDERS																	
ORD. DATE/ INIT.	EXP. DATE	MEDICATION - DOSAGE FREQUENCY - ROUTE OF ADM.	PRN MEDICATIONS														
			DATE														
			TIME														
			SITE														
			INIT														
			DATE														
			TIME														
			SITE														
			INIT														
			DATE														
			TIME														
			SITE														
			INIT														
			DATE														
			TIME														
			SITE														
			INIT														
			DATE														
			TIME														
			SITE														
			INIT														
			DATE														
			TIME														
			SITE														
			INIT														
			DATE														
			TIME														
			SITE														
			INIT														

St. Francis Hospital - MEDICATION ADMINISTRATION RECORD

ST FRANCIS HOSPITAL
Roslyn, New York

ADDRESSOGRAPH BELOW

Blake, Stanley Age 68
#1253478

INSULIN ADMINISTRATION AND DIABETIC RECORD

BEDISDE BLOOD GLUCOSE METER ORDERS:		PAGE #
☐ PERFOM LAB BACK-UP FOR RESULTS <60 OR >400		
☐ NO LAB BACK-UP ☐ BMP QD	RECOPIED BY	REVIEWED BY

SPECIAL INSTRUCTIONS:

SLIDING SCALES: Date and initial the scale according to physicians order. ***USE REGULAR INSULIN***

STANDARD		ALTERNATIVE		MODIFIED	
DATE FREQUENCY of BBGM		DATE FREQUENCY of BBGM		DATE FREQUENCY of BBGM	
INITIAL		INITIAL		INITIAL	
Route:______		Route:______		Route:______	
Blood Glucose	**Units**	**Blood Glucose**	**Units**	**Blood Glucose**	**Units**
200 – 250 mg/dl	2 units	150 – 200 mg/dl	2 units	______mg/dl	______units
251 – 300 mg/dl	4 units	200 – 250 mg/dl	4 units	______mg/dl	______units
301 – 350 mg/dl	6 units	251 – 300 mg/dl	6 units	______mg/dl	______units
351 – 400 mg/dl	8 units	301 – 350 mg/dl	8 units	______mg/dl	______units
> 400 mg/dl	Call MD	351 – 400 mg/dl	10 units	______mg/dl	______units
		> 400 mg/dl	Call MD	> 400 mg/dl	Call MD

DATE / INITIALS	SINGLE - STAT - PRE - OP INSULIN ORDERS	DATE / TIME TO BE GIVEN	INITIALS	DATE / INITIALS	INSULIN DRIP CONCENTRATION

AM DAILY INSULIN ORDERS			PM DAILY INSULIN ORDERS		
ORDER DATE / INITIALS	INSULIN Type - Dose - Route	TIME TO BE GIVEN	ORDER DATE / INITIALS	INSULIN Type - Dose - Route	TIME TO BE GIVEN
2/27/xx WP	Novolin N 25 U qd @ 7am sc	7am			

St. Francis Hospital
ROSLYN, NEW YORK

INSULIN / MEDICATION ADMINISRTATION RECORD

ADDRESSOGRAPH BELOW ➜

Blake, Stanley   Age 68
#1253478

BEDSIDE BLOOD GLUCOSE RESULTS <60 OR >400:
1-Assess / Treat Patient
2-Call Physician, and
3-Perfom Lab Back-up

INJECTION SITE CODE:
C = DELTOID R
D = DELTOID L
E = THIGH R LAT
F = THIGH L LAT

BLOOD GLUCOSE RESULTS				MEDICATIONS ADMINISTERED				
DATE	TIME	METER RESULT	SERUM RESULT	MEDICATION	DOSE	SITE / ROUTE	INIT	TIME
2/27	7am		178	Novolin N	25 U	sc	NEO	7⁰⁵AM
3/1	7am		192	Novolin N	25 U	sc	NEO	7¹⁰AM
3/2	7am		176	Novolin N	25 U	sc	CG	7²⁰AM
3/2	7am		185	Novolin N	25 U	sc	RG	7¹⁰AM

St. Francis Hospital - ROSLYN, NEW YORK
INITIALS - SIGNATURE VERIFICATION

Blake, Stanley   Age 68   #1253478

INITIAL	SIGNATURE / TITLE	INITIAL	SIGNATURE / TITLE
NEO	Norma E O'Neill		
CG	Colleen Glaumspiehs		
RG	Rita Gallo		

Example: The physician's orders for a patient admitted with acute pancreatitis are:

James, Henry 40 yrs
#24973862

NORTH SHORE - LONG ISLAND JEWISH HEALTH SYSTEM
DIRECT DOCTOR ORDER SHEET
DRUG ALLERGIES: **PLEASE PRINT - DO NOT USE LABEL**
WEIGHT: *145 lbs*
HEIGHT: *5'10"*

DATE & TIME	PROB NO.	ORDERS (BEFORE WRITING ORDERS BE SURE THERE IS A YELLOW COPY) →	SIGNATURE
2/20/xx		*Secrum amylase stat by lab*	
		Chest X-ray	
		Ultrasonogram and CT scan of pancreas	
		Pepcid 20 mg IVPB q12hr	
		Demerol 75 mg/Mq4hr prn for pain	
		IVD5/W 1000 mL c̄ KCl 20 mEq @ 100 ml/h	
		NPO	
		Bed rest	
		Nasogastric tube to low suction	
			L Jameson MD
2/21/xx		*Increase Pepcid to 40 mg IVPB q12h*	
10ᴬᴹ			
			L Jameson MD

On the day after admission, the notations on this patient's medication record, Stat-PRN medication record, IV medication drip record, and Kardex should be:

James, Henry 40 yrs
#24973862

NORTH SHORE - LONG ISLAND JEWISH HEALTH SYSTEM
MEDICATION RECORD
PLACE ALLERGY STICKER HERE

DATE OF ORDER	DATE OF EXP	MEDICATION DOSE ROUTE FREQUENCY	DATE: 2/20/xx	DATE: 2/21	DATE: 2/22	DATE: 2/23	DATE: 2/24	DATE: 2/25	DATE: 2/26
init		med *Pepcid* 20 mg dose	time/init	*6ᴬᴹ SS*	X		X		X
init		rte *IVPB* q12h freq	*6ᴾᴹ NEO*	*D/C*					
init									
init		*Pepcid* 40 mg	X	X					
init		*IVPB* q12h	X	*6ᴾᴹ NEO*					
init									

SIGNATURE	INIT						
Norma E O'Neill RN	*NEO*						
Shirley Schmidt RN	*SS*						

James, Henry 40 yrs
#24973862

NORTH SHORE - LONG ISLAND JEWISH HEALTH SYSTEM
STAT-PRN MEDICATION RECORD

PLACE ALLERGY STICKER HERE

DATE OF ORDER	DATE OF EXP	MEDICATION DOSE ROUTE FREQUENCY	DATE: 2/20	DATE:	DATE:	DATE:	DATE:	DATE:	DATE:
init		med *Demerol 75 mg* dose	time/init *3³⁰PM*						
init		rte *IM* *q4h prn for* freq *pain*	*NEO*						
init									

SIGNATURE	INIT						
Norma E O'Neill RN	*NEO*						

LIJ-HMC #522777   (OVER)

James, Henry 40 yrs
#24973862

NORTH SHORE - LONG ISLAND JEWISH HEALTH SYSTEM

IV MEDICATION DRIP RECORD

☐ IV MEDICATION DRIP
   -CONTINUOUS MED DRIPS
   -COMBINATION BOLUS/DRIP MEDS
☐ CHEMOTHERAPY PROTOCOL
   -USE ONE COLUMN FOR BOLUS MEDS
   -USE A SEPARATE COLUMN FOR EACH
                    CONTINUOUS DRIP

RECORD AT THE BEGINNING OF EACH SHIFT & ANY CHANGES MADE DURING THE SHIFT

DATE	TIME	INIT	MEDICATION	DATE	TIME	INIT	MEDICATION
			IV Drip				
2/20/XX	*3PM*	*DFS*	*20 mEqKCl in 1000 mL*				
			D5/W @ 100 mL/hr				

SIGNATURE	INIT	SIGNATURE	INIT	SIGNATURE	INIT
Dolores F. Saxton	*DFS*				

FORM NO. 22465 2/90   (OVER)

ST FRANCIS HOSPITAL
Roslyn, NY

NURSING CARE PLAN
KARDEX

James, Henry
#24973862

ADMISSION DATE / UNIT TRANSFERS (date / unit):

2/20/xx   *Age 40*

STATUS:
☐ DNR   ☐ HEALTH CARE PROXY

ADMITTING DIAGNOSIS (and or most current diagnosis)

acute pancreatitis

SURGICAL PROCEDURES / DATE   *1983*

appendectomy

PATIENT SAFETY:
RISK LEVEL   ☐ I   ☐ II   ☐ III   ☐ IV
       ☐ RESTRAINTS   ☐ POSEY VEST

ACTIVITY: ☐ BEDREST   ☐ BRP   ☐ OOB

TRANSFER: ☐ ASSIST   ☐ HOYER

DISABILITY OR LIMITATIONS:
Vision: ☐ Glasses   ☐ Contact lenses   ☐ Blind
Hearing: ☐ Deaf   ☐ HOH   ☐ Hearing aid
Dentures: ☐ Upper   ☐ Lower

PRIOR MEDICAL HISTORY

alcohol abuse

VITAL SIGNS:	**CARDIAC MONITORING:**	**PACEMAKERS:**	**NUTRITION:**
☐ Q SHIFT	☐ TRANSPORT WITH	☐ PERMANENT	☐ WEIGHT Q *D - 10^AM*
		type _____	☐ DIET *NPO*
☐ Q 4HR	☐ TRANSPORT WITHOUT	rate _____	
		☐ TEMPORARY ☐ on ☐ off	☒ I&O ☐ FLUID RESTRICTION
☐ PRN	☐ TREATMENT ORDERS	MA _____	☒ NGT ☐ PEG
		rate _____	☐ FEEDING
☐		☐ AICD ☐ on ☐ off	☐ FOLEY
		rate _____	☐ DRAINAGE

CONSULTATIONS (PHYSICIAN / DATE / SERVICE)

TREATMENTS

2/20 naso-gastric tube to low-suction

LAB STUDIES (PENDING) [DATE / STUDY]

2/20 serum amylase

TESTS (PENDING)   **[DATE / TEST]**

2/20 chest x-ray
2/20 ultrasonogram and CT scan of pancreas

IV THERAPY (DATE LINE INSERTED / SOLUTION)
☒ PERIPHERAL *2/20 D5/W 1000 mL c̄*
      KCL 20 mlq @ 100mL/h
☐ ARTERIAL
☐ SUBCLAVIAN
☐ SWAN GANZ
☐ RIJ
☐ MULTILUMEN
☐ PCA
☐ EPIDURAL

RESPIRATORY THERAPY
☐ TREATMENTS
☐ O2 _____
☐ VENTILATOR SETTINGS
   mode _____
   rate _____
   FIO2 _____
   TV _____
☐ CPT
☐ INCENTIVE SPIROMETER
☐ ET TUBE   size ___   date ___
☐ TRACH   size ___   date ___
☐ CHEST TUBES

PATIENT TEACHING: (DATE)
☐ CARDIAC MEDICAL
☐ DIABETES
☐ POST OP

DISCHARGE PLANNING:
☐ CASE WORKER

PLANS:
☐ HOME
☐ REHAB
☐ NSG HOME

James, Henry   40 yrs
#24973862

ALLERGIES: ☐ NO   ☐ YES

STANDING MEDICATIONS

ORD DATE	INIT	REORD DATE	INIT	MEDICATION	DOSAGE	ROUTE	FREQ	TIMES		DC DATE	INIT
2/20	NEO			Pepcid	20 mg	IVPB	q12h	6ᴬᴹ	6ᴾᴹ	2/21/xx	NEO
2/21	NEO			Pepcid	40 mg	IVPB	q12h	6ᴬᴹ	6ᴾᴹ		

PRN MEDICATIONS

ORD DATE	INIT	REORD DATE	INIT	MEDICATION	DOSAGE	ROUTE	FREQ	TIMES	DC DATE	INIT
2/20	NEO	2/23	NEO	Demerol	75 mg	IM	q4h prn			

Example: The physician's orders for a patient admitted with cellulitis of the left foot who is receiving maintenance chemotherapy for rheumatoid arthritis are:

Margolis, Henrick   Age 51
241793

NORTH SHORE - LONG ISLAND JEWISH HEALTH SYSTEM

DIRECT DOCTOR ORDER SHEET

DRUG ALLERGIES: **PLEASE PRINT - DO NOT USE LABEL**

WEIGHT: 150 lbs

HEIGHT: 5'10"

DATE & TIME	PROB NO.	ORDERS (BEFORE WRITING ORDERS BE SURE THERE IS A YELLOW COPY) →	SIGNATURE
2/20/xx		Methotrexate 10 mg po weekly	
9ᴬᴹ		Prednisone 40 mg po qod	
		Warm soaks to (L) foot q4h	
			Dr. Sanchez

On the day after admission, the notations on this patient's progress note should be:

Margolis, Henrick   Age 51

241793

LONG ISLAND JEWISH MEDICAL CENTER
PROGRESS NOTES

Format of Sample Entry:

Date   Problem No.

Subjective
Objective
Assessment | Signature, Title,
Plan | Dept.

PROGRESS NOTES

DATE/ TIME	PROB NO.	
2/20/xx		Prednisone given with milk. Warm soaks to left foot.
10ᴬᴹ		Area on left foot is reddened.
		Dolores F. Saxton RN
2/20/xx		Warm soaks to left foot.
2ᴾᴹ		Area is reddened and some edema is present.
		Dolores F. Saxton RN
2/20/xx		Warm soaks to left foot.
6ᴾᴹ		Edema is present and area is red.
		John Reynolds RN

Two weeks after admission, the notations on this patient's chemotherapy record should be:

Margolis, Henrick Age 51
241793

NORTH SHORE - LONG ISLAND JEWISH HEALTH SYSTEM
MEDICATION RECORD

PLACE ALLERGY STICKER HERE

DATE OF ORDER	DATE OF EXP	MEDICATION DOSE ROUTE FREQUENCY	DATE: 2/20/xx	DATE: 2/21/xx	DATE: 2/22/xx	DATE: 2/23/xx	DATE: 2/24/xx	DATE: 2/25/xx	DATE: 2/26/xx
2/20/xx init DFS		med Methotrexate 10 mg dose	time/init 10ᴬᴹ DFS	✗	✗	✗	✗	✗	✗
init		rte p.o. 1x weekly freq							
init									
init		Prednisone 40 mg	10ᴬᴹ DFS	✗	DFS	✗	MG	✗	JK
init		p.o. q.o.D.							
init									
init									
init									
init									
init									
init									
init									
init									
init									
init									
init									
init									
init									
init									
init									
init									
init									
init									
init									
init									
init									
init									

SIGNATURE	INIT				
Dolores F. Saxton	DFS				
Mildrid Guanty	MG				
Jerry Krammer	JK				

LIJ-HMC #522777   (OVER)

Problem Set 24.1

1.   Transpose the following physician's orders to the proper patient medication record:

Nichols, Ebenezer   Age 70
 # 230725

NORTH SHORE - LONG ISLAND JEWISH HEALTH SYSTEM		
DIRECT DOCTOR ORDER SHEET		
DRUG ALLERGIES: PLEASE PRINT - DO NOT USE LABEL		
WEIGHT: *165 lbs*		
HEIGHT: *5' 10"*		

DATE & TIME	PROB NO.	ORDERS (BEFORE WRITING ORDERS BE SURE THERE IS A YELLOW COPY) →	SIGNATURE
3/4/xx		*Heparin 5,000 U IVP stat*	
9ᴬᴹ		*Heparin 25,000 U in D5/W 500 mL @ 20 mL/h*	
		Nifedipine 30 mg po qid	
		F. Fender MD	

Nichols, Ebenezer   Age 70
#230725

NORTH SHORE - LONG ISLAND JEWISH HEALTH SYSTEM	
MEDICATION RECORD	
PLACE ALLERGY STICKER HERE	

DATE OF ORDER	DATE OF EXP	MEDICATION DOSE ROUTE FREQUENCY	DATE:	DATE:	DATE:	DATE:	DATE:	DATE:	DATE:
			time/init						
init		med dose							
init		rte freq							
init									
init									
init									
init									

SIGNATURE	INIT				

LIJ-HMC #522777   (OVER)

Nichols, Ebenezer Age 70
#230725

NORTH SHORE - LONG ISLAND JEWISH HEALTH SYSTEM

IV MEDICATION DRIP RECORD

☐ IV MEDICATION DRIP
   -CONTINUOUS MED DRIPS
   -COMBINATION BOLUS/DRIP MEDS
☐ CHEMOTHERAPY PROTOCOL
   -USE ONE COLUMN FOR BOLUS MEDS
   -USE A SEPARATE COLUMN FOR EACH
                        CONTINUOUS DRIP

RECORD AT THE BEGINNING OF EACH SHIFT & ANY CHANGES MADE DURING THE SHIFT

DATE	TIME	INIT	MEDICATION	DATE	TIME	INIT	MEDICATION

SIGNATURE	INIT	SIGNATURE	INIT	SIGNATURE	INIT

FORM NO. 22465 2/90   (OVER)

2. Transpose the following physician's orders to the proper patient medication record:

Walker, Peter Age 32
 # 235254

NORTH SHORE - LONG ISLAND JEWISH HEALTH SYSTEM

DIRECT DOCTOR ORDER SHEET

DRUG ALLERGIES: **PLEASE PRINT - DO NOT USE LABEL**

WEIGHT:

HEIGHT:

DATE & TIME	PROB NO.	ORDERS (BEFORE WRITING ORDERS BE SURE THERE IS A YELLOW COPY) →	SIGNATURE
3/4/xx		IVD5/W 2000 mL c̄ KCl 15 mEq in each liter	
8ᴬᴹ		Demerol 50 mg IM q4h prn for pain	
		Tobramycin 80 mg IVPB q8h	
			Dr. Jackson
3/5/xx		D/C Tobramycin	
9ᴬᴹ			Dr. Jackson

NORTH SHORE - LONG ISLAND JEWISH HEALTH SYSTEM

Walker, Peter Age 32
#235254

IV MEDICATION DRIP RECORD
☐ IV MEDICATION DRIP
-CONTINUOUS MED DRIPS
-COMBINATION BOLUS/DRIP MEDS
☐ CHEMOTHERAPY PROTOCOL
-USE ONE COLUMN FOR BOLUS MEDS
-USE A SEPARATE COLUMN FOR EACH
CONTINUOUS DRIP

RECORD AT THE BEGINNING OF EACH SHIFT & ANY CHANGES MADE DURING THE SHIFT

DATE	TIME	INIT	MEDICATION	DATE	TIME	INIT	MEDICATION

SIGNATURE	INIT	SIGNATURE	INIT	SIGNATURE	INIT

FORM NO. 22465 2/90   (OVER)

NORTH SHORE - LONG ISLAND JEWISH HEALTH SYSTEM
MEDICATION RECORD

Walker, Peter Age 32
 # 235254

PLACE ALLERGY STICKER HERE

DATE OF ORDER	DATE OF EXP	MEDICATION	DOSE	DATE:	DATE:	DATE:	DATE:	DATE:	DATE:	DATE:
		ROUTE	FREQUENCY							
init		med	dose	time/init						
init		rte	freq							
init										
init										
init										
init										

SIGNATURE	INIT		

LIJ-HMC #522777   (OVER)

Walker, Peter Age 32
235254

NORTH SHORE - LONG ISLAND JEWISH HEALTH SYSTEM
STAT-PRN MEDICATION RECORD

PLACE ALLERGY STICKER HERE

DATE OF ORDER	DATE OF EXP	MEDICATION DOSE ROUTE FREQUENCY	DATE:	DATE:	DATE:	DATE:	DATE:	DATE:	DATE:
			time/init						
init		med dose							
init		rte freq							
init									
init									
init									
init									

SIGNATURE	INIT					

LIJ-HMC #522777

(OVER)

3. Transpose the following physician's orders to the proper patient medication record:

USE BALLPOINT PEN - PRESS FIRMLY

St. Francis Hospital
ROSLYN, NEW YORK

PHYSICIAN ORDER RECORD

Chou, Susan   Age 39
125062

DOCTOR: PLEASE PRINT NAME & I.D. # AFTER EACH ORDER.
ALSO, PLEASE SIGN OFF ON ALL TELEPHONE AND P.A. ORDERS

DATE / TIME	
3/10/xx	Norvasc 10 mg po qd
	Calciferol 50,000 U po qd
	Epogen 3,000 U sc once weekly on Mondays
	Humulin L 26 U sc hs
	Check blood glucose with glucometer 1/2 hr AC
	Give 5 U Humulin R for 200–220 mg
	Give 10 U Humulin R for 221–230 mg
	Notify physician anytime reading is ↑ 230 mg
	Jane Brown MD ID# 157320

ST FRANCIS HOSPITAL
Roslyn, New York

MEDICATION ADMINISTRATION RECORD

REFER TO:
☐ RESPIRATORY FLOW SHEET
☐ INSULIN MAR
☐ HEPARIN FLOW SHEET
☐ PCA RECORD
☐ EPIDURAL RECORD

PAGE #	
	OF
YEAR	
20xx	

ADDRESSOGRAPH BELOW ➡

Chou, Susan   Age 39
 # 125062

Code to Chart Unadministered Meds:

HELD - See Patient Progress Notes
REF - Refused - See Patient Progress Notes
D/C - Discontinue Drug Use

SEE REVERSE SIDE FOR INJECTION SITE CODES

RECOPIED DATE	
RECOPIED BY	
REVIEWED BY	

DIAGNOSIS
CRF; diabetes

OPERATIVE PROCEDURE AND DATE

ALLERGIES:
☒ NONE

DATE ORD / INITIAL	EXP DATE	SCHEDULED MEDS DOSE - FREQ - ROUTE	HOUR / SITE	DATE	DATE	DATE	DATE	DATE	DATE	DATE	DATE	DATE
Medication Instruction Sheet Given												
Medication Instruction Sheet Given												
Medication Instruction Sheet Given												
Medication Instruction Sheet Given												

INITIAL	SIGNATURE/TITLE	INITIAL	SIGNATURE/TITLE	INITIAL	SIGNATURE/TITLE

FORM # 80080 REV. 3/28/97 MADISON BUSINESS SYSTEMS

ST FRANCIS HOSPITAL
Roslyn, New York

ADDRESSOGRAPH BELOW ➡

Chou, Susan Age 39
 # 125062

INSULIN ADMINISTRATION AND DIABETIC RECORD

BEDISDE BLOOD GLUCOSE METER ORDERS:

☐ PERFOM LAB BACK-UP FOR RESULTS <60 OR >400

☐ NO LAB BACK-UP

☐ BMP QD

PAGE #	
RECOPIED BY	REVIEWED BY

SPECIAL INSTRUCTIONS:

SLIDING SCALES: Date and initial the scale according to physicians order.   *USE REGULAR INSULIN*

STANDARD		ALTERNATIVE		MODIFIED	
DATE FREQUENCY of BBGM		DATE FREQUENCY of BBGM		DATE FREQUENCY of BBGM	
INITIAL		INITIAL		INITIAL	
Route:_____		Route:_____		Route:_____	
Blood Glucose	**Units**	**Blood Glucose**	**Units**	**Blood Glucose**	**Units**
200 – 250 mg/dl	2 units	150 – 200 mg/dl	2 units	_____mg/dl	_____units
251 – 300 mg/dl	4 units	200 – 250 mg/dl	4 units	_____mg/dl	_____units
301 – 350 mg/dl	6 units	251 – 300 mg/dl	6 units	_____mg/dl	_____units
351 – 400 mg/dl	8 units	301 – 350 mg/dl	8 units	_____mg/dl	_____units
> 400 mg/dl	Call MD	351 – 400 mg/dl	10 units	_____mg/dl	_____units
		> 400 mg/dl	Call MD	> 400 mg/dl	Call MD

DATE / INITIALS	SINGLE - STAT - PRE - OP INSULIN ORDERS	DATE / TIME TO BE GIVEN	INITIALS	DATE / INITIALS	INSULIN DRIP CONCENTRATION

AM DAILY INSULIN ORDERS			PM DAILY INSULIN ORDERS		
ORDER DATE / INITIALS	INSULIN Type - Dose - Route	TIME TO BE GIVEN	ORDER DATE / INITIALS	INSULIN Type - Dose - Route	TIME TO BE GIVEN

St. Francis Hospital
ROSLYN, NEW YORK

INSULIN / MEDICATION
ADMINISRTATION RECORD

ADDRESSOGRAPH BELOW ➡

Chou, Susan   Age 39
 # 125062

BEDSIDE BLOOD GLUCOSE
RESULTS <60 OR >400:
1-Assess / Treat Patient
2-Call Physician, and
3-Perfom Lab Back-up

⬇

INJECTION
SITE CODE:
C = DELTOID R
D = DELTOID L
E = THIGH R LAT
F = THIGH L LAT

BLOOD GLUCOSE RESULTS				MEDICATIONS ADMINISTERED				
DATE	TIME	METER RESULT	SERUM RESULT	MEDICATION	DOSE	SITE / ROUTE	INIT	TIME

St. Francis Hospital - ROSLYN, NEW YORK

INITIALS - SIGNATURE VERIFICATION

Chou, Susan   *Age 39*   *# 125062*

INITIAL	SIGNATURE / TITLE	INITIAL	SIGNATURE / TITLE

4. Transpose the following physician's orders and make the correct notations on this patient's medication records for the first three days of hospitalization:

Ruiz, Cynthia Age 65
 # 236709

		NORTH SHORE - LONG ISLAND JEWISH HEALTH SYSTEM	
		DIRECT DOCTOR ORDER SHEET	
		DRUG ALLERGIES: **PLEASE PRINT - DO NOT USE LABEL**	
		WEIGHT: *125 lb*	
		HEIGHT: *5'2"*	

DATE & TIME	PROB NO.	ORDERS (BEFORE WRITING ORDERS BE SURE THERE IS A YELLOW COPY) →	SIGNATURE
3/10/xx		*Continuous IV D5/W 1000 mL c̄ 20 mEq KCl @ 50 mL/hr*	
10ᴬᴹ		*Solu-medrol 100 mg IVPB q6h*	
		F. Reynolds MD	
3/11/xx		*Inderal 40 mg BID po*	
6ᴬᴹ		*D/C Solu-medrol IVPB*	
		Medrol 8 mg 2D po	
		MOM 7oz. stat po	
		F. Reynolds MD	

Ruiz, Cynthia Age 65
 # 236709

NORTH SHORE - LONG ISLAND JEWISH HEALTH SYSTEM
STAT-PRN MEDICATION RECORD

PLACE ALLERGY STICKER HERE

DATE OF ORDER	DATE OF EXP	MEDICATION DOSE ROUTE FREQUENCY	DATE:	DATE:	DATE:	DATE:	DATE:	DATE:	DATE:
			time/init						
init		med dose							
init		rte freq							
init									
init									
init									
init									

SIGNATURE	INIT					

LIJ-HMC #522777   (OVER)

Ruiz, Cynthia Age 65
 # 236709

NORTH SHORE - LONG ISLAND JEWISH HEALTH SYSTEM
MEDICATION RECORD

PLACE ALLERGY STICKER HERE

DATE OF ORDER	DATE OF EXP	MEDICATION DOSE ROUTE FREQUENCY	DATE:	DATE:	DATE:	DATE:	DATE:	DATE:	DATE:
			time/init						
init		med dose							
init		rte freq							
init									
init									
init									
init									

SIGNATURE	INIT				

LIJ-HMC #522777   (OVER)

NORTH SHORE - LONG ISLAND JEWISH HEALTH SYSTEM

Ruiz, Cynthia Age 65
#236709

IV MEDICATION DRIP RECORD

☐ IV MEDICATION DRIP
  -CONTINUOUS MED DRIPS
  -COMBINATION BOLUS/DRIP MEDS
☐ CHEMOTHERAPY PROTOCOL
  -USE ONE COLUMN FOR BOLUS MEDS
  -USE A SEPARATE COLUMN FOR EACH
    CONTINUOUS DRIP

RECORD AT THE BEGINNING OF EACH SHIFT & ANY CHANGES MADE DURING THE SHIFT

DATE	TIME	INIT	MEDICATION	DATE	TIME	INIT	MEDICATION

SIGNATURE	INIT	SIGNATURE	INIT	SIGNATURE	INIT

FORM NO. 22465 2/90   (OVER)

5. Transpose the following physician's orders and make the correct notations on this patient's medication records for the first four days of hospitalization:

Behr, Theodora Age 65	**NORTH SHORE - LONG ISLAND JEWISH HEALTH SYSTEM**	
# 234067	**DIRECT DOCTOR ORDER SHEET**	
	DRUG ALLERGIES: **PLEASE PRINT - DO NOT USE LABEL**	
	WEIGHT: 140 lb	
	HEIGHT: 5'10"	

DATE & TIME	PROB NO.	ORDERS (BEFORE WRITING ORDERS BE SURE THERE IS A YELLOW COPY) →	SIGNATURE
3/10/xx		D5/W 2000 mL c̄ MVI 5 mL in each liter daily x 4 days	
9³⁰AM		Decadron 40 mg IVPB qd	
		Dr. Tobias	
3/13/xx		DC Decadron IVPB	
11AM		Decadron 4 mg po q6h	
		Lasix 20 mg po qod	
		MOM 30 mL po stat	
		Dr. Tobias	

Behr, Theodora Age 65	**NORTH SHORE - LONG ISLAND JEWISH HEALTH SYSTEM**
# 234067	**STAT-PRN MEDICATION RECORD**
	PLACE ALLERGY STICKER HERE

DATE OF ORDER	DATE OF EXP	MEDICATION DOSE	DATE:	DATE:	DATE:	DATE:	DATE:	DATE:	DATE:	DATE:
		ROUTE FREQUENCY								
			time/init							
init		med dose								
init		rte freq								
init										
init										
init										
init										

SIGNATURE	INIT						

LIJ-HMC #522777   (OVER)

NORTH SHORE - LONG ISLAND JEWISH HEALTH SYSTEM

Behr, Theodora   Age 65
#234067

IV MEDICATION DRIP RECORD

☐ IV MEDICATION DRIP
  -CONTINUOUS MED DRIPS
  -COMBINATION BOLUS/DRIP MEDS
☐ CHEMOTHERAPY PROTOCOL
  -USE ONE COLUMN FOR BOLUS MEDS
  -USE A SEPARATE COLUMN FOR EACH
    CONTINUOUS DRIP

RECORD AT THE BEGINNING OF EACH SHIFT & ANY CHANGES MADE DURING THE SHIFT

DATE	TIME	INIT	MEDICATION	DATE	TIME	INIT	MEDICATION

SIGNATURE	INIT	SIGNATURE	INIT	SIGNATURE	INIT

FORM NO. 22465 2/90   (OVER)

Behr, Theodora Age 65
234067

NORTH SHORE - LONG ISLAND JEWISH HEALTH SYSTEM
MEDICATION RECORD

PLACE ALLERGY STICKER HERE

DATE OF ORDER	DATE OF EXP	MEDICATION DOSE ROUTE FREQUENCY	DATE:	DATE:	DATE:	DATE:	DATE:	DATE:	DATE:
init		med dose	time/init						
init		rte freq							
init									
init									
init									
init									

SIGNATURE	INIT				

LIJ-HMC #522777   (OVER)

Answers 1.

Nichols, Ebenezer Age 70
230725

NORTH SHORE - LONG ISLAND JEWISH HEALTH SYSTEM
MEDICATION RECORD

PLACE ALLERGY STICKER HERE

DATE OF ORDER	DATE OF EXP	MEDICATION DOSE ROUTE FREQUENCY	DATE: 3/4/XX	DATE: 3/5/xx	DATE: 3/6/xx	DATE: 3/7/xx	DATE: 3/8/xx	DATE: 3/9/xx	DATE: 3/10/xx
init		*Nifedipine* 30mg _{med} _{dose}	time/init 10ᴬᴹ NEO						
init		rte *po* *qid* freq	2ᴾᴹ						
init			6ᴾᴹ						
init			10ᴾᴹ						
init									
init									

SIGNATURE	INIT				
Norma E. O'Neill RN	*NEO*				

LIJ-HMC #522777   (OVER)

NORTH SHORE - LONG ISLAND JEWISH HEALTH SYSTEM

Nichols Ebenezer   Age 70
#230725

	IV MEDICATION DRIP RECORD
☐	IV MEDICATION DRIP
	-CONTINUOUS MED DRIPS
	-COMBINATION BOLUS/DRIP MEDS
☐	CHEMOTHERAPY PROTOCOL
	-USE ONE COLUMN FOR BOLUS MEDS
	-USE A SEPARATE COLUMN FOR EACH
	CONTINUOUS DRIP

RECORD AT THE BEGINNING OF EACH SHIFT & ANY CHANGES MADE DURING THE SHIFT

DATE	TIME	INIT	MEDICATION	DATE	TIME	INIT	MEDICATION
3/4/xx	9¹⁵AM	NEO	Heparin 5,000 U IVP				
3/4/xx	9³⁰AM	NEO	Heparin 25,000 U in D5/W 500 mL @ 20 mL/h				

SIGNATURE	INIT	SIGNATURE	INIT	SIGNATURE	INIT
Norma E. O'Neill	NEO				

FORM NO. 22465 2/90   (OVER)

2.

NORTH SHORE - LONG ISLAND JEWISH HEALTH SYSTEM

Walker, Peter   Age 32
#235254

	IV MEDICATION DRIP RECORD
☐	IV MEDICATION DRIP
	-CONTINUOUS MED DRIPS
	-COMBINATION BOLUS/DRIP MEDS
☐	CHEMOTHERAPY PROTOCOL
	-USE ONE COLUMN FOR BOLUS MEDS
	-USE A SEPARATE COLUMN FOR EACH
	CONTINUOUS DRIP

RECORD AT THE BEGINNING OF EACH SHIFT & ANY CHANGES MADE DURING THE SHIFT

DATE	TIME	INIT	MEDICATION	DATE	TIME	INIT	MEDICATION
3/4/XX	9AM	NEO	KCl 15 mEq in 1000 mL D5/W				
3/4/XX	9AM	DFS	KCl 15 mEq in 1000 mL D5/W				

SIGNATURE	INIT	SIGNATURE	INIT	SIGNATURE	INIT
Norma E. O'Neill	NEO				
Dolores F. Saxton	DFS				

FORM NO. 22465 2/90   (OVER)

Walker, Peter Age 32
 # 235254

NORTH SHORE - LONG ISLAND JEWISH HEALTH SYSTEM
MEDICATION RECORD

PLACE ALLERGY STICKER HERE

DATE OF ORDER	DATE OF EXP	MEDICATION DOSE / ROUTE FREQUENCY	DATE: 3/4/xx	DATE: 3/5/xx	DATE: 3/6/xx	DATE: 3/7/xx	DATE: 3/8/xx	DATE: 3/9/xx	DATE: 3/10/xx
init		*Tobramycin* 80 mg med dose	time/init	6PM DFS					
init		*IVPB* q8h rte freq	2PM NEO	DC					
init			10PM JA						
init									
init									
init									

SIGNATURE	INIT						
Norma E O'Neill RN	NEO						
Jason Adler RN	JA						
Dolores F. Saxton RN	DFS						

LIJ-HMC #522777   (OVER)

Walker, Peter Age 32
 # 235254

NORTH SHORE - LONG ISLAND JEWISH HEALTH SYSTEM
MEDICATION RECORD

PLACE ALLERGY STICKER HERE

DATE OF ORDER	DATE OF EXP	MEDICATION DOSE / ROUTE FREQUENCY	DATE:	DATE:	DATE:	DATE:	DATE:	DATE:	DATE:
init		*Demerol* 50 mg med dose	time/init						
init		*IM* qph prn rte freq							
init		*for pain*							
init									
init									
init									

SIGNATURE	INIT						

LIJ-HMC #522777   (OVER)

3.

ST FRANCIS HOSPITAL
Roslyn, New York

MEDICATION ADMINISTRATION RECORD

ADDRESSOGRAPH BELOW ➧

Chou, Susan   Age 39
#125062

REFER TO:
☐ RESPIRATORY FLOW SHEET
☐ INSULIN MAR
☐ HEPARIN FLOW SHEET
☐ PCA RECORD
☐ EPIDURAL RECORD

PAGE # OF *1*	
YEAR *20xx*	

Code to Chart Unadministered Meds:	RECOPIED DATE	DIAGNOSIS
HELD - See Patient Progress Notes	RECOPIED BY	OPERATIVE PROCEDURE AND DATE
REF - Refused - See Patient Progress Notes		
D/C - Discontinue Drug Use	REVIEWED BY	
SEE REVERSE SIDE FOR INJECTION SITE CODES		**ALLERGIES:** ☒ NONE

DATE ORD / INITIAL	EXP DATE	SCHEDULED MEDS DOSE - FREQ - ROUTE	HOUR / SITE	DATE 3/10	DATE 3/11	DATE 3/12	DATE 3/13	DATE 3/14	DATE 3/15	DATE 3/16	DATE 3/17	DATE 3/18
3/10/XX DFS		*Norvasc 10 mg qd po*	10^AM	DFS								
Medication Instruction Sheet Given												
3/10/XX DFS		*Calciferol 50,000 U qd po*	10^AM	DFS								
Medication Instruction Sheet Given												
3/10/XX DFS		*Epogen 3,000 U once weekly — Mondays sc*	10^AM	DFS	✗	✗	✗	✗	✗	✗		✗
Medication Instruction Sheet Given												

	Medication Instruction Sheet Given		

INITIAL	SIGNATURE/TITLE	INITIAL	SIGNATURE/TITLE	INITIAL	SIGNATURE/TITLE
DFS	*Dolores F. Saxton RN*				

FORM # 80080 REV. 3/28/97 MADISON BUSINESS SYSTEMS

ST FRANCIS HOSPITAL
Roslyn, New York

ADDRESSOGRAPH BELOW ➡

Chou, Susan   Age 39
#125062

INSULIN ADMINISTRATION AND DIABETIC RECORD

BEDISDE BLOOD GLUCOSE METER ORDERS:	PAGE #	
☐ PERFOM LAB BACK-UP FOR RESULTS <60 OR >400		
☐ NO LAB BACK-UP	RECOPIED BY	REVIEWED BY
☐ BMP QD		

SPECIAL INSTRUCTIONS:

SLIDING SCALES: Date and initial the scale according to physicians order.   *USE REGULAR INSULIN*

STANDARD		ALTERNATIVE		MODIFIED	
DATE	FREQUENCY of BBGM	DATE	FREQUENCY of BBGM	DATE *3/10/xx* FREQUENCY of BBGM	
INITIAL		INITIAL		INITIAL *NEO*	
Route:_____		Route:_____		Route: *sc*_____	
Blood Glucose	**Units**	**Blood Glucose**	**Units**	**Blood Glucose**	**Units**
200 – 250 mg/dl	2 units	150 – 200 mg/dl	2 units	*200 – 220* mg/dl *5* units	
251 – 300 mg/dl	4 units	200 – 250 mg/dl	4 units	*221 – 230* mg/dl *10* units	
301 – 350 mg/dl	6 units	251 – 300 mg/dl	6 units	_____ mg/dl _____ units	
351 – 400 mg/dl	8 units	301 – 350 mg/dl	8 units	_____ mg/dl _____ units	
> 400 mg/dl	Call MD	351 – 400 mg/dl	10 units	_____ mg/dl _____ units	
		> 400 mg/dl	Call MD	*>230 mg/dl* >400 mg/dl Call MD	

DATE / INITIALS	SINGLE - STAT - PRE - OP INSULIN ORDERS	DATE / TIME TO BE GIVEN	INITIALS	DATE / INITIALS	INSULIN DRIP CONCENTRATION

AM DAILY INSULIN ORDERS			PM DAILY INSULIN ORDERS		
ORDER DATE / INITIALS	INSULIN Type - Dose - Route	TIME TO BE GIVEN	ORDER DATE / INITIALS	INSULIN Type - Dose - Route	TIME TO BE GIVEN
			3/10/xx NEO	*Humulin L 26 U sc HS*	*9PM*

St. Francis Hospital
ROSLYN, NEW YORK

INSULIN / MEDICATION ADMINISRTATION RECORD

ADDRESSOGRAPH BELOW ➡

Chou, Susan Age 39
#125062

BEDSIDE BLOOD GLUCOSE RESULTS <60 OR >400:
1-Assess / Treat Patient
2-Call Physician, and
3-Perfom Lab Back-up

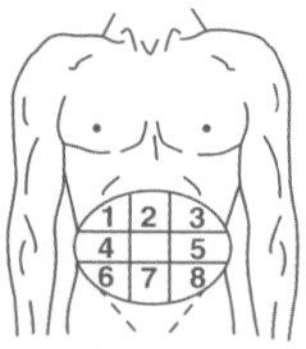

INJECTION SITE CODE:
C = DELTOID R
D = DELTOID L
E = THIGH R LAT
F = THIGH L LAT

BLOOD GLUCOSE RESULTS				MEDICATIONS ADMINISTERED				
DATE	TIME	METER RESULT	SERUM RESULT	MEDICATION	DOSE	SITE / ROUTE	INIT	TIME
3/10/xx	*8 30PM*	*186*		*Humulin*	*26 U*	*sc*	*NEO*	*9PM*

St. Francis Hospital - ROSLYN, NEW YORK

INITIALS - SIGNATURE VERIFICATION

INITIAL	SIGNATURE / TITLE	INITIAL	SIGNATURE / TITLE
NEO	*Norma E. O'Neill RN*		

4.

Ruiz, Cynthia Age 65
#236709

NORTH SHORE - LONG ISLAND JEWISH HEALTH SYSTEM
STAT-PRN MEDICATION RECORD

PLACE ALLERGY STICKER HERE

DATE OF ORDER	DATE OF EXP	MEDICATION DOSE ROUTE FREQUENCY	DATE: 3/11/xx	DATE:	DATE:	DATE:	DATE:	DATE:	DATE:
init		*MOM* med 1 oz. po STAT dose	time/init 6³⁰PM						
init		rte freq	*NEO*						
init									
init									
init									
init									

SIGNATURE	INIT							
Norma E O'Neill RN	*NEO*							

LIJ-HMC #522777   (OVER)

NORTH SHORE - LONG ISLAND JEWISH HEALTH SYSTEM

Ruiz, Cynthia   Age 65
#236709

IV MEDICATION DRIP RECORD
☒ IV MEDICATION DRIP
  -CONTINUOUS MED DRIPS
  -COMBINATION BOLUS/DRIP MEDS
☐ CHEMOTHERAPY PROTOCOL
  -USE ONE COLUMN FOR BOLUS MEDS
  -USE A SEPARATE COLUMN FOR EACH
                    CONTINUOUS DRIP

RECORD AT THE BEGINNING OF EACH SHIFT & ANY CHANGES MADE DURING THE SHIFT

DATE	TIME	INIT	MEDICATION	DATE	TIME	INIT	MEDICATION
3/10/xx	10³⁰AM	NEO	¹Continuous IV				
			¹KCl 20 mEq in D5/W				
			1000 mL @ 50 mL/h				

SIGNATURE	INIT	SIGNATURE	INIT	SIGNATURE	INIT
Norma E. O'Neill	*NEO*				

FORM NO. 22465 2/90   (OVER)

Ruiz, Cynthia Age 65
#236709

PLACE ALLERGY STICKER HERE

DATE OF ORDER	DATE OF EXP	MEDICATION DOSE ROUTE FREQUENCY	DATE: 3/10	DATE: 3/11	DATE: 3/12	DATE: 3/13	DATE: 3/14	DATE: 3/15	DATE: 3/16
3/10/xx init LAP		Solu-medrol 100 mg med	time/init 6^AM	6^AM D9S					
init		rte IVPB q6h freq	12^N NEO	12^N NEO					
init			6^PM NEO	6^PM D/C					
init			12^M D9S	12^M					
init									
3/12/xx init LAP		Medrol 8 mg			10^AM D9S				
init		p.o. qd							
init									
3/12/xx init LAP		Inderal 40 mg			10^AM D9S				
init		p.o. bid			6^PM				
init									
init									
init									
init									
init									
init									
init									
init									
init									
init									
init									
init									
init									
init									
init									
init									

SIGNATURE	INIT					
Norma E. O'Neill	NEO					
Dolores F. Saxton	D9S					

5.

					NORTH SHORE - LONG ISLAND JEWISH HEALTH SYSTEM
					STAT-PRN MEDICATION RECORD

Behr, Theodora   Age 65
#234067

PLACE ALLERGY STICKER HERE

DATE OF ORDER	DATE OF EXP	MEDICATION DOSE	DATE:	DATE:	DATE:	DATE:	DATE:	DATE:	DATE:
		ROUTE FREQUENCY	3/3/xx						
init		med *MOM* 30 mL dose	time/init *11 AM*						
init		rte *po* *STAT* freq	*DFS*						
init									
init									
init									
init									

SIGNATURE	INIT				
Dolores F. Saxton	*DFS*				

LIJ-HMC #522777   (OVER)

Behr, Theodora   Age 65
#234067

NORTH SHORE - LONG ISLAND JEWISH HEALTH SYSTEM

IV MEDICATION DRIP RECORD
☐ IV MEDICATION DRIP 　　-CONTINUOUS MED DRIPS 　　-COMBINATION BOLUS/DRIP MEDS ☐ CHEMOTHERAPY PROTOCOL 　　-USE ONE COLUMN FOR BOLUS MEDS 　　-USE A SEPARATE COLUMN FOR EACH 　　　　　　CONTINUOUS DRIP

RECORD AT THE BEGINNING OF EACH SHIFT & ANY CHANGES MADE DURING THE SHIFT

DATE	TIME	INIT	MEDICATION MVI IV Drip	DATE	TIME	INIT	MEDICATION
3/10/xx	10^AM	NEO	MVI 5 ml in D5/W				
			1000 ml				
3/10/xx	10^PM	RG	MVI 5 ml in D5/W				
			1000 ml				
3/11/xx	10^AM	NEO	MVI 5 ml in D5/W				
			1000 ml				
3/11/xx	10^PM	RG	MVI 5 ml in D5/W				
			1000 ml				
3/12/xx	10^AM	DW	MVI 5 ml in D5/W				
			1000 ml				
3/12/xx	10^PM	DFS	MVI 5 ml in D5/W				
			1000 ml				
3/13/xx	10^AM	DW	MVI 5 ml in D5/W				
			1000 ml				
3/13/xx	10^PM	DFS	MVI 5 ml in D5/W				
			1000 ml				

SIGNATURE	INIT	SIGNATURE	INIT	SIGNATURE	INIT
Norma E. O'Neill RN	NEO	Dolores F. Saxton RN	DFS		
Rita Gregory RN	RG				
Dave Waheed RN	DW				

FORM NO. 22465 2/90   (OVER)

Behr, Theodora   Age 65
#234067

NORTH SHORE - LONG ISLAND JEWISH HEALTH SYSTEM
MEDICATION RECORD

PLACE ALLERGY STICKER HERE

DATE OF ORDER	DATE OF EXP	MEDICATION DOSE ROUTE FREQUENCY	DATE: 3/10/xx	DATE: 3/11/xx	DATE: 3/12/xx	DATE: 3/13/xx	DATE: 3/14/xx	DATE: 3/15/xx	DATE: 3/16/xx
3/10/xx init *LAP*		med *Decadron* 40 mg dose	time/init 10^AM *LG*	10^AM *NEO*	10^AM *DFS*	10^AM *NEO*	✕	✕	✕
init		rte *IVPB* qd freq				D/C			
init									
3/12/xx init *LAP*		*Decadron* 4 mg	✕	✕	✕	6^AM			
init		p.o. q6d	✕	✕	✕	12^PM			
init			✕	✕	6^PM *LG*	6^PM			
init			✕	✕	12^AM *LG*	12^AM			
init									
3/13/xx init *LAP*		*Lasix* 20 mg	✕	✕	✕	11^AM *NEO*	✕	10^AM	✕
init		p.o. qod							
init									
init									
init									
init									
init									
init									
init									
init									
init									
init									
init									
init									
init									
init									
init									
init									

SIGNATURE	INIT		
Larry Grey RN	*LG*		
Norma E. O'Neill RN	*NEO*		
Dolores F. Saxton RN	*DFS*		

LIJ-HMC #522777   (OVER)

ERRORS IN THE ADMINISTRATION OF MEDICATIONS

A surprisingly high number of errors are made in the administration of medication. Some unconfirmed studies report that one out of every four to one out of every six medications given are incorrect. Most of these errors occur as a result of carelessness, interruptions, distractions, rushing, and/or stress in the workplace rather than lack of knowledge. These errors include:

- wrong patient
- wrong medication
- wrong dose
- wrong time
- wrong form
- wrong route

Some of the most common errors occur because the nurse fails to:

- Verify unclear, incomplete, or questionable physicians' orders.
- Verify medication order with the physician's order sheet rather than the Medex or Kardex.
- Check medication supply received from the pharmacy with the physician's order sheet.
- Recognize that an ordered dose of a given medication is unsafe.
- Recognize an unusual order for a given medication.
- Compute the dose correctly.
- Follow the manufacturer's instruction for mixing, storing, or administering a drug.
- Recognize that an excessive amount of medication would be necessary to administer a prescribed dose.
- Read carefully and recognize that labels or orders in mg, mL, g, minims, mcg, and/or mEq must be converted to equal measurements.

Situation:

The physician writes the following order for a patient:

Bell, Susan   Age 56
#2469384279

CRANIS HOSPITAL

DOCTOR'S ORDER SHEET

DATE	TIME	ORDERS	SIGNATURE
3/3/xx	8am	Codeine 30 mg tid po x 3 days	
			j bowman
			md

Identification of Error:

The nurse transcribing the order to the medication sheet probably was interrupted a number of times with questions from staff members, physicians, or visitors. Being somewhat rushed to give the 10:00 a.m. medication, the nurse writes the order as:

MEDICATION RECORD - STANDING ORDERS

PAGE ___1___   WEIGHT ___186 lb___

KNOWN ALERGIES ___None___

Bell, Susan   Age 56
#2469384279

Addressograph

DATE:			Fri.	Sat.	Sun.	Mon. 3/3	Tues. 3/4	Wed. 3/5	Thurs. 3/6
Date Order	Renew Date	Medication; Dosage; Route; Frequency; Physician; Nurse	Time Initial	Time Initial	Time Initial	Time Initial	Time Initial	Time Initial	Time Initial
3/3/xx	3/5/xx	Codeine 30 mg po TID Dr. Brown/Jerry Kusman RN				10AM JK 2PM JK 6PM	10AM 2PM 6PM	10AM 2PM 6PM	

SIGNATURE	INIT	SIGNATURE	INIT	SIGNATURE	INIT
Jerry Kusman RN	JK				

LIJ-HMC #522777   (OVER)

The patient receives the codeine at 10:00 a.m. and 2:00 p.m. before another nurse, preparing to administer the 6:00 p.m. dose, checks the medication with the doctor's order because the tid order for codeine seems unusual. On checking the order, this nurse finds that the drug name is unclear and calls the physician to clarify the order. The physician states that the order is for Cardene 30 mg tid po × 3 days.

Evaluation:

1. The first nurse should have been in a quiet area while transcribing orders, to avoid distractions.

2. The first nurse should have questioned the physician immediately when difficulty in reading the name of the drug prescribed was noted. Any time there is doubt, the physician must be called.

3. The first nurse should have recognized that an order for codeine tid was unusual because this medication is usually given q 4–6 h prn for pain.

Situation:

The physician writes the following order for a patient:

Klein, Alex   Age 28
#579264

CRANIS HOSPITAL

DOCTOR'S ORDER SHEET

DATE	TIME	ORDERS	SIGNATURE
3/22/xx	9AM	Prednisone 20 mg po qod c̄ milk	
		Brian McCanna MD	

Identification of Error:

The nurse transcribing the order to the medication sheet writes the order on the medication record as a daily order rather than an every-other-day order:

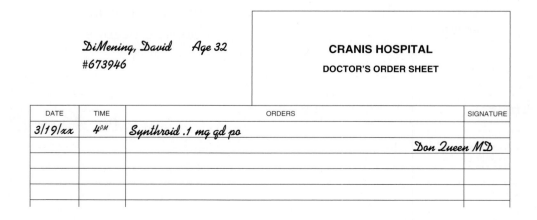

MEDICATION RECORD - STANDING ORDERS				Fri.	Sat. 3/22	Sun. 3/23	Mon. 3/24	Tues. 3/25	Wed. 3/26	Thurs. 3/27

PAGE 1   WEIGHT 160 lb

Klein, Alex   Age 28
#579264

KNOWN ALERGIES   None

Addressograph

DATE:				Fri.	Sat. 3/22	Sun. 3/23	Mon. 3/24	Tues. 3/25	Wed. 3/26	Thurs. 3/27
Date Order	Renew Date	Medication; Dosage; Route; Frequency; Physician; Nurse		Time Initial	Time Initial	Time Initial	Time Initial	Time Initial	Time Initial	Time Initial
3/22		Prednisone 20 mg po qd Dr. McCannal/Helen Kruger		✗	10ᴬᴹ HK	10ᴬᴹ RP	10ᴬᴹ JL	10ᴬᴹ	10ᴬᴹ	10ᴬᴹ

SIGNATURE	INIT	SIGNATURE	INIT	SIGNATURE	INIT
Helen Kruger RN	HK				
Rita Putman RN	RP				
Jane Little RN	JL				

LIJ-HMC #522777

(OVER)

Evaluation:

1. The nurse transcribing the physician's order interpreted the abbreviation for "every other day" incorrectly and thought it was the abbreviation for "every day."

2. The nurse did not write "with milk" on the medication record.

3. Any time there is the slightest doubt about an order, the nurse should clarify the order with the physician.

4. The nurses giving the medication on succeeding days were in error because they never checked the original order on the doctor's order sheet, therefore, the error was continued without correction.

Situation:

The physician writes the following order for a patient:

DiMening, David   Age 32
#673946

CRANIS HOSPITAL

DOCTOR'S ORDER SHEET

DATE	TIME	ORDERS	SIGNATURE
3/19/xx	4ᴾᴹ	Synthroid .1 mg qd po	
			Don Queen MD

Identification of Error:

The nurse transcribes the order on the patient's medication record as Synthroid 1 mg and sends a request to the hospital pharmacy for this strength drug. The pharmacist calls both the nurse and the physician and the error was corrected before the medication was administered.

Evaluation:

1. The physician was incorrect for writing .1 mg rather than 0.1 mg to avoid confusion. The decimal error could have been avoided if the physician had prescribed the drug in micrograms (0.1 mg = 100 mcg), as the drug is labeled in both micrograms and milligrams.

2. The nurse transcribing the order should have looked more carefully at the dose and realized that a 1 mg or 1000 mcg dose would be unusual and should be questioned.

Situation:

The physician writes the following order for a patient:

| | | CRANIS HOSPITAL | |
| | | DOCTOR'S ORDER SHEET | |

Levy, Hannah   *Age 45*
#232984

DATE	TIME	ORDERS	SIGNATURE
3/13/xx	10^AM	*IV infusion of D5/W 1000 mL c̄*	
		potassium chloride 30 mEq @ 100 mL/h Dr. Jones	

Identification of Error:

The nurse transcribes the order as potassium chloride 30 mL instead of 30 mEq and prepares to add the potassium chloride to the prescribed IV solution. On hand is a vial of potassium chloride labeled:

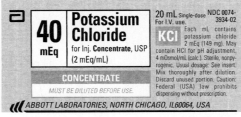

06-7193-4/R15-4/92

The nurse, using 2 vials of potassium chloride, withdraws 30 mL, adds it to the 1000 mL of D5/W, and sets the electronic pump controller to deliver 100 mL/hr. The nurse, in charting the medication, refers to the physician's order sheet and recognizes that an error had been made. The nurse immediately stops the IV and calls the physician.

Evaluation:

1. The nurse transcribing the physician's order copied the abbreviation for mEq as mL. This error could have been avoided by carefully transcribing the physician's order.

2. The nurse should have recognized that parenteral medications are never ordered in mL. If any parenteral medication is ordered in this manner, the physician should be questioned before administering the medication.

Situation:

The physician writes the following order for a 10-year-old who weighs 70 pounds:

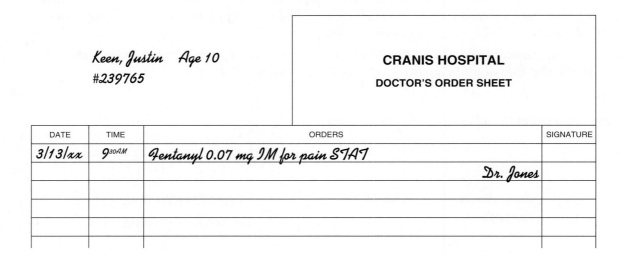

Keen, Justin   Age 10
#239765

CRANIS HOSPITAL

DOCTOR'S ORDER SHEET

DATE	TIME	ORDERS	SIGNATURE
3/13/xx	9³⁰AM	Fentanyl 0.07 mg IM for pain STAT	
			Dr. Jones

Identification of Error:

The manufacturer's instructions state that the recommended safe dosage for a child is 0.001 mg per kg. The child weighs 70 pounds or 32 kg (31.8 kg), meaning that the safe dose for this child would be 0.03 mg, not the 0.07 mg ordered. The nurse notifies the physician, who immediately realizes that the child's weight in pounds (not kilograms) was used, and changed the order to 0.03 mg.

Evaluation:

1. Although the physician made the error in prescribing, the nurse would have been just as culpable if the medication had been administered as ordered.

2. The nurse must remember at all times to calculate the safe dosage of medication for a child and never assume that the physician's prescribed dose is the safe, recommended dose suggested by the manufacturer.

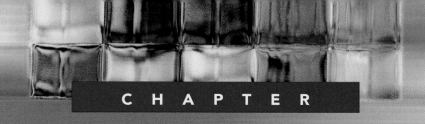

25

Posttest in Computation of Drugs and Solutions

To evaluate your ability and skill in computing proper dosage, it is important that you spend the necessary time doing the problems included in this posttest.

Answer the question or questions in each set. If, after scoring your paper, you find you have incorrectly answered questions in any set, work through the section that applies to that set. If you have correctly answered 90% of the questions, you can feel confident of your basic knowledge and should have little trouble with the task of administering medications.

Remember, the physician usually specifies the amount of drug and the mL of IV fluid to be used. Whether the volume of IV fluid ordered includes the volume of medication is a hospital policy, and may vary from hospital to hospital. For consistency, the problems on this posttest subtract the medication volume from the total volume of IV fluid ordered.

Set 25.1

Give the equivalents for the following.

1. 1 kg = _____ lb = _____ g

2. 1 fluid ounce = _____ fluid drams = _____ mL

3. gr $\dfrac{1}{100}$ = _____ mg = _____ mcg

4. gr $\dfrac{1}{2}$ = _____ mg = _____ g

5. gr $\dfrac{1}{60}$ = _____ mg = _____ g

Set 25.2

Circle the dosage with the greater value.

1. gr $\frac{1}{6}$, gr $\frac{1}{8}$, gr $\frac{1}{12}$ _____

2. 0.125 mg, 0.25 mg, 0.05 mg _____

3. gr $\frac{1}{32}$, gr $\frac{1}{64}$, gr $\frac{1}{60}$ _____

4. 0.004 g, 0.006 g, 0.01 g _____

5. gr $\frac{1}{200}$, gr $\frac{1}{150}$, gr $\frac{1}{100}$ _____

Set 25.3

Convert the following temperatures as indicated.

1. 39°C = _____ °F

2. 22°C = _____ °F

3. 70°F = _____ °C

4. 103°F = _____ °C

5. 101°F = _____ °C

Set 25.4

The physician has prescribed secobarbitol (Seconal) 0.2 g. Each capsule is labeled 100 mg.

The nurse should administer _____ capsules.

Set 25.5

The physician has prescribed phenytoin (Dilantin) 300 mg od. On hand are capsules labeled 0.1 gram.

The nurse should administer _____ capsules.

Set 25.6

The physician has prescribed acyclovir (Lovirax) 0.8 g po q4h. Available are Lovirax tablets labeled 200 mg.

The nurse should administer _____ tablets.

Set 25.7

The physician has prescribed alprazolam (Xanax) 1 mg po tid. Available are Xanax tablets labeled 0.5 mg.

The nurse should administer _____ tablets.

Set 25.8

The physician has prescribed liothyronine sodium (Cytomel) 12.5 mcg po daily. Available are Cytomel tablets labeled 5 mcg.

The nurse should administer _____ tablets.

Set 25.9

The physician has prescribed Elixir of Lanoxin (digoxin) 125 mcg. The bottle is labeled 0.05 mg = 1 mL.

The nurse should administer _____ mL.

Set 25.10

The physician has ordered nafcillin sodium (Unipen) oral solution 500 mg. Available is a bottle labeled 250 mg = 5 mL.

The nurse should administer _____ mL.

Set 25.11

The physician has ordered furosemide (Lasix) oral solution 35 mg. The bottle is labeled 10 mg = 1 mL.

The nurse should administer _____ mL.

Set 25.12

The physician has prescribed ranitidine hydrochloride (Zantax) syrup 150 mg bid. Available is a container labeled Zantax syrup 15 mg per 1 mL.

The nurse should administer _____ mL.

Set 25.13

The physician has prescribed potassium chloride oral solution 20 mEq po daily. Available is a bottle of potassium chloride oral solution labeled 15 mEq per 11.25 mL.

The nurse should administer _____ mL.

Set 25.14

The physician has prescribed furosemide (Lasix) 25 mg IM. The vial is labeled 40 mg = 4 mL.

The nurse should administer _____ mL.

Set 25.15

The physician has prescribed nafcillin sodium (Unipen) 750 mg IM q6h. On hand is a 2 gram vial that states: "Add 6.8 mL of diluent to provide a total solution of 8 mL."

The nurse should administer _____ mL.

Set 25.16

The physician has prescribed hydromorphine hydrochloride (Dilaudid) 1 mg IM q4h. Available is a multidose vial labeled Dilaudid 2 mg = 1 mL.

The nurse should administer _____ mL.

Set 25.17

The physician has prescribed morphine sulfate 8 mg IM q4h prn. On hand is a vial of morphine sulfate labeled 10 mg/1 mL.

The nurse should administer _____ mL.

Set 25.18

The physician has prescribed Humulin R Insulin 25 units sc stat. On hand is a vial labeled Humulin R Insulin 100 units per 1 mL.

How many mL of insulin should the nurse administer? _____ mL

Set 25.19

The physician has prescribed epoetin alfa recombitant (Epogen) 50 units per kg of body weight subcutaneously. The patient weighs 50 kg. Available is a vial labeled Epogen 3000 units per 1 mL.

1. How many units of Epogen should this patient receive? _____ Units
2. The nurse should administer _____ mL.

Set 25.20

The physician has prescribed 7500 units of heparin sodium subcutaneously. The vial is labeled 5000 U = 1 mL.

Using a tuberculin syringe, the nurse should administer _____ mL.

Set 25.21

The physician has prescribed heparin sodium 18,000 units sc stat. Available is a vial that is labeled heparin sodium 20,000 units = 1 mL.

Using a tuberculin syringe, the nurse should administer _____ mL.

Set 25.22

The physician has prescribed Lente human insulin (Humulin-L) 36 units sc od. Available is a vial that is labeled Humulin-L 100 units per 1 mL.

Using a tuberculin syringe, the nurse should administer _____ mL.

Set 25.23

The physician has prescribed heparin sodium 4500 units sc od. Available is a vial of heparin sodium that is labeled 5000 units per 1 mL.

Using a tuberculin syringe, the nurse should administer _____ mL.

Set 25.24

The physician has prescribed heparin sodium 3000 units sc. Available is a vial labeled heparin sodium 5000 units per 1 mL.

Using a tuberculin syringe, the nurse should administer _____ mL.

Set 25.25

The physician has prescribed clindamycin hydrochloride (Cleocin) oral solution 16 mg/kg/day po divided into four equal doses. The child weighs 66 lb or 30 kg. The available Cleocin oral solution is labeled 75 mg per 5 mL.

1. Based on the weight in kilograms, this child's daily dose would be _____ mg/day.
2. This should be divided into _____ mg q6h.
3. For each dose, the nurse should administer _____ mL.

Set 25.26

The physician has prescribed kanamycin sulfate (Kantrex) IM injection 15 mg/kg/day in two divided doses for an infant who weighs 11 lb or 5 kg. The available vial is labeled Kantrex Pediatric Injection 75 mg/2 mL.

1. Based on the weight in kilograms, this infant should receive _____ mg/day.
2. This should be divided into _____ mg q12h.
3. For each dose, the nurse should administer _____ mL.

Set 25.27

The physician has prescribed dronabinol (Marinol) 10 mg by mouth to be given 90 minutes prior to chemotherapy for a 10-year-old who weighs 32 kg (70.4 lb) and is 138 cm (54 inches) tall. The manufacturer's recommended average dose is 5 mg/m² before chemotherapy. Available are 5 mg capsules.

1. Using the pediatric BSA nomogram (see Figure 21.1), this child's BSA is determined to be _____ m².
2. Based on the manufacturer's recommended dose, the safe dose for this child would be _____ mg.
3. After determining the recommended dose, the nurse evaluates that this:

   Is a safe dose for this child and can be administered. _____ (a)

   Is an unsafe dose and the physician should be questioned. _____ (b)

Set 25.28

The physician has prescribed pegaspargase (Oncaspar) 1750 International Units (IU) IM every 14 days for a child whose BSA is 0.7 m². The manufacturer's recommended average dose for children with a BSA greater than 0.6 m² is 2500 IU per m² q14 days. Available is a 5 mL vial labeled Oncaspar 750 IU/1 mL.

1. Based on the manufacturer's recommended dose, the safe dose for this child would be _____ IU.

2. After determining the recommended dose, the nurse evaluates that this:

   Is a safe dose for this child and can be administered. _____ (a)

   Is an unsafe dose and the physician should be questioned. _____ (b)

Set 25.29

The physician has prescribed cytarabine (Cytosar) 80 mg in 100 mL of D5/W via a volume-controlled set to be given once daily over 120 minutes for a child whose BSA is 0.8 m². The Soluset, which is attached to an electronic infusion device, has a drop factor of 60. Available is a 100 mL vial labeled Cytosar 100 mg. The manufacturer's directions state: "Reconstitute with 5 mL of sterile water to yield a solution that contains Cytosar 20 mg/mL." The manufacturer's recommended average child's dose is 100 mg/m² per day.

1. Based on the manufacturer's recommended dose, the safe dose for this child would be _____ mg.

2. After determining the recommended dose, the nurse evaluates that this:

   Is a safe dose for this child and can be administered. _____ (a)

   Is an unsafe dose and the physician should be questioned. _____ (b)

3. How many mL of Cytosar 20 mg/mL will be needed? _____ mL

4. How many mL of D5/W should be added to the volume-controlled set? _____ mL

5. What is the total volume to be infused? _____ mL

6. What hourly rate should be set on the electronic infusion device? _____ mL/hr

Set 25.30

The physician has prescribed atropine 0.3 mg to be administered by IV bolus if cardiac arrhythmias develop. The vial of atropine is labeled 600 mcg = 1 mL.

How many mL should the nurse draw into the syringe? _____ mL

Set 25.31

The physician has prescribed 35 mEq of potassium chloride to be added to a primary intravenous infusion of 1000 mL of D5/W and run for 24 hours. The vial of potassium chloride is labeled 40 mEq = 10 mL. The drop factor of the infusion set is 10.

1. How many mL of potassium chloride 40 mEq/10 mL should be added to the 1000 mL of D5/W? _____ mL

2. The hourly rate of absorption should be _____ mL/hr.

3. How many drops per minute should infuse to deliver the required amount of drug and fluid in 24 hours? _____ gtt/min

4. What hourly rate should be set on the electronic infusion device? _____ mL/hr

Set 25.32

The physician has prescribed 1500 mL of D5/W to be infused over 24 hours. The infusion set has a drop factor of 15.

1. The hourly rate of the infusion should be _____ mL/hr.

2. How many mL per minute should infuse to deliver the required amount of fluid per hour? _____ mL/min

3. How many drops per minute should infuse to deliver the required amount of fluid per hour? _____ gtt/min

4. What hourly rate should be set on the electronic infusion device? _____ mL/hr

Set 25.33

The physician has written an order to keep the patient's vein open with an IV of 1000 mL of D5/W for 24 hours. Available is an IV set with a drop factor of 10 drops = 1 mL.

1. The nurse should set the IV at _____ gtt/min.

2. What hourly rate should be set on the electronic infusion device? _____ mL/hr

Set 25.34

The nurse is caring for a patient whose IV has been regulated to deliver 35 drops per minute of D5/NS. The drop factor of the infusion set is 15 drops/1 mL.

1. The nurse recognizes that the amount absorbed in 1 hour will be _____ mL.

2. At this rate, 1000 mL will be absorbed in _____ hours.

Set 25.35

The physician has written an IV order for D5/1/2NS to be given at 60 mL per hour. The available infusion set delivers 10 drops per mL.

1. How many drops per minute should infuse to deliver the required amount of solution per hour? _____ gtt/min

2. What hourly rate should be set on the electronic infusion device? _____ mL/hr

Set 25.36

The physician has prescribed a continuous secondary infusion of 50 units of Humulin R Insulin 100 units/mL in 500 mL of 1/2NS to run at a rate of 6 U/hr. The infusion set, which is attached to an electronic infusion device, has a drop factor of 60.

1. How many mL of Humulin R Insulin 100 units/mL should be added to the 500 mL of 1/2NS? _____ mL

2. How many units of insulin are in each mL of IV solution after mixing? _____ U/mL

3. How many mL of IV solution will contain 6 units? _____ mL

4. How many drops per minute should infuse to deliver the required amount of drug? _____ gtt/min

5. What hourly rate should be set on the electronic infusion device? _____ mL/hr

Set 25.37

The physician has prescribed a continuous secondary infusion of heparin sodium 20,000 units to be added to 1000 mL of 0.9% NaCl to be given at the rate of 1000 units/hr. Available is a vial labeled heparin sodium 20,000 units per 1 mL. The infusion set, which is attached to an electronic infusion device, has a drop factor of 60 drops/mL.

1. How many mL of heparin sodium 20,000 units per 1 mL should be added to the 1000 mL of 0.9% NaCl? _____ mL

2. How many units of heparin are present in 1 mL of the heparin sodium 20,000 units in 1000 mL of 0.9% NaCl? _____ units/mL

3. How many mL per minute must infuse to deliver the prescribed amount of the drug? _____ mL/min

4. How many mL per hour should the electronic infusion device be set to deliver? _____ mL/hr

Set 25.38

The patient is receiving TPN at a rate of 65 mL per hour via an electronic infusion device. The drop factor of the infusion set is 60 drops per mL.

1. How many drops per minute should infuse to deliver the required amount of TPN solution per hour? _____ gtt/min

2. What hourly rate should be set on the electronic infusion device? _____ mL/hr

3. The total amount of TPN solution that the patient will receive in 24 hours is _____ mL/24 hr.

Set 25.39

The physician has prescribed cefoxitin sodium (Mefoxin) 800 mg IVPB every 12 hours via an electronic infusion device. On hand is a 1 gram vial that reads: "Add 2 mL of diluent to provide a total solution of 2.5 mL." The instructions for IVPB administration suggest adding the Mefoxin to 100 mL of D5/W to be administered over 1 hour. The drop factor of the IV set is 60 drops per mL.

1. How many mL of Mefoxin 1 g/2.5 mL should be added to the 100 mL of D5/W? _____ mL

2. What will be the total volume of the IVPB solution? _____ mL

3. How many drops per minute should the IVPB infuse? _____ gtt/min

4. What hourly rate should be set on the electronic infusion device? _____ mL/hr

Set 25.40

The physician has prescribed 300 mg of cimetidine IVPB q6h. Available is a vial labeled cimetidine 300 mg/2 mL. The manufacturer's instructions state that each 300 mg should be diluted in 100 mL of D5/W and be administered over 20 minutes via an electronic infusion device. The drop factor of the infusion set is 10 gtt/mL.

1. How many mL of cimetidine 300 mg/2 mL should be added to the 100 mL of D5/W? _____ mL

2. What will be the total volume of the IVPB solution? _____ mL

3. How many drops per minute should the IVPB infuse? _____ gtt/min

4. What hourly rate should be set on the electronic infusion device? _____ mL/hr

Set 25.41

The physician has prescribed amikacin sulfate (Amikin) 500 mg IVPB every 12 hours. The manufacturer's instructions state: "Each 500 mg of Amikin should be diluted in 200 mL of D5/W to be administered over 60 minutes." Available are 2 mL vials labeled Amikin 250 mg/1 mL. The drop factor of the infusion set is 15 gtt/mL.

1. How many mL of Amikin 250 mg/1 mL should be added to the 200 mL of D5/W? _____ mL

2. What will be the total volume of the IVPB solution? _____ mL

3. How many drops per minute should the IVPB infuse? _____ gtt/min

4. What hourly rate should be set on the electronic infusion device? _____ mL/hr

Set 25.42

The physician has prescribed ciprofloxacin (Cipro) 200 mg in 100 mL D5/W IVPB via an electronic infusion device to be infused in 1 hour. Available is a 20 mL multidose vial labeled 10 mg/1 mL of Cipro. The drop factor of the set is 60 gtt/mL.

1. How many mL of Cipro 10 mg/1 mL will be needed? _____ mL

2. How many mL of Cipro should be added to the 100 mL bag of D5/W? _____ mL

3. What is the total volume to be infused? _____ mL

4. What hourly rate should be set on the electronic infusion device? _____ mL/hr

Set 25.43

The nurse is caring for a child whose volume-controlled IV has been regulated at 45 drops per minute. The pedidropper has a drop factor of 60 drops per mL.

1. The nurse recognizes that the amount absorbed in 1 hour will be _____ mL.

2. At this rate, 1000 mL will be absorbed in _____ hours.

Set 25.44

The physician has prescribed ofloxacin (Floxin IV) 300 mg in 75 mL of D5/W via a volume-controlled set to be given over 60 minutes. The Soluset, which is attached to an electronic infusion device, has a drop factor of 60. Available is a 10 mL vial labeled Floxin IV 400 mg/10 mL.

1. How many mL of Floxin IV 400 mg/10 mL will be needed? _____ mL

2. How many mL of D5/W should be added to the volume-controlled set? _____ mL

3. What is the total volume to be infused? _____ mL

4. What hourly rate should be set on the electronic infusion device? _____ mL/hr

Set 25.45

The physician has prescribed ondansetron HCl (Zofran) 32 mg in 50 mL of D5/W via a volume-controlled set to be given over 20 minutes. The Soluset, which is attached to an electronic infusion device, has a drop factor of 60. Available is a 20 mL vial labeled Zofran 2 mg/1 mL.

1. How many mL of Zofran 2 mg/1 mL will be needed? _____ mL

2. How many mL of D5/W should be added to the volume-controlled set? _____ mL

3. What is the total volume to be infused? _____ mL

4. What hourly rate should be set on the electronic infusion device? _____ mL/hr

Set 25.46

The physician has prescribed a continuous IV of heparin sodium 25,000 units in 500 mL of D5/W to infuse at a rate of 18 units/kg/hour. The patient weighs 83.6 pounds.

1. How many kilograms does the patient weigh? _____ kg

2. How many units of heparin should the patient receive per hour? _____ units

3. What will be the hourly rate to deliver the ordered dose of heparin? _____ mL/hr

Set 25.47

The physician has prescribed isoproterenol hydrochloride 1:5000 solution (Isuprel 1:5000 solution) 2 mg to be added to 500 mL D5/W and given as a secondary IV at a rate of 5 mcg/minute. Available are ampules that are labeled Isuprel 1:5000 solution 1 mg/5 mL. The infusion set, which is attached to an electronic infusion device, has a drop factor of 60 drops/mL.

1. How many mL of Isuprel 1:5000 solution 1 mg/5 mL should be added to the 500 mL of D5/W? _____ mL

2. How many mg of drug are present in 1 mL of the Isuprel 1:5000 2 mg in 500 mL of D5/W solution? _____ mg/mL

3. Convert this value to mcg/mL. _____ mcg/mL

4. How many mL per minute must infuse to deliver the prescribed amount of the drug? _____ mL/min

5. How many mL per hour should the electronic infusion device be set to deliver? _____ mL/hr

Set 25.48

The physician has prescribed lidocaine hydrochloride (Xylocaine) 120 mg to be added to 100 mL of D5/W and given at a rate of 20 mcg/kg/min for a child who weighs 35 kg. The available vial is labeled Xylocaine 10 mg/mL. The infusion set, which is attached to an electronic infusion device, has a drop factor of 60 drops/mL.

1. How many mL of Xylocaine solution 10 mg/mL should be added to the 100 mL of D5/W? _____ mL

2. How many mg of drug are present in 1 mL of the Xylocaine 120 mg in 100 mL of D5/W solution? _____ mg/mL

3. Convert this value to mcg/mL. _____ mcg/mL

4. How many mcg/min should this child, who weighs 35 kg, receive? _____ mcg/min

5. How many mL per minute must infuse to deliver the prescribed amount of the drug?

_____ mL/min

6. How many mL per hour should the electronic infusion device be set to deliver?

_____ mL/hr

Set 25.49

A patient is receiving 700 units per hour of heparin sodium 25,000 units in 500 mL of D5/W by IV continuous infusion. Lab results indicate that the patient has a partial thromboplastin time (PTT) that is 35. According to sliding-scale protocol, the patient should recieve a bolus of 80 units per kg intravenous push. The continuous IV infusion should also be increased by 4 units per kg of body weight per hour. The patient weighs 38 kg.

1. How many units of heparin should the patient receive for a bolus?

_____ units

2. How many additional units of heparin should the patient receive per hour?

_____ units

3. How many total units of heparin should the patient receive per hour?

_____ units

4. What will be the new hourly rate for delivery of the ordered dose of heparin?

_____ mL/hr

Set 25.50

The physician has prescribed aminophylline 500 mg to be added to 250 mL of D5/W to be given at a rate of 0.5 mg/kg/hr for a patient who weighs 80 kg. The available vial contains aminophylline 500 mg/20 mL. The infusion set, which is attached to an electronic infusion device, has a drop factor of 60 drops/mL.

1. How many mL of aminophylline 500 mg/20 mL should be added to the 250 mL of D5/W?

_____ mL

2. How many mg of drug are present in 1 mL of the aminophylline 500 mg in 250 mL of D5/W solution?

_____ mg/mL

3. How many mg/hr should this patient, who weighs 80 kg, receive?

_____ mg/hr

4. How many mL per hour should the electronic infusion device be set to deliver?

_____ mL/hr

ANSWERS TO POSTTEST

Set 25.1

1. 2.2 lb; 1000 g 2. 8 fluid drams; 30 or 32 mL
3. 0.6 mg; 600 mcg 4. 30 mg; 0.03 g 5. 1 mg; 0.001 g

Set 25.2

1. gr $\frac{1}{6}$ 2. 0.25 mg 3. gr $\frac{1}{32}$ 4. 0.01 g

5. gr $\frac{1}{100}$

Set 25.3

1. 102.2°F 2. 71.6°F 3. 21.1 or 21°C 4. 39.4°C 5. 38.3 or 38.4°C

Set 25.4

2 capsules

Set 25.5

3 capsules

Set 25.6

4 tablets

Set 25.7

2 tablets

Set 25.8

$2\frac{1}{2}$ tablets

Set 25.9

2.5 mL

Set 25.10

10 mL

Set 25.11

3.5 mL

Set 25.12

10 mL

Set 25.13

15 mL

Set 25.14

2.5 mL

Set 25.15

3 mL

Set 25.16

0.5 mL

Set 25.17

0.8 mL

Set 25.18

0.25 mL

Set 25.19

1. 2500 units   2. 0.83 mL

Set 25.20

1.5 mL

Set 25.21

0.9 mL

Set 25.22

0.36 mL

Set 25.23

0.9 mL

Set 25.24

0.6 mL

Set 25.25

1. 480 mg per day   2. 120 mg q6h   3. 8 mL

Set 25.26

1. 75 mg per day   2. 37.5 mg/12 hr   3. 1 mL

Set 25.27

1. 1.1 m²   2. 5.5 mg   3. b

Set 25.28

1. 1750 IU   2. a

Set 25.29

1. 80 mg   2. a   3. 4 mL   4. 96 mL   5. 115 mL
6. 57.5 or 58 mL/hr

Set 25.30

0.5 mL

Set 25.31

1. 8.75 or 8.8 mL   2. 42 mL/hr   3. 7 gtt/min
4. 42 mL/hr

Set 25.32

1. 62.5 mL/hr or 63 mL/hr   2. 1.04 mL/min   3.
15.6 or 16 gtt/min   4. 62.5 or 63 mL/hr

Set 25.33

1. 6.9 or 7 gtt/min   2. 41.6 or 42 mL/hr

Set 25.34

1. 139.9 or 140 mL   2. 7.14 hr (7 hr, 8 min)

Set 25.35

1. 10 gtt/min   2. 60 mL/hr

Set 25.36

1. 0.5 mL   2. 0.1 unit per mL   3. 60 mL   4. 60
gtt/min   5. 60 mL/hr

Set 25.37

1. 1 mL   2. 20 units/mL   3. 50 mL/min   4. 50
mL/hr

Set 25.38

1. 65 gtt/min   2. 65 mL/hr   3. 1560 mL/24 hr

Set 25.39

1. 2 mL   2. 102 mL   3. 102 gtt/min   4. 102
mL/hr

Set 25.40

1. 2 mL   2. 102 mL   3. 51 gtt/min   4. 306
mL/hr

Set 25.41

1. 2 mL   2. 202 mL   3. 50.5 or 51 gtt/min   4.
202 mL/hr

Set 25.42

1. 20 mL   2. 20 mL   3. 120 mL   4. 120 mL/hr

Set 25.43

1. 45 mL   2. 22.22 hr (22 hr, 13 min)

Set 25.44

1. 7.5 mL   2. 67.5 mL   3. 90 mL   4. 90 mL/hr

Set 25.45

1. 16 mL   2. 34 mL   3. 65 mL   4. 195 mL/hr

Set 25.46

1. 38 kg   2. 684 units   3. 14 mL/hr

Set 25.47

1. 10 mL   2. 0.004 mg/mL   3. 4 mcg/mL   4.
1.25 mL/min   5. 75 mL/hr

Set 25.48

1. 12 mL   2. 1.2 mg/mL   3. 1200 mcg/mL   4.
700 mcg/min   5. 0.58 mL/min   6. 34.8 or 35
mL/hr

Set 25.49

1. 3040 units   2. 152 units   3. 852 units   4. 17
mL/hr

Set 25.50

1. 20 mL   2. 2 mg/mL   3. 40 mg/hr   4. 20
mL/hr

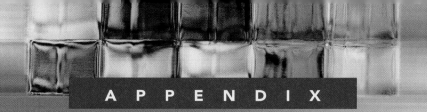

Solutions for Self-Evaluation and Review Tests

Self-Evaluation Test 9.1

1. $4 = 1.8°C + 32$
$4 - 32 = 1.8°C + 32 - 32$
$-28 = 1.8°C$
$C = -15.55 = -15.6°C$

2. $42 = 1.8°C + 32$
$42 - 32 = 1.8°C + 32 - 32$
$10 = 1.8°C$
$C = 5.6°C$

3. $50 = 1.8°C + 32$
$50 - 32 = 1.8°C + 32 - 32$
$18 = 1.8°C$
$C = 10°C$

4. $70 = 1.8°C + 32$
$70 - 32 = 1.8°C + 32 - 32$
$38 = 1.8°C$
$C = 21.1°C$

5. $102 = 1.8°C + 32$
$102 - 32 = 1.8°C + 32 - 32$
$70 = 1.8°C$
$C = 38.9°C$

6. $103 = 1.8°C + 32$
$103 - 32 = 1.8°C + 32 - 32$
$71 = 1.8°C$
$C = 39.4°C$

7. $98.6 = 1.8°C + 32$
$98.6 - 32 = 1.8°C - 32$
$66.6 = 1.8°C$
$C = 37°C$

8. $F = 1.8°C + 32$
$F = 1.8 \times 18 + 32$
$F = 32.4 + 32$
$F = 64.4°F$

9. $F = 1.8°C + 32$
$F = 1.8 \times 20 + 32$
$F = 36 + 32$
$F = 68°F$

10. $F = 1.8°C + 32$
$F = 1.8 \times 21 + 32$
$F = 37.8 + 32$
$F = 69.8°F$

11. $F = 1.8°C + 32$
    $F = 1.8 \times 32 + 32$
    $F = 57.6 + 32$
    $F = 89.6°F$

12. $F = 1.8°C + 32$
    $F = 1.8 \times 72 + 32$
    $F = 129.6 + 32$
    $F = 161.6°F$

13. $F = 1.8°C + 32$
    $F = 1.8 \times 96 + 32$
    $F = 172.8 + 32$
    $F = 204.8°F$

14. $F = 1.8°C + 32$
    $F = 1.8 \times 37.5 + 32$
    $F = 67.5 + 32$
    $F = 99.5°F$

15. $F = 1.8°C + 32$
    $F = 1.8 \times 39.6 + 32$
    $F = 71.28 + 32$
    $F = 103.3°F$

Self-Evaluation Test 9.2

1. $40 = 1.8°C + 32$
   $40 - 32 = 1.8°C + 32 - 32$
   $8 = 1.8°C$
   $C = 4.4°C$

2. $60 = 1.8°C + 32$
   $60 - 32 = 1.8°C + 32 - 32$
   $28 = 1.8°C$
   $C = 15.6°$

3. $81 = 1.8°C + 32$
   $81 - 32 = 1.8°C + 32 - 32$
   $49 = 1.8°C$
   $C = 27.2°C$

4. $97 = 1.8°C + 32$
   $97 - 32 = 1.8°C + 32 - 32$
   $65 = 1.8°C$
   $C = 36.1°C$

5. $101 = 1.8°C + 32$
   $101 - 32 = 1.8°C + 32 - 32$
   $69 = 1.8°C$
   $C = 38.3°C$

6. $99.8 = 1.8°C + 32$
   $99.8 - 32 = 1.8°C + 32 - 32$
   $67.8 = 1.8°C$
   $C = 37.7°C$

7. $-12 = 1.8°C + 32$
   $-12 - 32 = 1.8°C + 32 - 32$
   $-44 = 1.8°C$
   $C = -24.4°C$

8. $F = 1.8°C + 32$
   $F = 1.8 \times 15 + 32$
   $F = 27 + 32$
   $F = 59°F$

9. $F = 1.8°C + 32$
   $F = 1.8 \times 19 + 32$
   $F = 34.2 + 32$
   $F = 66.2°C$

10. $F = 1.8°C + 32$
    $F = 1.8 \times 29 + 32$
    $F = 52.2 + 32$
    $F = 84.2°F$

11. $F = 1.8°C + 32$
    $F = 1.8 \times 36 + 32$
    $F = 64.8 + 32$
    $F = 96.8°F$

12. $F = 1.8°C + 32$
    $F = 1.8 \times 39 + 32$
    $F = 70.2 + 32$
    $F = 102.2°F$

13. $F = 1.8°C + 32$
    $F = 1.8 \times 64 + 32$
    $F = 115.2 + 32$
    $F = 147.2°F$

14. $F = 1.8°C + 32$
    $F = 1.8 \times 22.2 + 32$
    $F = 39.96 + 32$
    $F = 71.96 = 72°F$

15. $F = 1.8°C + 32$
    $F = 1.8 \times 37.6 + 32$
    $F = 67.68 + 32$
    $F = 99.7°F \ (99.68)$

Self-Evaluation Test 10.1

1. 75 drops = 1 tsp

2. 3 tsp = 1 Tbs

$$\frac{3 \text{ tsp}}{1 \text{ Tbs}} = \frac{8 \text{ tsp}}{\text{x Tbs}}$$

$$3x = 8$$

$$x = 2\frac{2}{3} \text{ Tbs}$$

3. 8 oz = 1 cup

$$\frac{8 \text{ oz}}{1 \text{ cup}} = \frac{24 \text{ oz}}{\text{x cup}}$$

$$8x = 24$$

$$x = 3 \text{ cups}$$

4. 6 oz = 1 teacup

$$\frac{6 \text{ oz}}{1 \text{ teacup}} = \frac{24 \text{ oz}}{\text{x teacup}}$$

$$6x = 24$$

$$x = 4 \text{ teacups}$$

5. 2 Tbs = 1 oz

$$\frac{2 \text{ Tbs}}{1 \text{ oz}} = \frac{3 \text{ Tbs}}{\text{x oz}}$$

$$2x = 3$$

$$x = 1\frac{1}{2} \text{ oz}$$

6. 3 tsp = 1 Tbs

$$\frac{3 \text{ tsp}}{1 \text{ Tbs}} = \frac{8 \text{ tsp}}{\text{x Tbs}}$$

$$3x = 8$$

$$x = 2\frac{2}{3} \text{ Tbs}$$

then:

2 Tbs = 1oz

$$\frac{2 \text{ Tbs}}{1 \text{ oz}} = \frac{2\frac{2}{3} \text{ Tbs}}{\text{x oz}}$$

$$2x = 2\frac{2}{3}$$

$$x = 1\frac{1}{3} \text{ oz}$$

7. 1 cup = 8 oz

$$\frac{1 \text{ cup}}{8 \text{ oz}} = \frac{4 \text{ cups}}{\text{x oz}}$$

$$x = 32 \text{ oz}$$

8. 2 Tbs = 1 oz

$$\frac{2 \text{ Tbs}}{1 \text{ oz}} = \frac{8 \text{ Tbs}}{\text{x oz}}$$

$$2x = 8$$

$$x = 4 \text{ oz}$$

9. 75 gtt = 1 tsp

$$\frac{75 \text{ gtt}}{1 \text{ tsp}} = \frac{\text{x gtt}}{\frac{1}{2} \text{ gtt}}$$

$$x = 37\frac{1}{2} \text{ gtt}$$

10. 1 Tbs = 3 tsp

$$\frac{1 \text{ Tbs}}{3 \text{ tsp}} = \frac{4 \text{ Tbs}}{\text{x tsp}}$$

$$x = 12 \text{ tsp}$$

Self-Evaluation Test 10.2

1. 16 oz = 1 pound

$$\frac{16 \text{ oz}}{1 \text{ pound}} = \frac{\text{x oz}}{2 \text{ pounds}}$$

$$x = 32 \text{ oz}$$

2. 6 oz = 1 teacup

$$\frac{6 \text{ oz}}{1 \text{ teacup}} = \frac{\text{x oz}}{8 \text{ teacups}}$$

$$x = 48 \text{ oz}$$

3. $16 \text{ oz} = 1 \text{ pound}$

$$\frac{16 \text{ oz}}{1 \text{ pound}} = \frac{48 \text{ oz}}{\text{x pound}}$$

$$16x = 48$$

$$x = 3 \text{ pounds}$$

4. $8 \text{ oz} = 1 \text{ cup}$

$$\frac{8 \text{ oz}}{1 \text{ cup}} = \frac{32 \text{ oz}}{\text{x cups}}$$

$$8x = 32$$

$$x = 4 \text{ cups}$$

5. $2 \text{ Tbs} = 1 \text{ oz}$

$$\frac{2 \text{ Tbs}}{1 \text{ oz}} = \frac{\text{x Tbs}}{10 \text{ oz}}$$

$$x = 20 \text{ oz}$$

6. $75 \text{ gtt} = 1 \text{ tsp}$

$$\frac{75 \text{ gtt}}{1 \text{ tsp}} = \frac{45 \text{ gtt}}{\text{x tsp}}$$

$$75x = 45$$

$$x = \frac{3}{5} \text{ tsp}$$

7. $75 \text{ gtt} = 1 \text{ tsp}$

$$75 \times 2 = 150 \text{ gtt}$$

8. $8 \text{ oz} = 1 \text{ glass}$

$$\frac{8 \text{ oz}}{1 \text{ glass}} = \frac{16 \text{ oz}}{\text{x glass}}$$

$$8x = 16$$

$$x = 2 \text{ glasses}$$

9. $8 \text{ oz} = 1 \text{ cup}$

$$\frac{8 \text{ oz}}{1 \text{ cup}} = \frac{\text{x oz}}{3 \text{ cups}}$$

$$x = 24 \text{ oz}$$

10. $2 \text{ Tbs} = 1 \text{ oz}$

$$\frac{2 \text{ Tbs}}{1 \text{ oz}} = \frac{\text{x Tbs}}{3 \text{ oz}}$$

$$x = 6 \text{ Tbs}$$

Self-Evaluation Test 11.1

1. 80 drams   (8 drams = 1 oz $8 \times 10 = 80$)

2. 20 quarts   (4 quarts = 1 gallon $4 \times 5 = 20$)

3. 600 grains   (60 grains = 1 dram $10 \times 60 = 600$)

4. $\frac{3}{4}$ ounce $\left(8 \text{ drams} = 1 \text{ oz} \quad 6 \div 8 = \frac{3}{4}\right)$

5. 48 fluid ounces   (16 oz = 1 pt $3 \times 16 = 48$)

6. 30 grains $\left(60 \text{ gr} = 1 \text{ dr} \quad \frac{1}{2} \times 60 = 30\right)$

7. 90 grains $\left(60 \text{ gr} = 1 \text{ dr} \quad 1\frac{1}{2} \times 60 = 90\right)$

8. 480 grains   (60 gr = 1 dr $8 \times 60 = 480$)

9. 120 minims   (60 M = 1 dr $2 \times 60 = 120$)

10. 32 fluid drams   (8 fl dr = 1 fl oz $4 \times 8 = 32$)

11. 8 fluid ounces $\left(16 \text{ oz} = 1 \text{ pt} \quad \frac{1}{2} \times 16 = 8\right)$

12. $1\frac{1}{2}$ pints $\left(16 \text{ oz} = 1\text{pt} \quad 24 \div 16 = 1\frac{1}{2}\right)$

13. $\frac{1}{2}$ gallon $\left(4 \text{ qt} = 1 \text{ gal} \quad 2 \div 4 = \frac{1}{2}\right)$

14. 4 fluid ounces   (8 fl dr = 1 fl oz $32 \div 8 = 4$)

15. 2 drams   (60 gr = 1 dr $120 \div 60 = 2$)

Self-Evaluation Test 11.2

1. 80 fluid ounces $(16 \text{ fl oz} = 1 \text{ pt} \qquad 16 \times 5 = 80)$

2. 48 pints $(2 \text{ pts} = 1 \text{ qt}, 4 \text{ qt} = 1 \text{ gal} \qquad 2 \times 1 \times 4 \times 6 = 48)$

3. 40 drams $(8 \text{ dr} = 1 \text{ oz} \qquad 8 \times 5 = 40)$

4. 96 fluid ounces $(16 \text{ oz} = 1 \text{ pt}, 2 \text{ pt} = 1 \text{ qt} \qquad 16 \times 2 \times 3 = 96)$

5. $2\frac{1}{2}$ ounces $\left(8 \text{ dr} = 1 \text{ oz} \qquad 20 \div 8 = 2\frac{1}{2}\right)$

6. 40 pints $(2 \text{ pt} = 1 \text{ qt} \qquad 20 \times 2 = 40)$

7. 4 quarts $(1 \text{ qt} = 2 \text{ pt} \qquad 8 \div 2 = 4)$

8. $\frac{1}{2}$ fluid drams $\left(60 \text{ M} = 1 \text{ dr} \qquad 30 \div 60 = \frac{1}{2}\right)$

9. 16 quarts $(2 \text{ pts} = 1 \text{ qt} \qquad 32 \div 2 = 16)$

10. 2 fluid ounces $(8 \text{ dr} = 1 \text{ oz} \qquad 16 \div 8 = 2)$

11. 200 fluid drams $(1 \text{ oz} = 8 \text{ dr} \qquad 25 \times 8 = 200)$

12. 3 fluid ounces $(8 \text{ dr} = 1 \text{ oz} \qquad 24 \div 8 = 3)$

13. 45 grains $\left(1 \text{ dr} = 60 \text{ gr} \qquad \frac{3}{4} \times 60 = 45\right)$

14. 20 quarts $(1 \text{ gal} = 4 \text{ qt} \qquad 5 \times 4 = 20)$

15. 32 drams $(1 \text{ oz} = 8 \text{ dr} \qquad 4 \times 8 = 32)$

Self-Evaluation Test 12.1

1. $5 \text{ L} = 5000 \text{ mL}$ $5{,}000.$

2. $7 \text{ kg} = 7000 \text{ g}$ $7{,}000.$

3. $15 \text{ L} = 15{,}000 \text{ mL}$ $15{,}000.$

4. $10 \text{ g} = 10{,}000 \text{ mg}$ $10{,}000.$

5. $0.5 \text{ g} = 500 \text{ mg}$ $0{,}500.$

6. $375 \text{ g} = 0.375 \text{ kg}$ $0.375{,}$

7. $0.4 \text{ mg} = 400 \text{ mcg}$ $0{,}400.$

8. $750 \text{ mL} = 0.75 \text{ L}$ $0.750{,}$ delete extra 0

9. $250 \text{ mL} = 0.25 \text{ L}$ $0.250{,}$ delete extra 0

10. $100 \text{ mg} = 0.1 \text{ g}$ $0.100{,}$

11. $0.02 \text{ kg} = 20 \text{ g}$ $0{,}020.$

12. $45 \text{ mcg} = 0.045 \text{ mg}$ $0.045{,}$

13. $0.33 \text{ g} = 330 \text{ mg}$ $0{,}330.$

14. $0.01 \text{ mg} = 10 \text{ mcg}$ $0{,}010.$

15. $0.125 \text{ mg} = 125 \text{ mcg}$ $0{,}125.$

Self-Evaluation Test 12.2

1. 0.5 L = 500 mL $0\overset{\rightarrow}{.500.}$

2. 200 g = 0.2 kg $0.\overset{\leftarrow}{200.}_x$ delete extra 0

3. 0.25 g = 250 mg $0\overset{\rightarrow}{.250.}$

4. 90 mg = 0.09 g $0.\overset{\leftarrow}{090.}_x$ delete extra 0

5. 9.5 kg = 9500 g $9\overset{\rightarrow}{.500.}$

6. 100 μg = 0.1 mg $0.\overset{\leftarrow}{100.}_x$ delete extra 0

7. 850 mL = 0.850 L $0.\overset{\leftarrow}{850.}_x$ delete extra 0

8. 650 mg = 0.650 L $0.\overset{\leftarrow}{650.}_x$ delete extra 0

9. 60 mcg = 0.06 mg $0.\overset{\leftarrow}{060.}_x$ delete extra 0

10. 750 mg = 0.75 g $0.\overset{\leftarrow}{750.}_x$

11. 0.025 L = 25 mL $0\overset{\rightarrow}{.025.}$

12. 0.325 g = 325 mg $0\overset{\rightarrow}{.325.}$

13. 0.02 mg = 20 mcg $0\overset{\rightarrow}{.020.}$

14. 0.006 kg = 6 g $0\overset{\rightarrow}{.006.}$

15. 0.75 mcg = 750 mg $0\overset{\rightarrow}{.750.}$

Self-Evaluation Test 13.1

1. $\dfrac{1\,g}{16\,gr} = \dfrac{x\,g}{10\,gr}$

   $16x = 10$

   $x = 0.625\ (0.6)\ grams$

2. $\dfrac{30\,g}{1\,oz} = \dfrac{x\,g}{5\,oz}$ *or* $\dfrac{32\,g}{1\,oz} = \dfrac{x\,g}{5\,oz}$

   $x = 150\ grams$ $x = 160\ grams$

3. $\dfrac{15\,gr}{1\,g} = \dfrac{x\,gr}{0.5\,g}$

   $x = 7.5 \left(7\dfrac{1}{2}\right)\ grains$

4. $\dfrac{1\,oz}{30\,g} = \dfrac{x\,oz}{250\,g}$

   $30x = 250$

   $x = 8\ ounces$

5. $\dfrac{1\,dr}{4\,g} = \dfrac{x\,dr}{240\,g}$

   $4x = 240$

   $x = 60\ drams$

6. $\dfrac{1\,oz}{32\,g} = \dfrac{x\,oz}{640\,g}$

   $32x = 640$

   $x = 20\ ounces$

7. $\dfrac{1\,gr}{60\,mg} = \dfrac{x\,gr}{0.6\,mg}$

   $60x = 0.6$

   $x = gr\ \dfrac{1}{100}$

8. First, change 100 μg to mg by moving the decimal 3 places to the left or calculating

   $0.\overset{\leftarrow}{100.}_x = 0.1\ mg$ $\dfrac{1\,mg}{1000\,\mu g} = \dfrac{x\,mg}{100\,\mu}$

   $1000x = 100$

   $x = 0.1\ mg$

   then:

   $\dfrac{1\,gr}{60\,mg} = \dfrac{x\,gr}{0.1\,mg}$

   $60x = 0.1$

   $x = gr\ \dfrac{1}{600}$

9. $\dfrac{1\,gr}{60\,mg} = \dfrac{x\,gr}{180\,mg}$

   $60x = 180$

   $x = 3\ grains$

10. First, convert $gr\dfrac{1}{200}$ to mg:

$$\dfrac{60\,mg}{1\,gr} = \dfrac{x\,mg}{gr\dfrac{1}{200}}$$

x = 0.3 milligrams

Then convert 0.3 mg to mcg by moving the decimal three places to the

right $0{.}\overset{\longrightarrow}{300}.$ = 300 mcg or calculating:

$$\dfrac{1000\,\mu g}{1\,mg} = \dfrac{x\,\mu g}{0.3\,mg}$$

x = 300 micrograms

11. $\dfrac{60\,mg}{1\,gr} = \dfrac{x\,mg}{gr\dfrac{1}{6}}$

x = 10 milligrams

12. $\dfrac{15\,gr}{1\,g} = \dfrac{x\,gr}{10\,g}$ *or* $\dfrac{16\,gr}{1\,g} = \dfrac{x\,gr}{10\,g}$

x = 150 grains   x = 160 grains

13. $\dfrac{1\,kg}{2.2\,lb} = \dfrac{x\,kg}{8\,lb}$

2.2x = 8

x = 3.6 kilograms

14. $\dfrac{60\,mg}{1\,gr} = \dfrac{x\,mg}{60\,gr}$

x = 3600 milligrams

15. First, convert $gr\dfrac{1}{150}$ to mg:

$$\dfrac{gr\dfrac{1}{150}}{1\,gr} = \dfrac{x\,mg}{60\,mg}$$

x = 0.4 mg

Then convert 0.4 mg to mcg by moving the decimal three places to the right

$0{.}\overset{\longrightarrow}{400}.$ = 400 mcg or by calculating:

$$\dfrac{1000\,mcg}{1\,mg} = \dfrac{x\,mcg}{0.4\,mg}$$

x = 400 micrograms

Self-Evaluation Test 13.2

1. $\dfrac{30\,g}{1\,oz} = \dfrac{x\,g}{10\,oz}$ *or* $\dfrac{32\,g}{1\,oz} = \dfrac{x\,g}{10\,oz}$

x = 300 grams   x = 320 grams

2. $\dfrac{15\,gr}{1\,g} = \dfrac{x\,gr}{25\,g}$ *or* $\dfrac{16\,gr}{1\,g} = \dfrac{x\,gr}{25\,g}$

x = 375 grains   x = 400 grains

3. $\dfrac{30\,g}{1\,oz} = \dfrac{x\,g}{16\,oz}$

x = 480 grains

4. $\dfrac{30\,g}{1\,oz} = \dfrac{x\,g}{25\,oz}$

x = 750 grains

5. $\dfrac{60\,mg}{1\,gr} = \dfrac{x\,mg}{\dfrac{3}{4}\,gr}$

x = 45 milligrams

6. $\dfrac{1\,kg}{2.2\,lb} = \dfrac{x\,kg}{10\,lb}$

2.2x = 10

x = 4.5 kilograms

7. $\dfrac{60\,mg}{1\,gr} = \dfrac{x\,mg}{gr\dfrac{1}{8}}$

x = 7.5 = 8 milligrams

8. $\dfrac{1\,gr}{60\,mg} = \dfrac{x\,gr}{0.2\,mg}$

60x = 0.2

$x = gr\dfrac{1}{300}$

9. First change 600 μg to mg by moving the decimal three places to the left:

$0{.}\overset{\longleftarrow}{600}_x$ = 0.6 mg

$$\dfrac{1\,gr}{60\,mg} = \dfrac{x\,gr}{0.6\,mg}$$

60x = 0.6

$x = gr\dfrac{1}{100}$

10. $\dfrac{1\,gr}{60\,mg} = \dfrac{x\,gr}{0.4\,mg}$

60x = 0.4

$x = gr\dfrac{1}{150}$

11. $\dfrac{4\,g}{1\,dr} = \dfrac{x\,g}{4\,dr}$

x = 16 grams

12. $\dfrac{1\,g}{16\,gr} = \dfrac{x\,g}{8\,gr}$

16x = 8

x = 0.5 grams

13. $\dfrac{60\,mg}{1\,gr} = \dfrac{x\,mg}{25\,gr}$

x = 1500 milligrams

14. $\dfrac{4\,g}{1\,dr} = \dfrac{x\,g}{100\,dr}$

x = 400 grams

15. First convert $gr\,\dfrac{1}{300}$ to mg:

$\dfrac{gr\,\dfrac{1}{300}}{1\,gr} = \dfrac{x\,mg}{60\,mg}$

x = 0.2 mg

Then convert 0.2 mg to mcg by moving the decimal three places to the

$\longrightarrow$

right 0.200. = 200 mcg

Self-Evaluation Test 13.3

1. $\dfrac{15\,M}{1\,mL} = \dfrac{x\,M}{8\,mL}$ *or* $\dfrac{16\,M}{1\,mL} = \dfrac{x\,M}{8\,mL}$

x = 120 minims   x = 128 minims

2. $\dfrac{15\,M}{1\,mL} = \dfrac{x\,M}{15\,mL}$ *or* $\dfrac{16\,M}{1\,mL} = \dfrac{x\,M}{15\,mL}$

x = 225 minims   x = 240 minims

3. $\dfrac{1\,fl\,oz}{30\,mL} = \dfrac{x\,fl\,oz}{45\,mL}$

30x = 45

x = $1\dfrac{1}{2}$ fluid ounces

4. $\dfrac{30\,mL}{1\,fl\,oz} = \dfrac{x\,mL}{2\,fl\,oz}$ *or* $\dfrac{32\,mL}{1\,fl\,oz} = \dfrac{x\,mL}{2\,fl\,oz}$

x = 60 milliliters   x = 64 milliliters

5. $\dfrac{1\,fl\,oz}{30\,mL} = \dfrac{x\,fl\,oz}{600\,mL}$

30x = 600

x = 20 fluid ounces

6. $\dfrac{1000\,mL}{1\,qt} = \dfrac{x\,mL}{6\,qt}$

x = 6000 mL

7. $\dfrac{1\,pt}{500\,mL} = \dfrac{x\,pts}{1000\,mL}$

500x = 1000

x = 2 pints

8. $\dfrac{1\,qt}{1000\,mL} = \dfrac{x\,qt}{4500\,mL}$

1000x = 4500

x = $4\dfrac{1}{2}$ quarts

9. $\dfrac{1\,mL}{15\,M} = \dfrac{x\,mL}{8\,M}$

15x = 8

x = 0.5 milliliter

10. $\dfrac{1\,mL}{15\,M} = \dfrac{x\,mL}{6\,M}$

15x = 6

x = 0.4 milliliter

11. $\dfrac{4\,mL}{1\,dr} = \dfrac{x\,mL}{2\,dr}$

x = 8 milliliters

12. $\dfrac{4\,mL}{1\,dr} = \dfrac{x\,mL}{28\,dr}$

x = 112 milliliters

13. $\dfrac{1\,qt}{1000\,mL} = \dfrac{x\,qt}{5000\,mL}$

1000x = 5000

x = 5 quarts

14. $\dfrac{30\,mL}{1\,fl\,oz} = \dfrac{x\,mL}{48\,fl\,oz}$ *or* $\dfrac{32\,mL}{1\,fl\,oz} = \dfrac{x\,mL}{48\,fl\,oz}$

x = 1440 mL   x = 1536 mL

15. $\dfrac{0.5\,L}{16\,fl\,oz} = \dfrac{x\,L}{250\,fl\,oz}$

16x = 125

x = 7.8 (8) L

Self-Evaluation Test 13.4

1. $\dfrac{15\,M}{1\,mL} = \dfrac{x\,M}{10\,mL}$ *or* $\dfrac{16\,M}{1\,mL} = \dfrac{x\,M}{10\,mL}$

   x = 150 minims   x = 160 minims

2. $\dfrac{8\,fl\,dr}{32\,mL} = \dfrac{x\,fl\,dr}{60\,mL}$

   32x = 480

   x = 15 fluid drams

3. $\dfrac{15\,M}{1\,mL} = \dfrac{x\,M}{0.2\,mL}$

   x = 3 minims

4. $\dfrac{30\,mL}{1\,fl\,oz} = \dfrac{x\,mL}{4\,fl\,oz}$ *or* $\dfrac{32\,mL}{1\,fl\,oz} = \dfrac{x\,mL}{4\,fl\,oz}$

   x = 120 milliliters   x = 128 milliliters

5. $\dfrac{500\,mL}{1\,pt} = \dfrac{x\,mL}{4\,pt}$

   x = 2000 mL

6. $\dfrac{5\,L}{1\,L} = \dfrac{x\,fl\,oz}{32\,fl\,oz}$

   x = 160 fluid ounces

7. $\dfrac{4\,qt}{1\,qt} = \dfrac{x\,mL}{1000\,mL}$

   x = 4000 mL

8. $\dfrac{30\,mL}{1\,fl\,oz} = \dfrac{x\,mL}{30\,fl\,oz}$ *or* $\dfrac{32\,mL}{1\,fl\,oz} = \dfrac{x\,mL}{30\,fl\,oz}$

   x = 900 mL   x = 960 mL

9. $\dfrac{1\,qt}{1000\,mL} = \dfrac{x\,qt}{2500\,mL}$

   1000x = 2500

   $x = 2\dfrac{1}{2}$ quarts

10. $\dfrac{1\,mL}{15\,M} = \dfrac{x\,mL}{45\,M}$

    15x = 45

    x = 3 mL

11. $\dfrac{1\,mL}{15\,M} = \dfrac{x\,mL}{10\,M}$ *or* $\dfrac{1\,mL}{16\,M} = \dfrac{x\,mL}{10\,M}$

    15x = 10   16x = 10

    x = 0.66 = 0.7 mL   x = 0.6 mL

12. $\dfrac{15\,M}{1\,mL} = \dfrac{x\,M}{12\,mL}$ *or* $\dfrac{16\,M}{1\,mL} = \dfrac{x\,M}{12\,mL}$

    x = 180 minims   x = 192 minims

13. $\dfrac{1\,oz}{30\,mL} = \dfrac{x\,fl\,oz}{225\,mL}$

    30x = 225

    $x = 7.5\left(7\dfrac{1}{2}\right)$ fluid ounces

14. $\dfrac{4\,mL}{1\,fl\,dr} = \dfrac{x\,mL}{8\,fl\,dr}$

    x = 32 mL

15. $\dfrac{30\,mL}{1\,fl\,oz} = \dfrac{x\,mL}{64\,fl\,oz}$ *or* $\dfrac{32\,mL}{1\,fl\,oz} = \dfrac{x\,mL}{64\,fl\,oz}$

    x = 1920 mL   x = 2048 mL

Self-Evaluation Test 13.5

1. 5000 mL   (move decimal three places to the right) $5\overset{\rightarrow}{,}000.$

2. 300 gtt   (75 gtt = 1 teaspoon,   4 × 75 = 300)

3. 3 glasses   (8 oz = 1 glass,   24 ÷ 8 = 3)

4. 0.01 mg   (move decimal three places to the left) $\overset{\leftarrow}{.010}_x$

5. $\dfrac{1}{2}$ dram $\left(60\,grains = 1\,dram,\quad 30 \div 60 = \dfrac{1}{2}\right)$

6. 250 mL   (move the decimal three places to the right) $0\overset{\rightarrow}{,}250.$

7. 1250 mg   (move the decimal three places to the right) $\overrightarrow{1,250.}$

8. 1.5 kg   (move the decimal three places to the left) $\overleftarrow{1.500}_x$

9. 0.3 L   (move the decimal three places to the left) $\overleftarrow{0.300}_x$

10. 0.75 g   (move the decimal three places to the left) $\overleftarrow{0.750}_x$

11. 2.5 L   (move the decimal three places to the left) $\overleftarrow{2.500}_x$

12. 6 ounces   (8 dr = 1 oz,   48 ÷ 8 = 6)

13. 4 μg   (move decimal three places to the right) $\overrightarrow{0,004.}$

14. 4 teacups   (16 oz = 1 teacup,   24 ÷ 6 = 4)

15. 2 pt   (16 oz = 1 pt,   32 ÷ 16 = 2)

Self-Evaluation Test 13.6

1. 4000 mL   (move decimal three places to the right) $\overrightarrow{4,000.}$

2. 0.005 mg   (move decimal three places to the left) $\overleftarrow{.005}_x$

3. 7500 mg   (move decimal three places to the right) $\overrightarrow{7,500.}$

4. 6700 g   (move decimal three places to the right) $\overrightarrow{6,700.}$

5. 30 minims   (1 fl dr = 60 M,   60 ÷ 2 = 30)

6. 0.5 L   (move decimal three places to the left) $\overleftarrow{0.500}_x$

7. 2 fluid ounces   (8 dr = 1 fl oz,   16 ÷ 8 = 2)

8. 0.15 g   (move decimal three places to the left) $\overleftarrow{.150}_x$

9. 325 mg   (move decimal three places to the right) $\overrightarrow{0,325.}$

10. 15 μg   (move decimal three places to the right) $\overrightarrow{0,015.}$

11. 3.5 g   (move decimal three places to the left) $\overleftarrow{3.500}_x$

12. 4 fl oz $\left(1 \text{ glass} = 8 \text{ oz}, \quad \dfrac{1}{2} \times 8 = 4\right)$

13. 64 drams   (8 dr = 1 oz,   8 × 8 = 64)

14. 3 quarts   (32 oz = 1 qt,   96 ÷ 32 = 3)

15. 9 ounces $\left(6 \text{ oz} = 1 \text{ teacup}, \quad 1\dfrac{1}{2} \times 6 = 9\right)$

Review Test 16.1

1. $\dfrac{\dfrac{1}{100}\text{ gr}}{\dfrac{1}{200}\text{ gr}} = \dfrac{x \text{ tablets}}{1 \text{ tablet}}$

$\dfrac{1}{200}x = \dfrac{1}{100}$

x = 2 tablets

2. $\dfrac{0.75 \text{ mg}}{0.25 \text{ mg}} = \dfrac{x \text{ tablets}}{1 \text{ tablet}}$

0.25x = 0.75

x = 3 tablets

3. $\dfrac{0.5 \text{ mg}}{0.25 \text{ mg}} = \dfrac{x \text{ tablets}}{1 \text{ tablet}}$

0.25x = 0.5

x = 2 tablets

4. First convert 0.5 g to mg by moving the decimal three places to the right

$\overrightarrow{0,500.}$ = 500 mg or calculate:

$\dfrac{0.5 \text{ g}}{1 \text{ g}} = \dfrac{x \text{ mg}}{1000 \text{ mg}}$

x = 500 mg

then

$\dfrac{500 \text{ mg}}{250 \text{ mg}} = \dfrac{x \text{ mL}}{5 \text{ mL}}$

250x = 2500

x = 10 mL

5. First, convert 0.1 g to mg by moving the decimal three places to the right

$\overrightarrow{0,100.}$ = 100 mg or calculate:

$\dfrac{0.1 \text{ g}}{1 \text{ g}} = \dfrac{x \text{ mg}}{1000 \text{ mg}}$

x = 100 mg

then

$\dfrac{100 \text{ mg}}{50 \text{ mg}} = \dfrac{x \text{ tablets}}{1 \text{ tablet}}$

50x = 100

x = 2 tablets

6. First convert gr $1\frac{1}{2}$ to mg

$\dfrac{1\frac{1}{2}\text{ gr}}{1 \text{ gr}} = \dfrac{x \text{ mg}}{60 \text{ mg}}$

x = 90 mg

then

$\dfrac{90 \text{ mg}}{100 \text{ mg}} = \dfrac{x \text{ capsules}}{1 \text{ capsule}}$

100x = 90

x = 0.9 (give 1 capsule as you can't give 0.9 cap)

7. $\dfrac{10 \text{ mg}}{7.5 \text{ mg}} = \dfrac{x \text{ mL}}{15 \text{ mL}}$ $\qquad$ $\dfrac{667 \text{ mg}}{500 \text{ mg}} = \dfrac{x \text{ mL}}{15 \text{ mL}}$

$\qquad$ 7.5x = 150 $\qquad\qquad$ 500x = 10005

$\qquad\quad$ x = 20 mL $\qquad\qquad$ x = 20 mL

This documents that 20 mL of the drug will contain both 10 mg of hydrocodone and 667 mg of acetaminophen.

8. First, convert gr 5 to mg

$\dfrac{5 \text{ gr}}{1 \text{ gr}} = \dfrac{x \text{ mg}}{60 \text{ mg}}$

x = 300 mg

then

$\dfrac{300 \text{ mg}}{100 \text{ mg}} = \dfrac{x \text{ capsules}}{1 \text{ capsule}}$

100x = 300

x = 3 capsules

9. 1 gr = 60 mg

$\dfrac{60 \text{ mg}}{20 \text{ mg}} = \dfrac{x \text{ tablets}}{1 \text{ tablet}}$

20x = 60

x = 3 tablets

10. $\dfrac{0.25 \text{ mg}}{0.125 \text{ mg}} = \dfrac{x \text{ tablets}}{1 \text{ tablet}}$

0.125x = 0.25

x = 2 tablets

11. $\dfrac{12 \text{ mEq}}{8 \text{ mEq}} = \dfrac{x \text{ mL}}{5 \text{ mL}}$

$8x = 60$

$x = 7.5 \text{ mL}$

12. First convert 0.01 g to mg by moving the decimal three places to the right

$\overrightarrow{0.010.} = 10 \text{ mg}$ or calculate:

$\dfrac{0.01 \text{ g}}{1 \text{ g}} = \dfrac{x \text{ mg}}{1000 \text{ mg}}$

$x = 10 \text{ mg}$

then

$\dfrac{10 \text{ mg}}{5 \text{ mg}} = \dfrac{x \text{ tablets}}{1 \text{ tablet}}$

$5x = 10$

$x = 2 \text{ tablets}$

13. $\dfrac{6 \text{ mg}}{4 \text{ mg}} = \dfrac{x \text{ tablets}}{1 \text{ tablet}}$

$4x = 6$

$x = 1\dfrac{1}{2} \text{ tablets}$

14. First convert 0.3 g to mg by moving the decimal three places to the right

$\overrightarrow{0.300.} = 300 \text{ mg}$ or calculate:

$\dfrac{0.3 \text{ g}}{1 \text{ g}} = \dfrac{x \text{ mg}}{1000 \text{ mg}}$

$x = 300 \text{ mg}$

then

$\dfrac{300 \text{ mg}}{150 \text{ mg}} = \dfrac{x \text{ tablets}}{1 \text{ tablet}}$

$150x = 300$

$x = 2 \text{ tablets}$

15. $\dfrac{37.5 \text{ mg}}{25 \text{ mg}} = \dfrac{x \text{ tablets}}{1 \text{ tablet}}$

$25x = 37.5$

$x = 1\dfrac{1}{2} \text{ tablets}$

Review Test 16.2

1. $\dfrac{75 \text{ mg}}{50 \text{ mg}} = \dfrac{x \text{ tablets}}{1 \text{ tablet}}$

$50x = 75$

$x = 1.5 \left(1\dfrac{1}{2}\right) \text{ tablets}$

2. First convert 0.5 g to mg by moving the decimal three places to the right

$\overrightarrow{0.500.} = 500 \text{ mg}$

$\dfrac{500 \text{ mg}}{250 \text{ mg}} = \dfrac{x \text{ tablets}}{1 \text{ tablet}}$

$250x = 500$

$x = 2 \text{ tablets}$

3. $\dfrac{300 \text{ mg}}{15 \text{ mg}} = \dfrac{x \text{ mL}}{1 \text{ mL}}$

$15x = 300$

$x = 20 \text{ mL}$

4. $60 \text{ mg} = 1 \text{ grain}$

$\dfrac{60 \text{ mg}}{15 \text{ mg}} = \dfrac{x \text{ mL}}{5 \text{ mL}}$

$15x = 300$

$x = 20 \text{ mL}$

5. $\dfrac{10 \text{ mg}}{2.5 \text{ mg}} = \dfrac{x \text{ tablets}}{1 \text{ tablet}}$

$2.5x = 10$

$x = 4 \text{ tablets}$

6. $\dfrac{2 \text{ mg}}{4 \text{ mg}} = \dfrac{x \text{ tablets}}{1 \text{ tablet}}$

$4x = 2$

$x = \dfrac{1}{2} \text{ tablet}$

7. $\dfrac{3.75 \text{ mg}}{1.25 \text{ mg}} = \dfrac{x \text{ tablets}}{1 \text{ tablet}}$

$1.25x = 3.75$

$x = 3 \text{ tablets}$

8. First, convert 0.375 g to mg by moving the decimal three places to the right

$\overrightarrow{0.375.}$ = 375 mg or calculate:

$$\frac{0.375 \text{ g}}{1 \text{ g}} = \frac{x \text{ mg}}{1000 \text{ mg}}$$

x = 375 mg

then

$$\frac{375 \text{ mg}}{250 \text{ mg}} = \frac{x \text{ tablets}}{1 \text{ tablet}}$$

250x = 375

$x = 1.5 \left(1\frac{1}{2}\right)$ tablets

9. $$\frac{1{,}000{,}000 \text{ U}}{500{,}000 \text{ U}} = \frac{x \text{ tablets}}{1 \text{ tablet}}$$

500,000x = 1,000,000

x = 2 tablets

10. $$\frac{10 \text{ mg}}{5 \text{ mg}} = \frac{x \text{ mL}}{5 \text{ mL}}$$

5x = 50

x = 10 mL

11. First convert gr $\frac{1}{4}$ to mg

$$\frac{\frac{1}{4} \text{ gr}}{1 \text{ gr}} = \frac{x \text{ mg}}{60 \text{ mg}}$$

x = 15 mg

then

$$\frac{15 \text{ mg}}{20 \text{ mg}} = \frac{x \text{ mL}}{10 \text{ mL}}$$

20x = 150

x = 7.5 mL

12. First, convert 0.2 g to mg by moving the decimal three places to the right

$\overrightarrow{0.200.}$ = 200 mg or calculate:

$$\frac{0.2 \text{ g}}{1 \text{ g}} = \frac{x \text{ mg}}{1000 \text{ mg}}$$

x = 200 mg

then

$$\frac{200 \text{ mg}}{100 \text{ mg}} = \frac{x \text{ tablets}}{1 \text{ tablet}}$$

100x = 200

x = 2 tablets

13. $$\frac{600 \text{ mg}}{300 \text{ mg}} = \frac{x \text{ mL}}{5 \text{ mL}}$$

300x = 3000

x = 10 mL

14. $$\frac{30 \text{ mg}}{20 \text{ mg}} = \frac{x \text{ mL}}{5 \text{ mL}}$$

20x = 150

$x = 7.5 \left(7\frac{1}{2}\right)$ mL

15. $$\frac{12.5 \text{ mg}}{5 \text{ mg}} = \frac{x \text{ tablets}}{1 \text{ tablet}}$$

5x = 12.5

$x = 2.5 \left(2\frac{1}{2}\right)$ tablets

Review Test 17.1

1. $\dfrac{12\,mg}{15\,mg} = \dfrac{x\,mL}{1\,mL}$

   $15x = 12$

   $x = 0.8\,mL$

2. $\dfrac{60\,mg}{80\,mg} = \dfrac{x\,mL}{2\,mL}$

   $80x = 120$

   $x = 1.5\,mL$

3. $\dfrac{50\,mg}{100\,mg} = \dfrac{x\,mL}{1\,mL}$

   $100x = 50$

   $x = 0.5\,mL$

4. $1\,gram = 1000\,mg$

   $\dfrac{500\,mg}{1000\,mg} = \dfrac{x\,mL}{3\,mL}$

   $1000x = 1500$

   $x = 1.5\,mL$

5. $\dfrac{75\,mg}{50\,mg} = \dfrac{x\,mL}{1\,mL}$

   $50x = 75$

   $x = 1.5\,mL$

6. 40 units

   $\dfrac{40\,U}{100\,U} = \dfrac{x\,mL}{1\,mL}$

   $100x = 40$

   $x = 0.4\,mL$

7. 5 units

   $\dfrac{5\,U}{100\,U} = \dfrac{x\,mL}{1\,mL}$

   $100x = 5$

   $x = 0.05\,mL$

8. $\dfrac{750,000\,U}{500,000\,U} = \dfrac{x\,mL}{1\,mL}$

   $500,000x = 750,000$

   $x = 1.5\,mL$

9. $\dfrac{0.17\,mg}{0.1\,mg} = \dfrac{x\,mL}{1\,mL}$

   $0.1x = 0.17$

   $x = 1.7\,mL$

10. $\dfrac{4000\,U}{5000\,U} = \dfrac{x\,mL}{1\,mL}$

    $5000x = 4000$

    $x = 0.8\,mL$

11. $\dfrac{7500\,U}{10,000\,U} = \dfrac{x\,mL}{1\,mL}$

    $10,000x = 7500$

    $x = 0.75\,mL$

12. 85 units

    $\dfrac{85\,U}{100\,U} = \dfrac{x\,mL}{1\,mL}$

    $100x = 85$

    $x = 0.85\,mL$

13. $\dfrac{0.5\,mg}{2\,mg} = \dfrac{x\,mL}{1\,mL}$

    $2x = 0.5$

    $x = 0.25\,mL$

14. $\dfrac{240\,mg}{125\,mg} = \dfrac{x\,mL}{1\,mL}$

    $125x = 240$

    $x = 1.9\,mL$

15. $\dfrac{750\,mg}{285\,mg} = \dfrac{x\,mL}{1\,mL}$

    $285x = 750$

    $x = 2.6\,mL$

Review Test 17.2

1. $\dfrac{65\,mg}{100\,mg} = \dfrac{x\,mL}{2\,mL}$

   $100x = 130$

   $x = 1.3\ mL$

2. $1\ gram = 1000\ mg$

   $\dfrac{800\,mg}{1000\,mg} = \dfrac{x\,mL}{2.5\,mL}$

   $1000x = 2000$

   $x = 2\ mL$

3. $\dfrac{25\,mg}{40\,mg} = \dfrac{x\,mL}{4\,mL}$

   $40x = 100$

   $x = 2.5\ mL$

4. $\dfrac{0.5\,g}{1\,g} = \dfrac{x\,mL}{2\,mL}$

   $x = 1\ mL$

5. First, change 0.1 mg to mcg by moving the decimal three places to the right

   $\overrightarrow{0.100.}$ = 100 mcg or calculate:

   $\dfrac{0.1\,mg}{1\,mg} = \dfrac{x\,mcg}{1000\,mcg}$

   $x = 100\ mcg$

   then

   $\dfrac{100\,mcg}{50\,mcg} = \dfrac{x\,mL}{1\,mL}$

   $50x = 100$

   $x = 2\ mL$

6. First, change gr $\dfrac{3}{4}$ to mg

   $\dfrac{\frac{3}{4}\,gr}{1\,gr} = \dfrac{x\,mg}{60\,mg}$

   $x = 45\ mg$

   then

   $\dfrac{45\,mg}{60\,mg} = \dfrac{x\,mL}{1\,mL}$

   $60x = 45$

   $x = 0.75\ (0.8)\ mL$

7. $\dfrac{750,000\,U}{500,000\,U} = \dfrac{x\,mL}{1\,mL}$

   $500,000x = 750,000$

   $x = 1.5\ mL$

8. $\dfrac{5000\,U}{7500\,U} = \dfrac{x\,mL}{1\,mL}$

   $7500x = 5000$

   $x = 0.66\ (0.7)\ mL$

9. $\dfrac{150,000\,U}{100,000\,U} = \dfrac{x\,mL}{1\,mL}$

   $100,000x = 150,000$

   $x = 1.5\ mL$

10. $\dfrac{8000\,U}{10,000\,U} = \dfrac{x\,mL}{1\,mL}$

    $10,000x = 8000$

    $x = 0.8\ mL$

11. 20 units

    $\dfrac{20\,U}{100\,U} = \dfrac{x\,mL}{1\,mL}$

    $100x = 20$

    $x = 0.2\ mL$

12. 70 units

    $\dfrac{70\,U}{100\,U} = \dfrac{x\,mL}{1\,mL}$

    $100x = 70$

    $x = 0.7\ mL$

13. $\dfrac{750\,mg}{270\,mg} = \dfrac{x\,mL}{1\,mL}$

    $270x = 750$

    $x = 2.77\ (2.8)\ mL$

14. $\dfrac{250\,mg}{100\,mg} = \dfrac{x\,mL}{1\,mL}$

    $100x = 250$

    $x = 2.5\ mL$

15. $\dfrac{2.5\,mg}{1\,mg} = \dfrac{x\,mL}{0.5\,mL}$

    $x = 1.25\ mL$

Review Test 18.1

1. a) $\dfrac{10\,g}{100\,mL} = \dfrac{x\,g}{500\,mL}$

   $100x = 5000$

   $x = 50$ g of dextrose

   b) $\dfrac{0.9\,g}{100\,mL} = \dfrac{x\,g}{500\,mL}$

   $100x = 450$

   $x = 4.5$ g of sodium chloride

2. $\dfrac{5\,g}{100\,mL} = \dfrac{x\,g}{1000\,mL}$

   $100x = 5000$

   $x = 50$ g dextrose

3. a) 3000 mL ÷ 24 hr = 125 mL/hr

   b) $\dfrac{1\,min}{60\,min} = \dfrac{x\,mL}{125\,mL}$

   $60x = 125$

   $x = 2.08$ mL/min

   c) 2.08 mL/min

   $\underline{\times\ 10\ \text{drop factor}}$

   20.8 = 21 gtt/min

4. a) 1500 mL ÷ 24 hr = 62.5 mL/hr

   b) $\dfrac{1\,min}{60\,min} = \dfrac{x\,mL}{62.5\,mL}$

   $60x = 62.5$

   $x = 1.04$ mL/min

   c) 1.04 mL/min

   $\underline{\times\ 60\ \text{drop factor}}$

   62.4 = 62 gtt/min

5. a) 2000 mL ÷ 24 hr = 83.3 mL/hr

   b) $\dfrac{1\,min}{60\,min} = \dfrac{x\,mL}{83.3}$

   $60x = 83.3$

   $x = 1.388 = 1.39$ mL/min

   c) 1.39 mL/min

   $\underline{\times\ 20\ \text{drop factor}}$

   27.8 = 28 gtt/min

6. a) 1000 mL ÷ 24 hr = 41.6 mL/hr

   b) $\dfrac{1\,min}{60\,min} = \dfrac{x\,mL}{41.6\,mL}$

   $60x = 41.6$

   $x = 0.69$ mL/min

   c) 0.69 mL/min

   $\underline{\times\ 10\ \text{drop factor}}$

   6.9 = 7 gtt/min

7. a) 75 ml ÷ 1 hr = 75 mL/hr

   b) $\dfrac{1\,min}{60\,min} = \dfrac{x\,mL}{75\,mL}$

   $60x = 75$

   $x = 1.25$ mL/min

   c) 1.25 mL/min

   $\underline{\times\ 60\ \text{drop factor}}$

   75 gtt/min

8. a) $\dfrac{1\,min}{60\,min} = \dfrac{x\,mL}{80\,mL}$

   $60x = 80$

   $x = 1.33$ mL/min

   b) 1.33 mL/min

   $\underline{\times\ 60\ \text{drop factor}}$

   79.9 = 80 gtt/min

   c) $\dfrac{1\,hr}{80\,mL} = \dfrac{x\,hr}{1500\,mL}$

   $80x = 1500$

   $x = 18.75 = 18$ hr, 45 min

9. a) $\dfrac{1\,min}{60\,min} = \dfrac{x\,mL}{60\,mL}$

   $60x = 60$

   $x = 1$ mL/min

   b) 1 × 60 = 60 gtt/min

   c) $\dfrac{1\,hr}{60\,mL} = \dfrac{x\,hr}{750\,mL}$

   $60x = 750$

   $x = 12.5 = 12$ hr, 30 min

10. a) $\dfrac{1\,min}{60\,min} = \dfrac{x\,mL}{75\,mL}$

    $60x = 75$

    $x = 1.25$ mL/min

    b) 1.25

    $\underline{\times\ 20}$

    25 gtt/min

    c) $\dfrac{1\,hr}{75\,mL} = \dfrac{x\,hr}{1000\,mL}$

    $75x = 1000$

    $x = 13.3 = 13$ hours 20 min

Review Test 18.2

1. $\dfrac{5\,g}{100\,mL} = \dfrac{x\,g}{1500\,mL}$

   a) $100x = 7500$

   $x = 75$ g of dextrose

   b) $\dfrac{0.45\ g}{100\ mL} = \dfrac{x\,g}{1500\,mL}$

   $100x = 675$

   $x = 6.75$ g of sodium chloride

2. $\dfrac{20\,g}{100\,mL} = \dfrac{x\,g}{1000\,mL}$

   $100x = 2000$

   $x = 200$ g of dextrose

3. a) $1000\ ml \div 12\ hr = 83.3$ mL/hr

   $\dfrac{1\,min}{60\,min} = \dfrac{x\ mL}{83.3\ mL}$

   b) $60x = 83.3$

   $x = 1.39$ mL/min

   c) 1.39 mL/min

   $\underline{\times\ 15\ \text{drop factor}}$

   $20.82 = 21$ gtt/min

4. a) $2500\ mL \div 24\ hr = 104.16$ mL/hr

   b) $\dfrac{1\,min}{60\,min} = \dfrac{x\ mL}{104.16\ mL}$

   $60x = 104.16$

   $x = 1.736$ or 1.74 mL/min

   c) 1.74 mL/min

   $\underline{\times\ 10\ \text{drop factor}}$

   $17.36 = 17$ gtt/min

5. a) $1000\ mL \div 24\ hr = 41.67$ mL/hr

   b) $\dfrac{1\,min}{60\,min} = \dfrac{x\ mL}{41.67 mL}$

   $60x = 41.7$

   $x = 0.69$ mL/min

   c) 0.69 mL/min

   $\underline{\times\ 60\ \text{drop factor}}$

   $41.67 = 42$ gtt/min

6. a) $500\ mL \div 24\ hr = 20.83$ mL/hr

   b) $\dfrac{1\,min}{60\,min} = \dfrac{x\ mL}{20.83\ mL}$

   $60x = 20.83$

   $x = 0.347 = 0.35$ mL/min

   c) 0.347 mL/min

   $\underline{\times\ 20\ \text{drop factor}}$

   6.94 (7 gtt/min)

   or

   0.35 mL/min

   $\underline{\times\ 20\ \text{drop factor}}$

   7 gtt/min

7. a) 50 mL/hr

   b) $\dfrac{1\,min}{60\,min} = \dfrac{x\,mL}{50\,mL}$

   $60x = 50$

   $x = 0.83$ mL/min

   c) 0.83 mL/min

   $\underline{\times\ 60\ \text{drop factor}}$

   $49.9 = 50$ gtt/min

8. a) $\dfrac{1\,min}{60\,min} = \dfrac{x\ mL}{125\,mL}$

   $60x = 125$

   $x = 2.08$ mL/min

   b) 2.08 mL/min

   $\underline{\times\ 10\ \text{drop factor}}$

   $20.8 = 21$ gtt/min

   c) $\dfrac{1\,hr}{125\,mL} = \dfrac{x\ hr}{1500\ mL}$

   $125x = 1500$

   $x = 12$ hours

9. a) $\dfrac{1\,\text{min}}{60\,\text{min}} = \dfrac{x\,\text{mL}}{60\,\text{mL}}$

$60x = 60$

$x = 1\ \text{mL/min}$

b) $1\ \text{mL/min}$

$\underline{\times\ 10\ \text{drop factor}}$

$10\ \text{gtt/min}$

c) $\dfrac{1\,\text{hr}}{60\,\text{mL}} = \dfrac{x\,\text{hr}}{1000\,\text{mL}}$

$60x = 1000$

$x = 16.67 = 16\ \text{hr},\ 40\ \text{min}$

10. $\dfrac{1\,\text{min}}{60\,\text{min}} = \dfrac{x\,\text{mL}}{50\,\text{mL}}$

a) $60x = 50$

$x = 0.83\ \text{mL/min}$

b) $0.83\ \text{mL/min}$

$\underline{\times\ 60\ \text{drop factor}}$

$49.8 = 50\ \text{gtt/min}$

c) $\dfrac{1\,\text{hr}}{50\,\text{mL}} = \dfrac{x\,\text{hr}}{1500\,\text{mL}}$

$50x = 1500$

$x = 30\ \text{hours}$

Review Test 19.1

1. $\dfrac{500\,\text{mg}}{500\,\text{mg}} = \dfrac{x\,\text{mL}}{1\,\text{mL}}$

$500x = 500$

a) $x = 1\ \text{mL}$

b) $1001 \div 8 = 125.1 \div 6 = 20.8$
$= 21\ \text{gtt/min}$

c) $1001 \div 8 = 125.1 = 125\ \text{mL/hr}$

2. $\dfrac{45\,\text{mEq}}{40\,\text{mEq}} = \dfrac{x\,\text{mL}}{20\,\text{mL}}$

$40x = 900$

a) $x = 22.5\ \text{mL}$

b) $\dfrac{1.5\,\text{mL}}{1\,\text{mL}} = \dfrac{x\,\text{gtts}}{60\,\text{gtts}}$

$x = 90\ \text{gtt/min}$

c) $90 \times 1 = 90\ \text{mL/hr}$

3. $\dfrac{300\,\text{mg}}{300\,\text{mg}} = \dfrac{x\,\text{mL}}{2\,\text{mL}}$

$300x = 600$

a) $x = 2\ \text{mL}$

b) $100 + 2 = 102\ \text{mL}$

c) $102 \div 6 = 17\ \text{gtt/min}$

d) $102 \times 1 = 102\ \text{mL/hr}$

e) $3000 \div 20 = 150 \div 6 = 25\ \text{gtt/min}$

f) $3000 \div 20 = 150\ \text{mL/hr}$ (24 hr $-$ 4 hr for IVPB = 20 hr)

4. $\dfrac{375\,\text{mg}}{250\,\text{mg}} = \dfrac{x\,\text{mL}}{5\,\text{mL}}$

a) $250x = 1875$

$x = 7.5\ \text{mL}$

b) $100 + 7.5 = 107.5$

c) $107.5 \div 1 = 107.5 = 108\ \text{gtt/min}$

d) $107.5 \times 1 = 107.5 = 108\ \text{mL/hr}$

5. $\dfrac{8000\,\text{U}}{10{,}000\,\text{U}} = \dfrac{x\,\text{mL}}{1\,\text{mL}}$

$10{,}000x = 8000$

a) $x = 0.8\ \text{mL}$

b) $500 \div 4 = 125\ \text{gtt/min}$

c) $125 \times 1 = 125\ \text{mL/hr}$

6. $\dfrac{4\,\text{g}}{4\,\text{g}} = \dfrac{x\,\text{mL}}{40\,\text{mL}}$

$4x = 160$

a) $x = 40\ \text{mL}$

b) $250 + 40 = 290\ \text{mL}$

c) $\dfrac{2\,\text{mL}}{290\,\text{mL}} = \dfrac{x\,\text{g}}{4\,\text{g}}$

$290x = 8$

$x = 0.02759\ \text{grams}$

d) $\dfrac{60\,\text{gtt}}{1\,\text{min}} = \dfrac{x\,\text{gtt}}{2\,\text{mL}}$

$x = 120\ \text{gtt/min}$

e) $\dfrac{60\,\text{min}}{1\,\text{min}} = \dfrac{x\,\text{mL}}{2\,\text{mL}}$

$x = 120\ \text{mL/hr}$

7. a) $\dfrac{100\,mg}{50\,mg} = \dfrac{x\,mL}{1\,mL}$

   $50x = 100$

   $x = 2\,mL$

   b) $150 - 2 = 148\,mL$

   c) $150 + 15 = 165\,mL$

   d) $165 \div 1 = 165\,mL/hr$

8. a) $\dfrac{5\,mg}{5\,mg} = \dfrac{x\,mL}{1\,mL}$

   $5x = 5$

   $x = 1\,mL$

   b) $\dfrac{5\,mg}{1\,mg} = \dfrac{x\,mg}{1000\,mcg}$

   $x = 5000\,mcg$

   $\dfrac{1\,mL}{1000\,mL} = \dfrac{x\,mcg}{5000\,mcg}$

   $1000x = 5000\,mcg$

   $x = 5\,mcg$

   c) $\dfrac{1\,hour}{12\,hours} = \dfrac{x\,mL}{1000\,mL}$

   $12x = 1000$

   $x = 83\,mL/hour$

   or

   $1000\,mL \div 12 = 83\,mL/hour$

   d) $83 \div 6 = 13.8$ or $14\,gtt/min$

   e) $\dfrac{1\,min}{60\,min} = \dfrac{x\,mL}{83\,mL}$

   $60x = 83$

   $x = 1.38$ or $1.4\,mL/min$

9. a) $\dfrac{20\,mg}{10\,mg} = \dfrac{x\,mL}{1\,mL}$

   $10x = 20$

   $x = 2\,mL$

   b) $50\,mL\,D5W + 2\,mL = 52\,mL$

   $\dfrac{1\,min}{20\,min} = \dfrac{x\,mL}{52\,mL}$

   $20x = 52$

   $x = 2.6\,mL / min$

   $\dfrac{2.6\,mL}{1\,mL} = \dfrac{x\,gtt}{10\,mL}$

   $x = 26\,gtt / min$

   c) $\dfrac{60\,min\,(1\,hr)}{20\,min} = \dfrac{x\,mL}{52\,mL}$

   $20x = 3120$

   $x = 156\,mL / hr$

10. a) $\dfrac{6\,mg}{2\,mg} = \dfrac{x\,mL}{1\,mL}$

    $2x = 6$

    $x = 3\,mL$

    b) $50\,mL\,D5W + 3\,mL = 53\,mL$

    $\dfrac{1\,min}{30\,min} = \dfrac{x\,mL}{53\,mL}$

    $30x = 53\,mL$

    $x = 1.8\,mL/min$

    $\dfrac{1.8\,mL}{1\,mL} = \dfrac{x\,gtt}{15\,gtt}$

    $x = 26.5$ or $27\,gtt/min$

    c) $\dfrac{60\,min\,(1\,hr)}{30\,min} = \dfrac{x\,mL}{53\,mL}$

    $30x = 3180$

    $x = 106\,mL / hr$

Review Test 19.2

1. a) $\dfrac{1\,mL}{1000\,mL} = \dfrac{x\,mEq}{20\,mEq}$

   $1000x = 20$

   $x = 0.02\,mEq/mL$

   b) $\dfrac{2\,mEq}{0.02\,mEq} = \dfrac{x\,mL}{1\,mL}$

   $0.02x = 2$

   $x = 100\,mL$

   c) $100 \times 1 = 100\,mL/hr$

2. a) $5\,mL$

   b) $1000 + 5 = 1005\,mL$

   c) $75 \div 6 = 12.5$ ($13\,gtt/min$)

   d) $75 \times 1 = 75\,mL/hr$

3. a) $3\,mL$

   b) $50 + 3 = 53\,mL$

   c) $53 \div 20 \times 60 = 159\,gtt/min$

   d) $53 \div 20 \times 60 = 159\,mL/hr$

4. $\dfrac{50\,\text{mg}}{50\,\text{mg}} = \dfrac{x\,\text{mL}}{2\,\text{mL}}$

$50x = 100$

a) $x = 2$ mL

b) $50 + 2 = 52$ mL

c) $52 \div 15 \times 10 = 34.6 = 35$ gtt/min

d) $52 \div 15 \times 60 = 207.9 = 208$ mL/hr

5. $\dfrac{100\,\text{U}}{100\,\text{U}} = \dfrac{x\,\text{mL}}{1\,\text{mL}}$

a) $100x = 100$

   $x = 1$ mL

b) $500 + 1 = 501$ mL

c) $\dfrac{1\,\text{mL}}{501\,\text{mL}} = \dfrac{x\,\text{U}}{100\,\text{U}}$

   $501x = 100$

   $x = 0.19 = 0.2$ U/mL

d) $\dfrac{12\,\text{U}}{0.2\,\text{U}} = \dfrac{x\,\text{mL}}{1\,\text{mL}}$

   $0.2x = 12$

   $x = 60$ mL

e) $60 \div 1 = 60$ gtt/min

f) $60 \times 1 = 60$ mL/hr

6. $\dfrac{900\,\text{mg}}{150\,\text{mg}} = \dfrac{x\,\text{mL}}{1\,\text{mL}}$

$150x = 900$

a) $x = 6$ mL

b) $1000 + 6 = 1006$ mL

c) $\dfrac{1\,\text{mL}}{1006\,\text{mL}} = \dfrac{x\,\text{mg}}{900\,\text{mg}}$

   $1006x = 900$

   $x = 0.89 = 0.9$ mg/mL

d) $\dfrac{37\,\text{mg}}{0.9\,\text{mg}} = \dfrac{x\,\text{mL}}{1\,\text{mL}}$

   $0.9x = 37$

   $x = 41.1$ mL

e) $41.1 \div 1 = 41$ gtt/min $= 41$ gtt/min

f) $41.1 \times 1 = 41.1$ mL/hr $= 41$ mL/hr

7. a) 3000 mL $= 3$ L

   $\dfrac{1\,\text{L}}{3\,\text{L}} = \dfrac{x\,\text{units}}{15{,}000{,}000\,\text{units}}$

   $3x = 15{,}000{,}000$

   $x = 5{,}000{,}000$ units

b) $\dfrac{5{,}000{,}000\,\text{units}}{1{,}000{,}000\,\text{units}} = \dfrac{x\,\text{mL}}{1\,\text{mL}}$

   $1{,}000{,}000x = 5{,}000{,}000$

   $x = 5$ mL

c) $\dfrac{1\,\text{L}}{3\,\text{L}} = \dfrac{x\,\text{hr}}{24\,\text{hr}}$

   $3x = 24$

   $x = 8$ hr to infuse 1 L

   1000 mL D5W $+ 5$ mL $= 1005$ mL

   $\dfrac{1\,\text{hr}}{8\,\text{hr}} = \dfrac{x\,\text{mL}}{1005\,\text{mL}}$

   $8x = \dfrac{1005}{126\,\text{mL/hr}}$

d) $\dfrac{1\,\text{min}}{60\,\text{min}} = \dfrac{x\,\text{mL}}{126\,\text{mL}}$

   $60x = 126$

   $x = 2.1$ mL/min

   $\dfrac{2.1\,\text{mL}}{1\,\text{mL}} = \dfrac{x\,\text{gtt}}{10\,\text{gtt}}$

   $x = 21$ gtt/min

e) $\dfrac{1\,\text{hr}}{8\,\text{hr}} = \dfrac{x\,\text{mL}}{1005\,\text{mL}}$

   $8x = 1005$

   $x = 126$ mL/hr

8. $\dfrac{200\,\text{mL}}{500\,\text{mL}} = \dfrac{x\,\text{mL}}{10\,\text{mL}}$

$500x = 2000$

a) $x = 4$ mL

b) $50 - 4 = 46$ mL

c) $50 + 15 = 65$ mL

d) $65 \times 1 = 65$ mL/hr

9. a) $\dfrac{85 \text{ mg}}{10 \text{ mg}} = \dfrac{x \text{ mL}}{1 \text{ mL}}$

$10x = 85$

$x = 8.5 \text{ mL}$

b) 100 mL D5/W + 8.5 mL Retrovir

= 108.5 or 109 mL

c) $\dfrac{1 \text{ min}}{60 \text{ min}} = \dfrac{x \text{ mL}}{109 \text{ mL}}$

$60x = 109$

$x = 1.8 \text{ mL/min}$

$\dfrac{1.8 \text{ mL}}{1 \text{ mL}} = \dfrac{x \text{ gtt}}{60 \text{ gtt}}$

$x = 108.5$ or 109 gtt/min

d) 100 mL D5/W + 8.5 mL Retrovir

= 108.5 or 109 mL

10. a) $\dfrac{70 \text{ mg}}{80 \text{ mg}} = \dfrac{x \text{ mL}}{2 \text{ mL}}$

$80x = 140$

$x = 1.75 \text{ mL}$

b) 100 mL D5/W + 1.75 mL Nebcin

= 101.75 or 102 mL

$\dfrac{60 \text{ min}}{75 \text{ min}} = \dfrac{x \text{ mL}}{102 \text{ mL}}$

$75 x = 6120$

$x = 81.6$ or 82 mL/hr

$82 \text{ mL} \div 1 = 82 \text{ gtt/min}$

c) 82 mL / hr or 164 mL/2 hr

Review Test 20.1

1. a) $\dfrac{60 \text{ kg}}{1 \text{ kg}} = \dfrac{x \text{ mg}}{15 \text{ mg}}$

$x = 900 \text{ mg}$

b) $\dfrac{900 \text{ mg}}{500 \text{ mg}} = \dfrac{x \text{ vials}}{1 \text{ vial}}$

$5x = 9$

$x = 1.8$ or 2 vials

c) $\dfrac{900 \text{ mg}}{100 \text{ mg}} = \dfrac{x \text{ mL}}{1 \text{ mL}}$

$100 x = 900$

$x = 9 \text{ mL}$

d) 100 mL + 9 mL = 109 mL

e) 109 mL

2. a) $\dfrac{38 \text{ kg}}{1 \text{ kg}} = \dfrac{x \text{ units}}{20 \text{ units}}$

$x = 760 \text{ units/hour}$

b) $\dfrac{1 \text{ mL}}{500 \text{ mL}} = \dfrac{x \text{ units}}{10,000 \text{ units}}$

$500x = 10,000$

$5x = 100$

$x = 20 \text{ units/mL}$

$\dfrac{760 \text{ units}}{20 \text{ units}} = \dfrac{x \text{ mL}}{1 \text{ mL}}$

$20x = 760$

$x = 38 \text{ mL/hour}$

c) 38 mL/ hr

3. a) 220 lb ÷ 2.2 = 100 kg

b) $\dfrac{100 \text{ kg}}{1 \text{ kg}} = \dfrac{x \text{ units}}{18 \text{ units}}$

$x = 1800 \text{ units}$

c) $\dfrac{1 \text{ mL}}{250 \text{ mL}} = \dfrac{x \text{ units}}{25,000 \text{ units}}$

$250x = 25,000$

$x = 100 \text{ units/mL}$

$\dfrac{1800 \text{ U}}{100 \text{ U}} = \dfrac{x \text{ mL}}{1 \text{ mL}}$

$100x = 1800$

$x = 18 \text{ mL/hr}$

4. a) $\dfrac{100 \text{ kg}}{1 \text{ kg}} = \dfrac{x \text{ units}}{40 \text{ units}}$

$x = 4000 \text{ units}$

b) $\dfrac{100 \text{ kg}}{1 \text{ kg}} = \dfrac{x \text{ units}}{2 \text{ units}}$

$x = 200 \text{ units}$

c) 1800 units per hour + 200 units =

2000 units

d) $\dfrac{2000 \text{ units}}{25,000 \text{ units}} = \dfrac{x \text{ mL}}{250 \text{ mL}}$

$25,000x = 500,000$

$25x = 500$

$x = 20 \text{ mL/hr}$

5. a) BSA = 1.7m^2

(determined by adult nomogram)

b) $\dfrac{1.7 \text{ m}^2}{1 \text{m}^2} = \dfrac{\text{x mg}}{10 \text{ mg}}$

x = 17 mg

c) $\dfrac{17 \text{ mg}}{10 \text{ mg}} = \dfrac{\text{x mL}}{1 \text{ mL}}$

10x = 17

x = 1.7 mL

d) 100 + 1.7 mL = 101.7 mL

e) $\dfrac{60 \text{ min}}{20 \text{ min}} = \dfrac{\text{x mL}}{101.7 \text{ mL}}$

20x = 6102

x = 305 mL/hr

6. a) 2.0 m^2

(determined on adult nomogram)

b) $\dfrac{2 \text{ m}^2}{1 \text{ m}^2} = \dfrac{\text{x mg}}{1000 \text{ mg}}$

x = 2000 mg

c) $\dfrac{2000 \text{ mg}}{1000 \text{ mg}} = \dfrac{\text{x mL}}{5 \text{ mL}}$

1000x = 10,000

x = 10 mL

d) 500 + 10 = 510 mL

e) 510 ÷ 63.75 or 64 mL/hr

7. a) 1.2 m^2

(determined on adult nomogram)

b) $\dfrac{1.2 \text{ m}^2}{1 \text{ m}^2} = \dfrac{\text{x mg}}{170 \text{ mg}}$

x = 204 mg

c) $\dfrac{204 \text{ m}}{150 \text{ mg}} = \dfrac{\text{x mL}}{25 \text{ mL}}$

150x = 5100

x = 34 mL

d) 180 mL + 34 mL = 214 mL

e) 214 mL ÷ 3 hours = 71 mL/hr

8. Change 25 mg to microns by moving decimal point 3 places to its right. 25 mg = 25,000. mcg

a) $\dfrac{1 \text{ mL}}{250 \text{ mL}} = \dfrac{\text{x mcg}}{25,000 \text{ mcg}}$

250x = 25,000

x = 100 mcg/mL

b) $\dfrac{5 \text{ mcg}}{100 \text{ mcg}} = \dfrac{\text{x mL}}{1 \text{ mL}}$

100x = 5

x = 0.05 mL

c) 0.05 × 60 min = 3 mL/hr

9. a) $\dfrac{10 \text{ U}}{10 \text{ U}} = \dfrac{\text{x mL}}{1 \text{ mL}}$

10x = 10

x = 1 mL

b) $\dfrac{1 \text{ mL}}{1000 \text{ mL}} = \dfrac{\text{x U}}{10 \text{ U}}$

1000x = 10

x = 0.01 units/mL

c) 0.01U = 10 mU/mL

(move decimal three spaces to right)

d) $\dfrac{1 \text{ mU}}{10 \text{ mU}} = \dfrac{\text{x mL}}{1 \text{ mL}}$

10x = 1

x = 0.1 mL/min

e) 0.1 × 60 = 6 mL/hr

10. a) $\dfrac{125 \text{ mg}}{25 \text{ mg}} = \dfrac{\text{x mL}}{5 \text{ mL}}$

25x = 625

x = 25 mL

b) $\dfrac{1 \text{ mL}}{(100 \text{ mL} + 25 \text{ mL})} = \dfrac{\text{x mg}}{125 \text{ mg}}$

$\dfrac{1 \text{ mL}}{125 \text{ mL}} = \dfrac{\text{x mg}}{125 \text{ mg}}$

125x = 125

x = 1 mg

c) $\dfrac{5 \text{ mg}}{1 \text{ mg}} = \dfrac{\text{x mL}}{1 \text{ mL}}$

x = 5 mL/hr

d)   5 mL/hour

Review Test 20.2

1. a) 165 lb ÷ 2.2 = 75 kg

b) $\dfrac{75 \text{ kg}}{1 \text{ kg}} = \dfrac{x \text{ mg}}{5 \text{ mg}}$

   x = 375 mg

c) $\dfrac{375 \text{ mg}}{50 \text{ mg}} = \dfrac{x \text{ mL}}{1 \text{ mL}}$

   50x = 375

   x = 7.5 mL

   $\dfrac{7.5 \text{ mL}}{5 \text{ mL}} = \dfrac{x \text{ vials}}{1 \text{ vial}}$

   5x = 7.5

   x = 1.5 vials or 2 vials

d) 7.5 mL

e) 100 mL + 7.5 mL = 107.5 or 108 mL

f) 108 mL ÷ 2 hours = 54 mL/hr

2. a) $\dfrac{50 \text{ kg}}{1 \text{ kg}} = \dfrac{x \text{ mcg}}{10 \text{ mcg}}$

   x = 500 mcg

b) $\dfrac{500 \text{ mcg}}{1000 \text{ mcg}} = \dfrac{x \text{ mL}}{1 \text{ mL}}$

   1000x = 500

   x = 0.5 mL

c) 50 mL + 0.5 mL = 50.5 mL or 51 mL

d) 50.5 ÷ 15 × 60 = 201.9 or 202 mL

   or

   51 mL ÷ 15 × 60 = 204 mL

3. a) 165 lb ÷ 2.2 = 75 kg

b) $\dfrac{75 \text{ kg}}{1 \text{ kg}} = \dfrac{x \text{ units}}{18 \text{ units}}$

   x = 1350 units

c) $\dfrac{1 \text{ mL}}{250 \text{ mL}} = \dfrac{x \text{ units}}{25,000 \text{ units}}$

   250x = 25,000

   x = 100 units/mL

   $\dfrac{1350 \text{ units}}{100 \text{ units}} = \dfrac{x \text{ mL}}{1 \text{ mL}}$

   100x = 1350

   x = 13.5 or 14 mL/hr

4. a) $\dfrac{75 \text{ kg}}{1 \text{ kg}} = \dfrac{x \text{ units}}{2 \text{ units}}$

   x = 150 units

b) 1200 units/hour − 150 units =

   1050 units

c) $\dfrac{1050 \text{ units}}{25,000 \text{ units}} = \dfrac{x \text{ mL}}{250 \text{ mL}}$

   2500x = 26250

   x = 10.5 or 11 mL/hr

5. a) $\dfrac{2.2 \text{ m}^2}{1 \text{ m}^2} = \dfrac{x \text{ mg}}{425 \text{ mg}}$

   x = 935 mg

b) $\dfrac{935 \text{ mg}}{500 \text{ mg}} = \dfrac{x \text{ mL}}{10 \text{ mL}}$

   500x = 9350

   x = 18.7 mL

c) 250 mL + 18.7 mL = 268.7 or 269 mL

d) 268.7 ÷ 6 = 44.7 or 45 mL/hr

6. a) 1.7 m²

   (determined on the adult nomogram)

b) $\dfrac{1.7 \text{ m}^2}{1 \text{ m}^2} = \dfrac{x \text{ mg}}{1.4 \text{ mg}}$

   x = 2.38 or 2.4 mg

c) $\dfrac{2.4 \text{ mL}}{5 \text{ mg}} = \dfrac{x \text{ mL}}{5 \text{ mL}}$

   5x = 12

   x = 2.4 mL

d) 50 mL + 2.4 mL = 52.4 mL

e) 52.4 ÷ 30 × 60 = 105

   or

   $\dfrac{60 \text{ min}}{30 \text{ min}} = \dfrac{x \text{ m}}{52.4 \text{ mL}}$

   3x = 314.4

   x = 104.8 or 105 mL/hr

7. a) 2 m^2

b) $\dfrac{2 \text{ m}^2}{1 \text{ m}^2} = \dfrac{x \text{ mg}}{100 \text{ mg}}$

$x = 200 \text{ mg}$

c) $\dfrac{200 \text{ mg}}{50 \text{ mg}} = \dfrac{x \text{ mL}}{50 \text{ mL}}$

$50x = 10,000 \text{ mL}$

$x = 200 \text{ mL}$

e) $2000 \text{ mL} + 200 \text{ mL} = 2200 \text{ mL}$

f) $2200 \text{ mL} \div 8 \text{ hr} = 275 \text{ mL/hr}$

8. a) $\dfrac{400 \text{ mg}}{400 \text{ mg}} = \dfrac{x \text{ mL}}{5 \text{ mL}}$

$400x = 2000$

$x = 5 \text{ mL}$

b) $\dfrac{1 \text{ mL}}{250 \text{ mL}} = \dfrac{x \text{ mg}}{400 \text{ mg}}$

$250x = 400$

$x = 1.6 \text{ mg/mL}$

c) Change 1.6 mg to mcg by moving the decimal three places to the right = 1600 mcg/mL

d) $\dfrac{100 \text{ mcg}}{x \text{ mcg}} = \dfrac{1 \text{ minute}}{60 \text{ min}}$

$x = 6000 \text{ mcg/60 min}$

$\dfrac{6000 \text{ mcg}}{1600 \text{ mcg}} = \dfrac{x \text{ mL}}{1 \text{ mL}}$

$1600x = 6000$

$x = 3.75 \text{ mL/hr}$

9. Change 0.5 g to mg by moving the decimal three places to the right = 500 mg

a) $\dfrac{500 \text{ mg}}{500 \text{ mg}} = \dfrac{x \text{ mL}}{1 \text{ mL}}$

$500x = 500$

$x = 1 \text{ mL}$

b) $\dfrac{1 \text{ mL}}{500 \text{ mL}} = \dfrac{x \text{ mg}}{500 \text{ mg}}$

$500x = 500$

$x = 1 \text{ mg/mL}$

c) $\dfrac{4 \text{ mg}}{500 \text{ mg}} = \dfrac{x \text{ mL}}{500 \text{ mL}}$

$500x = 2000$

$x = 4 \text{ mL/min}$

d) $\dfrac{4 \text{ mL}}{1 \text{ min}} = \dfrac{x \text{ mL}}{60 \text{ min}}$

$x = 240 \text{ mL/hr}$

10. a) $198 \text{ lb} \div 2.2 \text{ kg} = 90 \text{ kg}$

b) $\dfrac{800 \text{ mg}}{250 \text{ mL}} = \dfrac{x \text{ mg}}{1 \text{ mg}}$

$250x = 800$

$x = 3.2 \text{ mg/mL}$

c) $0.8 \text{ mg} \times 90 \text{ kg} = 72 \text{ mg/hr}$

d) $\dfrac{72 \text{ mg}}{800 \text{ mg}} = \dfrac{x \text{ mL}}{250 \text{ mL}}$

$800x = 18,000$

$x = 22.5 \text{ mL/hr}$

Review Test 21.1

1. Determine the child's weight in kilograms

$8 \text{ lb} \div 2.2 = 3.6 \text{ kg}$

Then determine the safe dose:

$\dfrac{2.5 \text{ mg}}{1 \text{ kg}} = \dfrac{x \text{ mg}}{3.6 \text{ kg}}$

$x = 9$ milligrams is a safe dosage

$\dfrac{9 \text{ mg}}{10 \text{ mg}} = \dfrac{x \text{ mL}}{1 \text{ mL}}$

$10x = 9$

$x = 0.9 \text{ mL}$

2. Determine the child's weight in kilograms:

$72.6 \text{ lb} \div 2.2 = 33 \text{ kg}$

Then determine the safe dose:

$\dfrac{30 \text{ mg}}{1 \text{ kg}} = \dfrac{x \text{ mg}}{33 \text{ kg}}$

$x = 990 \text{ mg} \div 4 \text{ doses} = 248 \text{ mg/dose}$ is a safe dose.

Then:

$\dfrac{248 \text{ mg}}{500 \text{ mg}} = \dfrac{x \text{ tab}}{1 \text{ tab}}$

$500x = 248$

$x = 0.49 \left(\dfrac{1}{2}\right)$ tablet

3. $\dfrac{40\,\text{mg}}{1\,\text{kg}} = \dfrac{x\,\text{mg}}{25\,\text{kg}}$

x = 1000 mg ÷ 4 doses = 250 mg/dose is a safe dose.

Then:

$\dfrac{250\,\text{mg}}{125\,\text{mg}} = \dfrac{x\,\text{pulvule}}{1\,\text{pulvule}}$

125x = 250

x = 2 pulvules

4. Determine the child's weight in kilograms:

99 ÷ 2.2 = 45 kg

$\dfrac{0.5\,\text{mg}}{1\,\text{kg}} = \dfrac{x\,\text{mg}}{45\,\text{kg}}$

x = 22.5 mg is a safe dose.

Then:

$\dfrac{22.5\,\text{mg}}{10\,\text{mg}} = \dfrac{x\,\text{tabs}}{1\,\text{tab}}$

10x = 22.5

x = 2.25 (2) tablets

5. Determine the child's safe dose:

$\dfrac{20\,\text{mg}}{1\,\text{kg}} = \dfrac{x\,\text{mg}}{37.5\,\text{kg}}$

x = 750 mg

which exceeds 600 mg/day recommended and is unsafe.

6.⎫ Require students
7.⎬ to read chart.
8.⎭ A worked-out
   solution is not required.

9. BSA is 1.15 m² × 25 mg × 6 doses = 172.5 mg daily ordered

Recommended is 150 mg/m² = 172.5 mg

Dose is safe; child should receive 1 tablet or 25 mg every 4 hours.

10. BSA is 0.91 m² × 6000 = 5460 IU

The child's BSA is below 1 m² and the ordered dose of 6000 IU would be higher than the 5400 IU recommended.

Review Test 21.2

1. $\dfrac{7.5\,\text{mg}}{1\,\text{kg}} = \dfrac{x\,\text{mg}}{37.7\,\text{kg}}$

x = 283 mg
therefore 296 mg would be a safe dose.

$\dfrac{296\,\text{mg}}{500\,\text{mg}} = \dfrac{x\,\text{mL}}{2\,\text{mL}}$

500x = 592

x = 1.1 mL

2. $\dfrac{2\,\text{mg}}{1\,\text{kg}} = \dfrac{x\,\text{mg}}{23\,\text{kg}}$ $\dfrac{2.5\,\text{mg}}{1\,\text{kg}} = \dfrac{x\,\text{mg}}{23\,\text{kg}}$

x = 46 mg   x = 57.5 (58) mg
(minimum dose)   (maximum dose)

The 50 mg would be a safe dose.

$\dfrac{50\,\text{mg}}{80\,\text{mg}} = \dfrac{x\,\text{mL}}{2\,\text{mL}}$

80x = 100

x = 1.25 mL

3. $\dfrac{40\,\text{mg}}{1\,\text{kg}} = \dfrac{x\,\text{mg}}{50\,\text{kg}}$

x = 2000 mg ÷ 4 (doses) = 500 mg/dose
The 500 mg 4 times a day would be a safe dose.

$\dfrac{500\,\text{mg}}{500\,\text{mg}} = \dfrac{x\,\text{mL}}{6\,\text{mL}}$

500x = 3000

x = 6 mL

4. min dose

$$\frac{8\,mg}{1\,kg} = \frac{x\,mg}{12.7\,kg}$$

$x = 101.6 = 102\ mg$

max dose

$$\frac{12\,mg}{1\,kg} = \frac{x\,mg}{12.7\,kg}$$

$x = 152.4 = 152\ mg$

The 135 mg (45 mg $\times$ 3) is between the minimum and maximum recommended dose and is a safe dose.

$$\frac{45\,mg}{75\,mg} = \frac{x\,mL}{5\,mL}$$

$75x = 225$

$x = 3\ mL$

5. min dose

$$\frac{35\,\mu g}{1\,kg} = \frac{x\,\mu g}{10\,kg}$$

$x = 350\ \mu g$

max dose

$$\frac{60\,\mu g}{1\,kg} = \frac{x\,\mu g}{10\,kg}$$

$x = 600\ \mu g$

The 360 mg (120 mg $\times$ 3) is between the minimum and maximum recommended dose and is a safe dose.

$$\frac{120\,\mu g}{50\,\mu g} = \frac{x\,mL}{1\,mL}$$

$50x = 120$

$x = 2.4\ mL$

6. 0.36 m^2 read from the Pediatric Body Surface Area nomogram

7. 0.5 m^2 read from the Pediatric Body Surface Area nomogram

8. $$\frac{50\,\mu g}{m^2} = \frac{x\,\mu g}{1.35\ m^2}$$

$x = 67.5\ (68)\mu g$

This is the recommended dose and is safe.

$$\frac{68\,mcg}{100\,mcg} = \frac{x\,mL}{0.5\,mL}$$

$100x = 34$

$x = 0.34\ mL$

9. $$\frac{30\,mg}{m^2} = \frac{x\,mg}{0.8\,m^2}$$

$x = 24\ mg$

This is the recommended dose and is safe.

$$\frac{24\,mg}{25\,mg} = \frac{x\,mL}{1\,mL}$$

$25x = 24$

$x = 0.96\ mL$

10. $$\frac{60\,mg}{m^2} = \frac{x\,mg}{1.2\,m^2}$$

$x = 72\ mg$

This is the recommended dose and the 70 mg ordered is safe.

Give 1 tablet 50 mg and 2 tablets 10 mg.

Review Test 22.1

1. First, convert 0.2 g to mg by moving the decimal three places to the right

$\overrightarrow{0.200.}$ = 200 mg or calculate:

$$\frac{0.2\,\text{g}}{1\,\text{g}} = \frac{x\ \text{mg}}{1000\ \text{mg}}$$

x = 200 mg

$$\frac{200\,\text{mg}}{100\,\text{mg}} \times 1\ \text{tab} = 2\ \text{tablets}$$

2. First convert gr $\dfrac{3}{4}$ to mg.

$$\frac{\frac{3}{4}\,\text{gr}}{1\,\text{gr}} = \frac{x\,\text{mg}}{60\,\text{mg}}$$

x = 45 mg

Then:

$$\frac{45\,\text{mg}}{15\,\text{mg}} \times 1\ \text{tab} = 3\ \text{tablets}$$

3. $\dfrac{500\,\text{mg}}{125\,\text{mg}} \times 5\ \text{mL} = 20\ \text{mL}$

4. $\dfrac{15\,\text{mg}}{7.5\,\text{mg}} \times 1\ \text{tab} = 2\ \text{tablets}$

5. First, change 200 mcg to mg by moving the decimal three places to the left

$\overleftarrow{0.200.}$ = 0.2 mg or calculate:

$$\frac{200\,\text{mcg}}{1000\,\text{mcg}} = \frac{x\,\text{mg}}{1\,\text{mg}}$$

1000x = 200

x = 0.2 mg

$$\frac{0.2\,\text{mg}}{0.2\,\text{mg}} \times 1\ \text{mL} = 1\ \text{mL}$$

6. $\dfrac{250\,\text{mg}}{225\,\text{mg}} \times 1\ \text{mL} = 1.1\ \text{mL}$

7. $\dfrac{5\,\text{mg}}{4\,\text{mg}} \times 1\ \text{mL} = 1.25\ \text{mL}$

8. $\dfrac{35\,\text{U}}{100\,\text{U}} \times 1\ \text{mL} = 0.35\ \text{mL}$

9. $\dfrac{8000\,\text{U}}{10000\,\text{U}} \times 1\ \text{mL} = 0.8\ \text{mL}$

10. First convert gr $\dfrac{1}{30}$ to mg:

$$\frac{\text{gr}\,\frac{1}{30}}{\text{gr}\,1} = \frac{x\,\text{mg}}{60\,\text{mg}}$$

x = 2 mg

Then:

$$\frac{2\,\text{mg}}{3\,\text{mg}} \times 1\ \text{mL} = 0.66\ \text{or}\ 0.7\ \text{mL}$$

Review Test 22.2

1. Change 0.8 g to mg by moving the decimal

3 places to the right $\overrightarrow{0.800.}$ = 800 mg and calculate:

$$\frac{800\,\text{mg}}{200\,\text{mg}} \times 5\ \text{mL} = 20\ \text{mL}$$

2. $\dfrac{1400\,\text{U}}{2000\,\text{U}} \times 1\ \text{mL} = 0.7\ \text{mL}$

3. $\dfrac{125\,\text{mg}}{50\,\text{mg}} \times 1\ \text{tab} = 2\dfrac{1}{2}\ \text{tablets}$

4. Change 0.75 g to mg by moving
   the decimal three places to the right
   $\overrightarrow{0.750.}$ = 750 mg and calculate:

   $\dfrac{750\,mg}{250\,mg} \times 5\,mL = 15\,mL$

5. Change 1 gr to 60 mg

   $\dfrac{60\,mg}{30\,mg} \times 1\,tab = 2\,tablets$

6. $\dfrac{270\,mg}{100\,mg} \times 1\,mL = 2.7\,mL$

7. Change 0.75 g to mg by moving
   the decimal three places to the right
   $\overrightarrow{0.750.}$ = 750 mg

   $\dfrac{750\,mg}{250\,mg} \times 1\,mL = 3\,mL$

8. $\dfrac{150\,mg}{50\,mg} \times 1\,mL = 3\,mL$

9. $\dfrac{400{,}000\,U}{500{,}000\,U} \times 1\,mL = 0.8\,mL$

10. Change 125 mcg to mg by moving the
    decimal three places to the left $\overleftarrow{0.125.}$ =
    0.125 mg

    $\dfrac{0.125\,mg}{0.5\,mg} \times 2\,mL = 0.5\,mL$

Review Test 23.1

1. tablets $= \dfrac{1\,tab}{0.3\,mg} \times \dfrac{1\,mg}{1000\,mg} \times 600\,mg =$

   $\dfrac{1 \times 1 \times 600}{300} = \dfrac{600}{300} = 2\,tablets$

2. tablets $= \dfrac{1\,tab}{240\,mg} \times 480\,mg =$

   $\dfrac{1 \times 480}{240} = \dfrac{480}{240} = 2\,tablets$

3. mL $= \dfrac{15\,mL}{20\,mg} \times 30\,mg =$

   $\dfrac{15 \times 30}{20} = \dfrac{450}{20} = 22.5\,mL$

4. mL $= \dfrac{5\,mL}{125\,mg} \times 400\,mg =$

   $\dfrac{5 \times 400}{125} = \dfrac{2000}{125} = 16\,mL$

5. tablets $= \dfrac{1\,tab}{50\,mg} \times 25\,mg =$

   $\dfrac{1 \times 25}{50} = \dfrac{25}{50} = 0.5$ or $\dfrac{1}{2}$ tablet

6. mL $= \dfrac{5\,mL}{12.5\,mg} \times 50\,mg =$

   $\dfrac{5 \times 50}{12.5} = \dfrac{250.0}{12.5} = 20\,mL$

7. mL $= \dfrac{1\,mL}{300{,}000\,U} \times 450{,}000\,U =$

   $\dfrac{1 \times 450{,}000}{300{,}000} = \dfrac{450{,}000}{300{,}000} = 1.5\,mL$

8. mL $= \dfrac{1\,mL}{0.4\,mg} \times 0.3\,mg =$

   $\dfrac{1 \times 0.3}{0.4} = \dfrac{0.3}{0.4} = 0.75\,mL$

9. mL $= \dfrac{3.6\,mL}{1\,G} \times \dfrac{1\,G}{1000\,mg} \times 500\,mg =$

   $\dfrac{3.6 \times 1 \times 500}{1 \times 1000} = \dfrac{1800}{1000} = 1.8\,mL$

10. mL $= \dfrac{4\,mL}{40\,mg} \times 20\,mg =$

    $\dfrac{4 \times 20}{40} = \dfrac{80}{40} = 2\,mL$

Review Test 23.2

1. $mL = \dfrac{5\ mL}{50\ mg} \times 200\ mg$

$\dfrac{5}{50} \times 200 = \dfrac{1000}{50} = 20\ mL$

2. $mL = \dfrac{5\ mL}{200\ mg} \times \dfrac{1000\ mg}{1\ G} =$

$\dfrac{5 \times 1000}{200} = \dfrac{5000}{200} = 25\ mL$

3. $tablets = \dfrac{1\ tab}{200\ mg} \times 800\ mg =$

$\dfrac{1 \times 800}{200} = \dfrac{800}{200} = 4\ tablets$

4. $capsules = \dfrac{1\ cap}{200\ mg} \times 600\ mg =$

$\dfrac{1 \times 600}{200} = \dfrac{6\cancel{00}}{2\cancel{00}} = 3\ capsules$

5. $tablets = \dfrac{1\ tab}{100\ mcg} \times \dfrac{1000\ mcg}{1\ mg} \times 0.2\ mg =$

$\dfrac{1 \times 1000 \times 0.2}{100} = \dfrac{2\cancel{00}}{1\cancel{00}} = 2\ tablets$

6. $mL = \dfrac{1\ mL}{1\ mg} \times 0.25\ mg =$

$\dfrac{1 \times 0.25}{1} = \dfrac{0.25}{1} = 0.25\ mL$

7. $mL = \dfrac{2.6\ mL}{1\ G} \times \dfrac{1\ G}{1000\ mg} \times 730\ mg =$

$\dfrac{2.6\ mL \times 1 \times 730}{1 \times 1000} = \dfrac{1898}{1000} = 1.89\ or\ 1.9\ mL$

8. $mL = \dfrac{2\ mL}{500\ mcg} \times \dfrac{1000\ mcg}{1\ mg} \times 0.125\ mg =$

$\dfrac{2 \times 1000 \times 0.125}{500} = \dfrac{25\cancel{0}}{50\cancel{0}} = 0.5\ mL$

9. $mL = \dfrac{3.6\ mL}{750\ mg} \times \dfrac{1000\ mg}{1\ G} \times 0.5\ G =$

$\dfrac{3.6 \times 1000 \times 0.5}{750 \times 1} = \dfrac{180\cancel{0}}{75\cancel{0}} = 2.4\ mL$

10. $mL = \dfrac{1\ mL}{150\ mg} \times 250\ mg =$

$\dfrac{1 \times 250}{150} = \dfrac{25\cancel{0}}{15\cancel{0}} = 1.66\ or\ 1.7\ mL$

CHAPTER 25 POSTTEST

Set 25.1

1. $\dfrac{1\ kg}{1\ kg} = \dfrac{x\ lb}{2.2\ lb}$ $\dfrac{1\ kg}{1\ kg} = \dfrac{x\ g}{1000\ g}$

$x = 2.2\ lb$ $x = 1000\ g$

2. $\dfrac{1\ fl\ oz}{1\ fl\ oz} = \dfrac{x\ dr}{8\ dr}$ $\dfrac{1\ fl\ oz}{1\ fl\ oz} = \dfrac{x\ mL}{30\ mL}$

$x = 8\ fluid\ drams$ $x = 30\ mL$

3. $\dfrac{gr\ \frac{1}{100}}{gr\ 1} = \dfrac{x\ mg}{60\ mg}$ $\dfrac{0.6\ mg}{1\ mg} = \dfrac{x\ mcg}{1000\ mcg}$

$x = \dfrac{1}{100} \times 60$ $x = 600\ mcg$

$x = 0.6\ mg$

4. $\dfrac{gr\ \frac{1}{2}}{gr\ 1} = \dfrac{x\ mg}{60\ mg}$ $\dfrac{30\ mg}{1000\ mg} = \dfrac{x\ g}{1\ g}$

$x = \dfrac{1}{2} \times 60$ $1000x = 30$

$x = 30\ mg$ $x = 0.03\ g$

5. $\dfrac{gr\ \frac{1}{60}}{gr\ 1} = \dfrac{x\ mg}{60\ mg}$ $\dfrac{1\ mg}{1000\ mg} = \dfrac{x\ g}{1\ g}$

$x = \dfrac{1}{60} \times 60$ $1000x = 1$

$x = 1\ mg$ $x = 0.001\ g$

Set 25.2

1. $gr \dfrac{1}{6} = \dfrac{4}{24}$

$gr \dfrac{1}{8} = \dfrac{3}{24}$ 　　　　Ans: $gr \dfrac{1}{6}$

$gr \dfrac{1}{12} = \dfrac{2}{24}$

2. $0.125 \text{ mg} = \dfrac{125}{1000} = \dfrac{1}{8}$

$0.25 \text{ mg} = \dfrac{25}{100} = \dfrac{1}{4}$ 　　Ans: 0.25 mg

$0.05 \text{ mg} = \dfrac{5}{100} = \dfrac{1}{20}$

3. $gr \dfrac{1}{32} = \dfrac{30}{960}$

$gr \dfrac{1}{64} = \dfrac{15}{960}$ 　　　Ans: $gr \dfrac{1}{32}$

$gr \dfrac{1}{60} = \dfrac{16}{960}$

4. $0.004 \text{ g} = \dfrac{4}{1000}$

$0.006 \text{ g} = \dfrac{6}{1000}$ 　　Ans: 0.01 g

$0.01 \text{ g} = \dfrac{1}{100}$

5. $gr \dfrac{1}{200} = \dfrac{3}{600}$

$gr \dfrac{1}{150} = \dfrac{4}{600}$ 　　Ans: $gr \dfrac{1}{100}$

$gr \dfrac{1}{100} = \dfrac{6}{600}$

Set 25.3

1. 39°C

$F = 1.8 \times 39°C + 32$

$F = 70.2 + 32$

$F = 102.2°F$

2. 22°C

$F = 1.8 \times 22°C + 32$

$F = 39.6 + 32$

$F = 71.6°F$

3. 70°F

$70 - 32 = 38 = 1.8°C + 32 - 32$

$38 = 1.8°C$

$C = 21.1°C \text{ or } 21°C$

4. 103°F

$103 - 32 = 71 = 1.8°C + 32 - 32$

$71 = 1.8°C$

$C = 39.4°C$

5. 101°F

$101 - 32 = 69 = 1.8°C + 32 - 32$

$69 = 1.8°C$

$C = 38.3° \text{ or } 38.4°C$

Set 25.4

Change 0.2 g to mg by moving the decimal three places to the right $0.200. = 200 \text{ mg}$

$\dfrac{200 \text{ mg}}{100 \text{ mg}} = \dfrac{x \text{ capsule}}{1 \text{ capsule}}$

$100x = 200$

$x = 2 \text{ capsules}$

Set 25.5

Change 0.1 g to 100 mg $(0.100.)$

$\dfrac{300 \text{ mg}}{100 \text{ mg}} = \dfrac{x \text{ capsule}}{1 \text{ capsule}}$

$100x = 300$

$x = 3 \text{ capsules}$

Set 25.6

Change 0.8 g to 800 mg $(0.800.)$

$\dfrac{800 \text{ mg}}{200 \text{ mg}} = \dfrac{x \text{ tab}}{1 \text{ tab}}$

$200x = 800$

$x = 4 \text{ tablets}$

Set 25.7

$$\frac{1\,mg}{0.5\,mg} = \frac{x\,tab}{1\,tab}$$

$0.5x = 1$

$x = 2$ tablets

Set 25.8

$$\frac{12.5\,mcg}{5\,mcg} = \frac{x\,tab}{1\,tab}$$

$5x = 12.5$

$x = 2.5 \left(2\frac{1}{2}\right)$ tablets

Set 25.9

Change 0.05 mg to 50 mcg $0.050.$

$$\frac{125\,mcg}{50\,mcg} = \frac{x\,mL}{1\,mL}$$

$50x = 125$

$x = 2.5$ mL

Set 25.10

$$\frac{500\,mg}{250\,mg} = \frac{x\,mL}{5\,mL}$$

$250x = 2500$

$x = 10$ mL

Set 25.11

$$\frac{35\,mg}{10\,mg} = \frac{x\,mL}{1\,mL}$$

$10x = 35$

$x = 3.5$ mg

Set 25.12

$$\frac{150\,mg}{15\,mg} = \frac{x\,mL}{1\,mL}$$

$15x = 150$

$x = 10$ mL

Set 25.13

$$\frac{20\,mEq}{15\,mEq} = \frac{x\,mL}{11.25\,mL}$$

$15x = 225$

$x = 15$ mL

Set 25.14

$$\frac{25\,mg}{40\,mg} = \frac{x\,mL}{4\,mL}$$

$40x = 100$

$x = 2.5$ mL

Set 25.15

Change 2 g to 2000 mg $2.000.$

$$\frac{750\,mg}{2000\,mg} = \frac{x\,mL}{8\,mL}$$

$2000x = 6000$

$x = 3$ mL

Set 25.16

$$\frac{1\,mg}{2\,mg} = \frac{x\,mL}{1\,mL}$$

$2x = 1$

$x = 0.5$ mL

Set 25.17

$$\frac{8\,mg}{10\,mg} = \frac{x\,mL}{1\,mL}$$

$10x = 8$

$x = 0.8$ mL

Set 25.18

$$\frac{25\,U}{100\,U} = \frac{x\,mL}{1\,mL}$$

$100x = 25$

$x = 0.25$ mL

Set 25.19

1. 50 U:1 Kg = xU:50 kg

   x = 2500 U

2. $\dfrac{2500\,U}{3000\,U} = \dfrac{x\,mL}{1\,mL}$

   3000x = 2500

   x = 0.83 mL

Set 25.20

$\dfrac{7500\,U}{5000\,U} = \dfrac{x\,mL}{1\,mL}$

5000x = 7500

x = 1.5 mL

Set 25.21

$\dfrac{18,000\,U}{20,000\,U} = \dfrac{x\,mL}{1\,mL}$

20,000x = 18,000

x = 0.9 mL

Set 25.22

$\dfrac{36\,U}{100\,U} = \dfrac{x\,mL}{1\,mL}$

100x = 36

x = 0.36 mL

Set 25.23

$\dfrac{4500\,U}{5000\,U} = \dfrac{x\,mL}{1\,mL}$

5000x = 4500

x = 0.9 mL

Set 25.24

$\dfrac{3000\,U}{5000\,U} = \dfrac{x\,mL}{1\,mL}$

5000x = 3000

x = 0.6 mL

Set 25.25

1. 16 mg:1 kg = x mg:30 kg

   x = 480 mg daily dose

2. 480 ÷ 4 = 120 mg q6h

3. $\dfrac{120\,mg}{75\,mg} = \dfrac{x\,mL}{5\,mL}$

   75x = 600

   x = 8 mL

Set 25.26

1. 15 mg:1 kg = x mg:5 kg

   x = 75 mg/day

2. 75 ÷ 2 = 37.5 mg q12h

3. $\dfrac{37.5\,mg}{75\,mg} = \dfrac{x\,mL}{2\,mL}$

   75x = 75

   x = 1 mL

Set 25.27

1. 1.1 m^2
2. 5 mg/m^2 × 1.1 m^2 = 5.5 mg
3. (b) unsafe—nearly two times as much as is safe

Set 25.28

1. 2500 U × 0.7 m^2 = 1750 IU

   recommended dose
2. (a) safe dose

Set 25.29

1. 100 mg/m^2 × 0.8 m^2 = 80 mg

   recommended dose
2. (a) safe dose
3. $\dfrac{80\,mg}{20\,mg} = \dfrac{x\,mL}{1\,mL}$

   20x = 80

   x = 4 mL

4. $100 - 4 = 96$ mL

5. $100 + 15 = 115$ mL

6. $115 \div 120 \times 60 = 57.5 = 58$ mL/hr

Set 25.30

Change 0.3 mg to mcg = 0.300. = 300 mcg

$$\frac{300\,\text{mcg}}{600\,\text{mcg}} = \frac{x\,\text{mL}}{1\,\text{mL}}$$

$600x = 300$

$x = 0.5$ mL

Set 25.31

1. $\dfrac{35\,\text{mEq}}{40\,\text{mEq}} = \dfrac{x\,\text{mL}}{10\,\text{mL}}$

   $40x = 350$

   $x = 8.75 = 8.8$ mL

2. 1000 mL $+ 9$ mL $= 1009 \div 24 = $
   42 mL/hr

3. $42 \div 6 = 7$ gtt/min

4. 42 mL/hr

Set 25.32

1. $1500 \div 24 = 62.5$ mL/hr

2. $62.5 \div 60 = 1.04$ mL/min

3. $62.4 \div 4 = 15.6 = 16$ gtt/min

4. 62.5 or 63 mL/hr

Set 25.33

1. $1000 \div 24 = 41.66 \div 6 = 6.9 = 7$ gtt/min

2. $1000 \div 24 = 41.6$ or 42 mL/hr

Set 25.34

1. $\dfrac{35\,\text{gtt}}{15\,\text{gtt}} = \dfrac{x\,\text{mL}}{1\,\text{mL}}$

   $15x = 35$

   $x = 2.33$

   $$\frac{\times\,60}{139.9} = 140\,\text{mL}$$

2. $1000 \div 140 = 7.14 = 7$ hr 8 min

Set 25.35

1. $60 \div 6 = 10$ gtt/min

2. 60 mL/hr

Set 25.36

1. $\dfrac{50\,\text{U}}{100\,\text{U}} = \dfrac{x\,\text{mL}}{1\,\text{mL}}$

   $100x = 50$

   $x = 0.5$ mL

2. $\dfrac{1\,\text{mL}}{500\,\text{mL}} = \dfrac{x\,\text{U}}{50\,\text{U}}$

   $500x = 50$

   $x = 0.1$ U/mL

3. $\dfrac{6\,\text{U}}{0.1\,\text{U}} = \dfrac{x\,\text{mL}}{1\,\text{mL}}$

   $0.1x = 6$

   $x = 60$ mL

4. 60 mL $\div 1 = 60$ gtt/min

5. $60 \times 1 = 60$ mL/hr

Set 25.37

1. $\dfrac{20{,}000\,\text{U}}{20{,}000\,\text{U}} = \dfrac{x\,\text{mL}}{1\,\text{mL}}$

   $20{,}000x = 20{,}000$

   $x = 1$ mL

2. $\dfrac{1\ \text{mL}}{1000\ \text{mL}} = \dfrac{x\ \text{U}}{20{,}000\ \text{U}}$

$1000x = 20{,}000$

$x = 20\ \text{U/mL}$

3. $\dfrac{1000\ \text{U}}{20\ \text{U}} = \dfrac{x\ \text{mL}}{1\ \text{mL}}$

$20x = 1000$

$x = 50\ \text{mL/min}$

4. $50 \times 1 = 50\ \text{mL/hr}$

Set 25.38

1. $65 \div 1 = 65\ \text{gtt/min}$

2. $65\ \text{mL/hr}$

3. $\dfrac{24\ \text{hrs}}{1\ \text{hr}} = \dfrac{x\ \text{mL}}{65\ \text{mL}}$

$x = 1560\ \text{mL/24 hr}$

Set 25.39

Change 1 g to 1000 mg $1{,}000.\overset{\longrightarrow}{}$

1. $\dfrac{2.5\ \text{mg}}{1000\ \text{mg}} = \dfrac{x\ \text{mL}}{800\ \text{mL}}$

$1000x = 2000$

$x = 2\ \text{mL}$

2. $100 + 2 = 102\ \text{mL}$

3. $102 \div 60 \times 60 = 102\ \text{gtt/min}$

4. $102 \times 1 = 102\ \text{mL/hr}$

Set 25.40

1. $\dfrac{300\ \text{mg}}{300\ \text{mg}} = \dfrac{x\ \text{mL}}{2\ \text{mL}}$

$300x = 600$

$x = 2\ \text{mL}$

2. $100 + 2 = 102\ \text{mL}$

3. $102 \div 20 \times 10 = 51\ \text{gtt/min}$

4. $\dfrac{102\ \text{mL}}{20\ \text{min}} = \dfrac{x\ \text{mL}}{60\ \text{min}}$

$20x = 6120$

$x = 306\ \text{mL/hr}$

Set 25.41

1. $\dfrac{500\ \text{mg}}{250\ \text{mg}} = \dfrac{x\ \text{mL}}{1\ \text{mL}}$

$250x = 500$

$x = 2\ \text{mL}$

2. $200 + 2 = 202\ \text{mL}$

3. $202 \div 60 \times 15 = 50.5 = 51\ \text{gtts/min}$

4. $\dfrac{202\ \text{mL}}{60\ \text{min}} = \dfrac{x\ \text{mL}}{60\ \text{min}}$

$60x = 12{,}120$

$x = 202\ \text{mL/hr}$

Set 25.42

1. $\dfrac{200\ \text{mg}}{10\ \text{mg}} = \dfrac{x\ \text{mL}}{1\ \text{mL}}$

$10x = 200$

$x = 20\ \text{mL}$

2. $20\ \text{mL}$

3. $120\ \text{mL}$

4. $120\ \text{mL}$

Set 25.43

1. $\dfrac{60\ \text{min}}{60\ \text{min}} = \dfrac{x\ \text{mL}}{45\ \text{mL}}$

$60x = 2700$

$x = 45\ \text{mL}$

2. $\dfrac{1000\ \text{mL}}{45\ \text{mL}} = \dfrac{x\ \text{hr}}{1\ \text{hr}}$

$45\ \text{mL} = 1000$

$x = 22.22\ \text{hr} = 22\ \text{hr and 13 min}$

Set 25.44

1. $\dfrac{300\ \text{mg}}{400\ \text{mg}} = \dfrac{x\ \text{mL}}{10\ \text{mL}}$

$400x = 3000$

$x = 7.5\ \text{mL}$

2. $75 - 7.5 = 67.5\ \text{mL}$

3. $75 + 15\ (\text{for flush}) = 90\ \text{mL}$

4. $\dfrac{90\,mL}{1\,hr} = \dfrac{x\,mL}{1\,hr}$

x = 90 mL/hr

Set 25.45

1. $\dfrac{32\,mg}{2\,mg} = \dfrac{x\,mL}{1\,mL}$

2x = 32

x = 16 mL

2. 50 − 16 = 34 mL

3. 50 + 15 (for flush) = 65 mL

4. $\dfrac{65\,mL}{20\,min} = \dfrac{x\,mL}{60\,min}$

20x = 3900

x = 195 mL/hr

Set 25.46

1. 83.6 ÷ 2.2 = 38 kg

2. $\dfrac{18\,U}{1\,kg} = \dfrac{x}{38\,kg}$

x = 684 U

3. $\dfrac{25,000\,U}{500\,mL} = \dfrac{684\,U}{x\,mL}$

25,000x = 342,000

x = 13.68 or 14 mL/hr

Set 25.47

1. $\dfrac{5\,mL}{1\,mg} = \dfrac{x\,mL}{2\,mg}$

x = 10 mL

2. $\dfrac{1\,mL}{500\,mL} = \dfrac{x\,mg}{2\,mg}$

500x = 2

x = 0.004 mg/mL

3. Change 0.004 mg to mcg by moving the decimal three places to the right = 4 mcg/mL

4. $\dfrac{5\,mcg}{4\,mcg} = \dfrac{x\,mL}{1\,mL}$

4x = 5

x = 1.25 mL/min

5. 1.25 × 60 = 75 mL/hr

Set 25.48

1. $\dfrac{120\,mg}{10\,mg} = \dfrac{x\,mL}{1\,mL}$

10x = 120

x = 12 mL

2. $\dfrac{1\,mL}{100\,mL} = \dfrac{x\,mg}{120\,mg}$

100x = 120

x = 1.2 mg/mL

3. Change 1.2 mg to mcg by moving the decimal three places to the right = 1200 mcg/mL

4. $\dfrac{20\,mcg}{1\,kg} = \dfrac{x\,mcg}{35\,kg}$

x = 700 mcg/min

5. $\dfrac{700\,mcg}{120,000\,mcg} = \dfrac{x\,mL}{100\,mL}$

120,000x = 70,000

x = 0.58 mL/min

6. $\dfrac{0.58\,mL}{1\,min} = \dfrac{x\,mL}{60\,min}$

x = 34.8 = 35 mL/hr

Set 25.49

1. $\dfrac{80\,U}{1\,kg} = \dfrac{x\,U}{38}$

x = 3040 U/bolus

2. $\dfrac{4\,U}{1\,kg} = \dfrac{x\,U}{38\,kg}$

x = 152 U

3. 700 U + 152 U = 852 U/hr

4. $\dfrac{25,000\,U}{500\,mL} = \dfrac{852\,U}{x\,mL}$

25,000x = 426,000

x = 17 mL/hr

Set 25.50

1. $\dfrac{500\,mg}{500\,mg} = \dfrac{x\,mL}{20\,mL}$

$500x = 10{,}000$

$x = 20$ mL

2. $\dfrac{1\ mL}{250\,mL} = \dfrac{x\,mg}{500\,mg}$

$250x = 500$

$x = 2$ mg/mL

3. 80 kg

$\underline{\times\ 0.5\ mg/kg\ ordered}$

40 mg/hr

4. $\dfrac{40\,mg}{500\,mg} = \dfrac{x\,mL}{250\,mL}$

$500x = 10{,}000$

$x = 20$ mL/hr

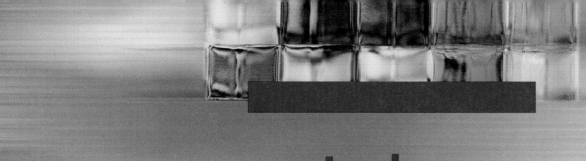

Index

Getting Started with the Math and Meds for Nurses, 2nd edition, Practice Software

System Requirements

Operating system: Microsoft Windows 98, ME, NT, 4.0, 2000, XP, or newer

Processor: Pentium II processor or faster

Memory: 32–64 MB

Hard disk space: 16 MB

Monitor: SVGA-compatible color

Graphics adapter: SVGA or higher: 800 × 600, true color (24-bit or 32-bit), or high color (16-bit) modes

CD-ROM drive: 8x or faster

An Internet connection and Netscape Navigator 6.2 or Microsoft Internet Explorer 5.5 or newer

Microsoft is a registered trademark, and Windows and Windows NT are trademarks of Microsoft Corporation.

Setup Instructions

1. Insert disc into CD-ROM drive. The program should start. If it does not, go to step 2.

2. From My Computer, double-click the icon for the CD drive.

3. Double-click the **index.htm** file to start the program.

Single User License Agreement

IMPORTANT! READ CAREFULLY: This End User License Agreement ("Agreement") sets forth the conditions by which Thomson Delmar Learning, a division of Thomson Learning Inc. ("Thomson") will make electronic access to the Thomson Delmar Learning-owned licensed content and associated media, software, documentation, printed materials, and electronic documentation contained in this package and/or made available to you via this product (the "Licensed Content"), available to you (the "End User"). BY CLICKING THE "I ACCEPT" BUTTON AND/OR OPENING THIS PACKAGE, YOU ACKNOWLEDGE THAT YOU HAVE READ ALL OF THE TERMS AND CONDITIONS, AND THAT YOU AGREE TO BE BOUND BY ITS TERMS, CONDITIONS, AND ALL APPLICABLE LAWS AND REGULATIONS GOVERNING THE USE OF THE LICENSED CONTENT.

1.0 SCOPE OF LICENSE

1.1 <u>Licensed Content.</u> The Licensed Content may contain portions of modifiable content ("Modifiable Content") and content which may not be modified or otherwise altered by the End User ("Non-Modifiable Content"). For purposes of this Agreement, Modifiable Content and Non-Modifiable Content may be collectively referred to herein as the "Licensed Content." All Licensed Content shall be considered Non-Modifiable Content, unless such Licensed Content is presented to the End User in a modifiable format and it is clearly indicated that modification of the Licensed Content is permitted.

1.2 Subject to the End User's compliance with the terms and conditions of this Agreement, Thomson Delmar Learning hereby grants the End User, a nontransferable, nonexclusive, limited right to access and view a single copy of the Licensed Content on a single personal computer system for noncommercial, internal, personal use only. The End User shall not (i) reproduce, copy, modify (except in the case of Modifiable Content), distribute, display, transfer, sublicense, prepare derivative work(s) based on, sell, exchange, barter or transfer, rent, lease, loan, resell, or in any other manner exploit the Licensed Content; (ii) remove, obscure, or alter any notice of Thomson Delmar Learning's intellectual property rights present on or in the Licensed Content, including, but not limited to, copyright, trademark, and/or patent notices; or (iii) disassemble, decompile, translate, reverse engineer, or otherwise reduce the Licensed Content.

2.0 TERMINATION

2.1 Thomson Delmar Learning may at any time (without prejudice to its other rights or remedies) immediately terminate this Agreement and/or suspend access to some or all of the Licensed Content, in the event that the End User does not comply with any of the terms and conditions of this Agreement. In the event of such termination by Thomson Delmar Learning, the End User shall immediately return any and all copies of the Licensed Content to Thomson Delmar Learning.

3.0 PROPRIETARY RIGHTS

3.1 The End User acknowledges that Thomson Delmar Learning owns all rights, title and interest, including, but not limited to all copyright rights therein, in and to the Licensed Content, and that the End User shall not take any action inconsistent with such ownership. The Licensed Content is protected by U.S., Canadian and other applicable copyright laws and by international treaties, including the Berne Convention and the Universal Copyright Convention. Nothing contained in this Agreement shall be construed as granting the End User any ownership rights in or to the Licensed Content.

3.2 Thomson Delmar Learning reserves the right at any time to withdraw from the Licensed Content any item or part of an item for which it no longer retains the right to publish, or which it has reasonable grounds to believe infringes copyright or is defamatory, unlawful, or otherwise objectionable.

4.0 PROTECTION AND SECURITY

4.1 The End User shall use its best efforts and take all reasonable steps to safeguard its copy of the Licensed Content to ensure that no unauthorized reproduction, publication, disclosure, modification, or distribution of the Licensed Content, in whole or in part, is made. To the extent that the End User becomes aware of any such unauthorized use of the Licensed Content, the End User shall immediately notify Thomson Delmar Learning. Notification of such violations may be made by sending an e-mail to delmarhelp@thomson.com.

5.0 MISUSE OF THE LICENSED PRODUCT

5.1 In the event that the End User uses the Licensed Content in violation of this Agreement, Thomson Delmar Learning shall have the option of electing liquidated damages, which shall include all profits generated by the End User's use of the Licensed Content plus interest computed at the maximum rate permitted by law and all legal fees and other expenses incurred by Thomson Delmar Learning in enforcing its rights, plus penalties.

6.0 FEDERAL GOVERNMENT CLIENTS

6.1 Except as expressly authorized by Thomson Delmar Learning, Federal Government clients obtain only the rights specified in this Agreement and no other rights. The Government acknowledges that (i) all software and related documentation incorporated in the Licensed

Content is existing commercial computer software within the meaning of FAR 27.405(b)(2); and (2) all other data delivered in whatever form, is limited rights data within the meaning of FAR 27.401. The restrictions in this section are acceptable as consistent with the Government's need for software and other data under this Agreement.

7.0 DISCLAIMER OF WARRANTIES AND LIABILITIES

7.1 Although Thomson Delmar Learning believes the Licensed Content to be reliable, Thomson Delmar Learning does not guarantee or warrant (i) any information or materials contained in or produced by the Licensed Content, (ii) the accuracy, completeness or reliability of the Licensed Content, or (iii) that the Licensed Content is free from errors or other material defects. THE LICENSED PRODUCT IS PROVIDED "AS IS," WITHOUT ANY WARRANTY OF ANY KIND AND THOMSON DELMAR LEARNING DISCLAIMS ANY AND ALL WARRANTIES, EXPRESSED OR IMPLIED, INCLUDING, WITHOUT LIMITATION, WARRANTIES OF MERCHANTABILITY OR FITNESS OR A PARTICULAR PURPOSE. IN NO EVENT SHALL THOMSON DELMAR LEARNING BE LIABLE FOR: INDIRECT, SPECIAL, PUNITIVE OR CONSEQUENTIAL DAMAGES INCLUDING FOR LOST PROFITS, LOST DATA, OR OTHERWISE. IN NO EVENT SHALL THOMSON DELMAR LEARNING'S AGGREGATE LIABILITY HEREUNDER, WHETHER ARISING IN CONTRACT, TORT, STRICT LIABILITY OR OTHERWISE, EXCEED THE AMOUNT OF FEES PAID BY THE END USER HEREUNDER FOR THE LICENSE OF THE LICENSED CONTENT.

8.0 GENERAL

8.1 Entire Agreement. This Agreement shall constitute the entire Agreement between the Parties and supercedes all prior Agreements and understandings oral or written relating to the subject matter hereof.

8.2 Enhancements/Modifications of Licensed Content. From time to time, and in Thomson Delmar Learning's sole discretion, Thomson Delmar Learning may advise the End User of updates, upgrades, enhancements and/or improvements to the Licensed Content, and may permit the End User to access and use, subject to the terms and conditions of this Agreement, such modifications, upon payment of prices as may be established by Thomson Delmar Learning.

8.3 No Export. The End User shall use the Licensed Content solely in the United States and shall not transfer or export, directly or indirectly, the Licensed Content outside the United States.

8.4 Severability. If any provision of this Agreement is invalid, illegal, or unenforceable under any applicable statute or rule of law, the provision shall be deemed omitted to the extent that it is invalid, illegal, or unenforceable. In such a case, the remainder of the Agreement shall be construed in a manner as to give greatest effect to the original intention of the parties hereto.

8.5 Waiver. The waiver of any right or failure of either party to exercise in any respect any right provided in this Agreement in any instance shall not be deemed to be a waiver of such right in the future or a waiver of any other right under this Agreement.

8.6 Choice of Law/Venue. This Agreement shall be interpreted, construed, and governed by and in accordance with the laws of the State of New York, applicable to contracts executed and to be wholly preformed therein, without regard to its principles governing conflicts of law. Each party agrees that any proceeding arising out of or relating to this Agreement or the breach or threatened breach of this Agreement may be commenced and prosecuted in a court in the State and County of New York. Each party consents and submits to the nonexclusive personal jurisdiction of any court in the State and County of New York in respect of any such proceeding.

8.7 Acknowledgment. By opening this package and/or by accessing the Licensed Content on this Web site, THE END USER ACKNOWLEDGES THAT IT HAS READ THIS AGREEMENT, UNDERSTANDS IT, AND AGREES TO BE BOUND BY ITS TERMS AND CONDITIONS. IF YOU DO NOT ACCEPT THESE TERMS AND CONDITIONS, YOU MUST NOT ACCESS THE LICENSED CONTENT AND RETURN THE LICENSED PRODUCT TO DELMAR LEARNING (WITHIN 30 CALENDAR DAYS OF THE END USER'S PURCHASE) WITH PROOF OF PAYMENT ACCEPTABLE TO THOMSON DELMAR LEARNING, FOR A CREDIT OR A REFUND. Should the End User have any questions/comments regarding this Agreement, please contact Thomson Delmar Learning at delmarhelp@thomson.com.